Essentials in Clinical Anatomy of the Equine Locomotor System

Essentials in Clinical Anatomy of the Equine Locomotor System

BY JEAN-MARIE D

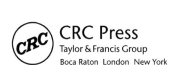

CRC Press
Taylor & Francis Group
Boca Raton London New York

CRC Press is an imprint of the
Taylor & Francis Group, an **informa** business

CRC Press
Taylor & Francis Group
6000 Broken Sound Parkway NW, Suite 300
Boca Raton, FL 33487-2742

© 2019 by Taylor & Francis Group, LLC
CRC Press is an imprint of Taylor & Francis Group, an Informa business

Library of Congress Cataloging-in-Publication Data

Names: Denoix, Jean-Marie, author. | Continuation of (work): Denoix, Jean-Marie. Equine distal limb.
Title: Essentials in clinical anatomy of the equine locomotor system / Jean-Marie Denoix.
Description: Boca Raton : Taylor & Francis, 2018. | This book continues The equine distal limb : an atlas of clinical anatomy and comparative imaging.
Identifiers: LCCN 2018034912| ISBN 9781498754415 (hardback : alk. paper) | ISBN 9780429755446 (pdf) | ISBN 9780429755439 (epub) | ISBN 9780429755422 (mobi/kindle)
Subjects: LCSH: Horses--Anatomy. | MESH: Horses--anatomy & histology | Musculoskeletal System--anatomy & histology | Locomotion--physiology | Atlases
Classification: LCC SF765 .D46 2018 | NLM SF 765 | DDC 636.10891--dc23
LC record available at https://lccn.loc.gov/2018034912

**Visit the Taylor & Francis Web site at
http://www.taylorandfrancis.com**

**and the CRC Press Web site at
http://www.crcpress.com**

CONTENTS

Introduction   **ix**
Author   **xi**

CHAPTER **A**   **THE PROXIMAL THORACIC LIMB**   **1**

A.1 PHYSICAL ASPECT   1
A.2 BONE AND RADIOGRAPHIC ANATOMY   2
A.3 DISSECTED SPECIMEN   7
A.4 CROSS-SECTIONS   13

CHAPTER **B**   **THE BRACHIUM AND ELBOW**   **19**

B.1 PHYSICAL ASPECT   19
B.2 BONES, JOINT AND RADIOGRAPHIC ANATOMY   21
B.3 DISSECTED SPECIMEN   25
B.4 CROSS-SECTIONS   31

CHAPTER **C**   **THE ANTEBRACHIUM**   **35**

C.1 PHYSICAL ASPECT   35
C.2 DISSECTED SPECIMEN   37
C.3 CROSS-SECTIONS   45

CHAPTER **D**   **THE CARPUS**   **49**

D.1 PHYSICAL ASPECT   49
D.2 RADIOGRAPHIC ANATOMY   50
D.3 DISSECTED SPECIMEN   59
D.4 CROSS-SECTIONS   70

CHAPTER **E**   **THE METACARPUS**   **77**

E.1 PHYSICAL ASPECT   77
E.2 RADIOGRAPHIC ANATOMY   78
E.3 DISSECTED SPECIMEN   80
E.4 CROSS-SECTIONS   87

CHAPTER **F**   **THE DIGITAL AREA**   **99**

F.1 PHYSICAL ASPECT   99
F.2 RADIOGRAPHIC ANATOMY   100
F.3 DISSECTED SPECIMEN   117
F.4 CROSS-SECTIONS   124

CHAPTER **G**   **THE NECK**   **131**

G.1 PHYSICAL ASPECT   131
G.2 NUCHAL AREA   132
  G.2.1 Radiographic anatomy   132
G.3 DISSECTED SPECIMEN   133
G.4 CROSS-SECTION   137
G.5 MIDDLE AND CAUDAL CERVICAL AREAS   138
  G.5.1 Radiographic anatomy   138
  G.5.2 Dissected specimen   141
  G.5.3 Cross-sections   147

CHAPTER **H**   **THE BACK (THORACOLUMBAR REGIONS)**   **151**

H.1 PHYSICAL ASPECT   151
H.2 RADIOGRAPHIC ANATOMY   152
H.3 DISSECTED SPECIMEN   156
H.4 CROSS-SECTIONS   164
  H.4.1 Median and paramedian sections   164
  H.4.2 Transverse sections   166

CHAPTER **I**   **THE PELVIS**   **171**

I.1 PHYSICAL ASPECT   171
I.2 BONES   172
I.3 DISSECTED SPECIMEN   177
I.4 CROSS-SECTIONS   185

CHAPTER **J**   **THE HIP AND THIGH**   **189**

J.1 PHYSICAL ASPECT   189
J.2 SUPERFICIAL STRUCTURES   190
J.3 THE HIP (COXOFEMORAL REGION) AND THIGH   191
  J.3.1 Physical aspect   191
  J.3.2 Radiographic anatomy   191
  J.3.3 Dissected specimen   192
  J.3.4 Cross-sections   199

CHAPTER **K**	**THE STIFLE**	**201**
	K.1 PHYSICAL ASPECT	201
	K.2 BONE AND RADIOGRAPHIC ANATOMY	202
	K.3 DISSECTED SPECIMEN	210
	K.4 CROSS-SECTIONS	217

CHAPTER **L**	**THE CRUS**	**221**
	L.1 PHYSICAL ASPECT	221
	L.2 BONE ANATOMY	222
	L.3 DISSECTED SPECIMEN	223
	L.4 CROSS-SECTIONS	227

CHAPTER **M**	**THE TARSUS**	**229**
	M.1 PHYSICAL ASPECT	229
	M.2 RADIOGRAPHIC ANATOMY	231
	M.3 DISSECTED SPECIMEN	238
	M.4 CROSS-SECTIONS	252

CHAPTER **N**	**THE METATARSUS**	**257**
	N.1 PHYSICAL ASPECT	257
	N.2 RADIOGRAPHIC ANATOMY	258
	N.3 DISSECTED SPECIMEN	260
	N.4 CROSS-SECTIONS	264

CHAPTER **O**	**THE DIGITAL AREA OF THE PELVIC LIMB**	**269**
	O.1 PHYSICAL ASPECT	269
	O.2 RADIOGRAPHIC ANATOMY	270
	O.3 DISSECTED SPECIMEN	271
	O.4 CROSS-SECTIONS	277

Index		**279**

INTRODUCTION

Anatomy is the mother science of a number of scientific fields and clinical procedures. Descriptive anatomy offers the foundation to understanding functional anatomy and biomechanics. In the clinical field, it is the basis of the physical examination, an important part of the evaluation of the horse's locomotor system. Understanding the strategy made by the horse to relieve biomechanical stresses on painful areas is essential in the diagnosis of lameness. Interpretation of diagnostic analgesic techniques and potential cross-reactions is also directly related to the knowledge of regional anatomic features. The need for precise information on descriptive anatomy and cross-sectional anatomy is increasingly important following the development and the clinical use of sophisticated diagnostic imaging techniques, including 3D representation. Anatomy and imaging techniques have also been incorporated in the therapeutic field with the development of real-time guided injections in precise structures, and biomechanics is gaining a paramount interest in the expanding field of rehabilitation.

This book continues on from *The Equine Distal Limb: An Atlas of Clinical Anatomy and Comparative Imaging*; in it, the complete thoracic limb, axial areas (neck, back and pelvis) and the complete pelvic limb are considered. For every area of the horse locomotor system, the superficial anatomy is presented to introduce the physical examination. Bone anatomy is considered through radiographic images (digital imaging facilitating the use of this technique). Dissections of the superficial and deep anatomical layers of each aspect of a specific area are presented and followed by cross-sections displaying the topographical aspect and relationships of anatomical structures.

The objective of this atlas is to provide the practitioner with all the clinically useful anatomical features needed to facilitate achievement and interpretation of diagnostic procedures, especially cross-sectional imaging such as ultrasonography and magnetic resonance imaging (MRI). It will also be useful to veterinary students who have little access to dissection, to complement their teaching material or provide a reference guide to help their access in the clinical sciences. In this book, trainers, riders and every person interested in horses will find illustrations of the detailed, and sometimes unexpected, constitution of the equine musculoskeletal system, which plays a key role in the horse's motion and needs to be an overriding consideration in training and rehabilitation.

J.-M. Denoix

JEAN-MARIE **Denoix** graduated from the Veterinary School of Lyon (France, 1977). He passed the *agrégation* in Veterinary Anatomy (1983) and defended a PhD thesis in Biomechanics (1987). In 1988 he moved to the Veterinary School of Alfort and became professor of Anatomy, head of the equine clinical unit (until 2005), and head of a research unit devoted to biomechanics and pathology of the locomotor system in horses (until 2003). He became head of CIRALE (Center of Imaging and Research in Equine Locomotor Pathology) in 1999. Since 2006, he has been President of the ISELP (International Society of Equine Locomotor Pathology), large animal imaging associate of the ECVDI (European College of Veterinary Diagnostic Imaging) since 2010, and President of the ALAPILE (South American Association of Pathology and Imaging of the Equine Locomotor System) since 2012. In 2013 he became Diplomate of the American College of Veterinary Sport Medicine and Rehabilitation (ACVSMR) and is a founding Diplomate of the European College of Veterinary Sport Medicine and Rehabilitation (ECVSMR).

THE PROXIMAL THORACIC LIMB

A.1 PHYSICAL ASPECT

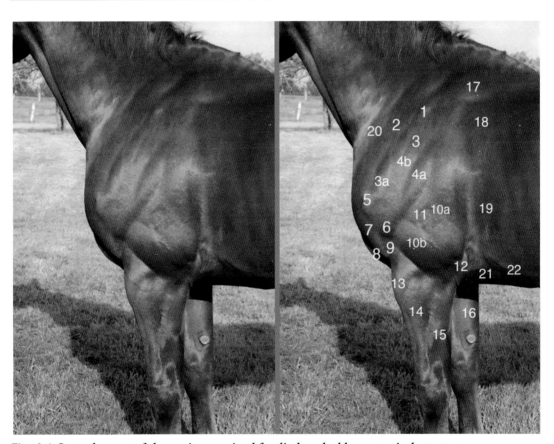

Fig. A.1 **Lateral aspect of the equine proximal forelimb: palpable anatomical structures.**

1- Spine of the scapula; 2- Supraspinatus muscle; 3- Infraspinatus muscle, 3a- tendon; 4- Deltoideus muscle, 4a- caudal muscle part, 4b- aponeurotic part; 5- Major tuberculum (caudal part or convexity); 6- Deltoid tuberosity; 7- Brachiocephalicus muscle covering the biceps brachii muscle; 8- Pectoralis descendens muscle; 9- Sulcus of the elbow and brachialis muscle; 10- Triceps brachii muscle, 10a- long head, 10b- lateral head; 11- Cutaneous omobrachialis muscle; 12- Point of the elbow (olecranon); 13- Extensor carpi radialis muscle; 14- Dorsal digital extensor muscle; 15- Ulnaris lateralis muscle; 16- Flexor carpi ulnaris muscle; 17- Trapezius muscle (thoracic part); 18- Latissimus dorsi muscle; 19- Serratus ventralis thoracis muscle; 20- Subclavius muscle; 21- Pectoralis ascendens muscle; 22- Lateral thoracic vein.

A.2 BONE AND RADIOGRAPHIC ANATOMY

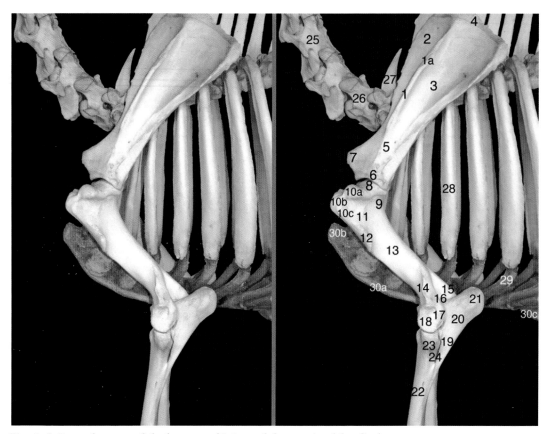

Fig. A.2 **Lateral aspect of the bones and joints of the proximal forelimb.**

Scapula: 1- Spine of the scapula, 1a- Tuberculum of the spine; 2- Supraspinatus fossa; 3- Infraspinatus fossa; 4- Proximal margin and cartilage of the scapula (partly ossified); 5- Neck of the scapula, 6- Glenoid cavity (lateral articular margin); 7- Tuberculum supraglenoidale;

Humerus: 8- Head; 9- Neck; 10- Major tuberculum, 10a- caudal part or convexity, 10a- cranial part or top, 10c- crest; 11- Tricipital line; 12- Deltoid tuberosity; 13- Brachial sulcus; 14- Supracondylar crest; 15- Medial epicondyle; 16- Olecranon fossa; 17- Lateral epicondyle; 18- Humeral condyle;

Ulna: 19- Body; 20- Olecranon; 21- Tuber olecrani;

Radius: 22- Body; 23- Lateral tuberosity (insertion of the lateral collateral ligament of the elbow joint); 24- Antebrachial interosseous space;

Vertebral column and thorax: 25- Fifth cervical vertebra; 26- Seventh cervical vertebra; 27- Spinous process of the first thoracic vertebra; 28- Fourth left rib; 29- Sixth costal cartilage; 30- Sternum, 30a- carina, 30b- manubrium, 30c- xiphoid process.

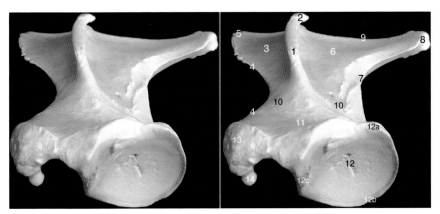

Fig. A.3 **Distolateral aspect of the scapula.**

1- Spine of the scapula; 2- Tuberculum of the spine; 3- Supraspinatus fossa; 4- Cranial margin; 5- Cranial angle; 6- Infraspinatus fossa; 7- Caudal margin; 8- Caudal angle; 9- Proximal margin; 10- Neck of the scapula; 11- Distal angle; 12- Glenoid cavity, 12a- lateral articular margin, 12b- medial articular margin, 12c- glenoid incisura; 13- Tuberculum supraglenoidale; 14- Coracoid process.

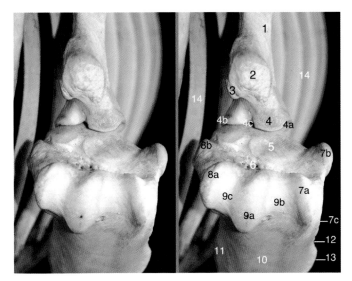

Fig. A.4 **Cranial aspect of the scapulohumeral joint.**

Scapula: 1- Neck of the scapula; 2- Tuberculum supraglenoidale; 3- Coracoid process; 4- Glenoid cavity, 4a- lateral articular margin, 4b- medial articular margin, 4c- glenoid incisura;

Humerus: 5- Head; 6- Synovial space between the head and tubercles of the humerus; 7- Major tuberculum, 7a- cranial part or top, 7b- caudal part or convexity, 7c- crest; 8- Minor tuberculum, 8a- cranial part or top, 8b- caudal part or convexity; 9- Sulcus intertubercularis, 9a- intermediate tuberculum, 9b- lateral groove, 9c- medial groove; 10- Body of the humerus; 11- Insertion tuberosity of the teres major and latissimus dorsi muscles; 12- Tricipital line; 13- Deltoid tuberosity;

Thorax: 14- Ribs.

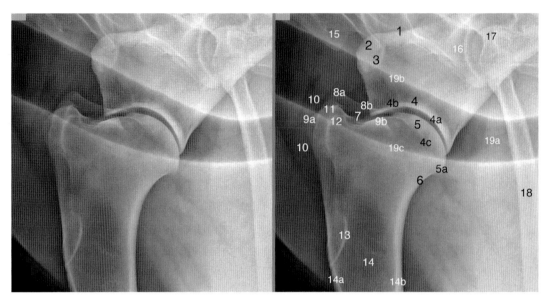

Fig. A.5 **Mediolateral radiographic image of the right scapulohumeral joint.**

Scapula: 1- Cranial border; 2- Tuberculum supraglenoidale; 3- Coracoid process; 4- Glenoid cavity, 4a- subchondral bone, 4b- glenoid incisura, 4c- articular margin;

Humerus: 5- Head, 5a- caudal articular margin; 6- Neck; 7- Synovial space between the head and tubercles of the humerus; 8- Minor tuberculum, 8a- cranial lobe (top), 8b- caudal lobe (convexity); 9- Major tuberculum, 9a- cranial lobe (top), 9b- caudal lobe (convexity); 10- Intermediate tuberculum; 11- Sulcus intertubercularis, medial groove; 12- Sulcus intertubercularis, lateral groove; 13- Deltoid tuberosity; 14- Body of the humerus, 14a- cranial cortex, 14b- caudal cortex;

Cervical vertebral column and thoracic structures: 15- Transverse process of the sixth cervical vertebra; 16- Vertebral fossa of the seventh cervical vertebra; 17- Head of the first thoracic vertebra; 18- First right rib; 19- Trachea, 19a- lumen, 19b- dorsal limit of the lumen, 19c- ventral limit of the lumen.

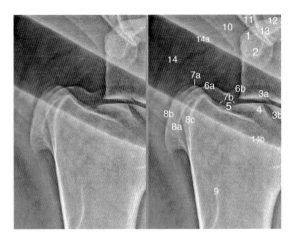

Fig. A.6 **Mediolateral radiographic image of the scapulohumeral joint.**

Scapula: 1- Tuberculum supraglenoidale; 2- Coracoid process; 3- Glenoid cavity, 3a- glenoid incisura, 3b- articular margin;

Humerus: 4- Head; 5- Synovial space between the head and tubercles of the humerus; 6- Major tuberculum, 6a- cranial lobe (top), 6b- caudal lobe (convexity); 7- Minor tuberculum, 7a- cranial lobe (top), 7b- caudal lobe (convexity); 8- Sulcus intertubercularis, 8a- medial groove, 8b- intermediate tuberculum, 8c- lateral groove; 9- Tricipital line (ending on the deltoid tuberosity);

Cervical vertebral column and thoracic structures: 10- Transverse process of the sixth cervical vertebra; 11- Vertebral fossa of the sixth cervical vertebra; 12- Head of the seventh cervical vertebra; 13- Intervertebral disc; 14- Trachea, 14a- dorsal limit of the lumen, 14b- ventral limit of the lumen.

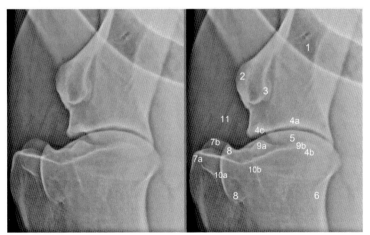

Fig. A.7 **Caudolateral oblique radiographic image of the scapulohumeral joint.**

Scapula: 1- Neck; 2- Tuberculum supraglenoidale; 3- Coracoid process; 4- Glenoid cavity, 4a- subchondral bone, 4b- articular margin;

Humerus: 5- Head; 6- Neck; 7- Major tuberculum, 7a- cranial lobe (top), 7b- caudal lobe (convexity); 8- Intermediate tuberculum; 9- Minor tuberculum, 9a- cranial lobe (top), 9b- caudal lobe (convexity); 10- Sulcus intertubercularis, 10a- lateral groove, 10b- medial groove, 11- Shadow of proximal tendon of the biceps brachii muscle.

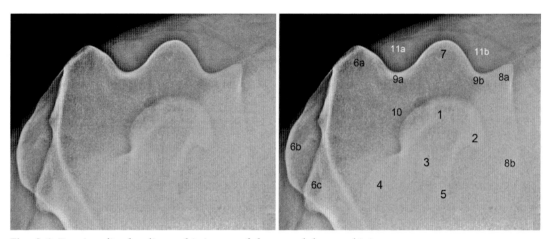

Fig. A.8 **Proximodistal radiographic image of the scapulohumeral joint.**

Scapula: 1- Tuberculum supraglenoidale; 2- Coracoid process; 3- Neck; 4- Glenoid cavity; 5- Subscapular fossa;

Humerus: 6- Major tuberculum, 6a- cranial lobe (top), 6b- caudal lobe (convexity), 6c- crest; 7- Intermediate tuberculum; 8- Minor tuberculum, 8a- cranial lobe (top), 8b- caudal lobe (convexity); 9- Sulcus intertubercularis, 9a- lateral groove, 9b- medial groove; 10- Synovial space between the head and tubercles of the humerus and vascular foramen; 11- Shadow of proximal tendon of the biceps brachii, 11a- lateral lobe, 11b- medial lobe.

A.3 DISSECTED SPECIMEN

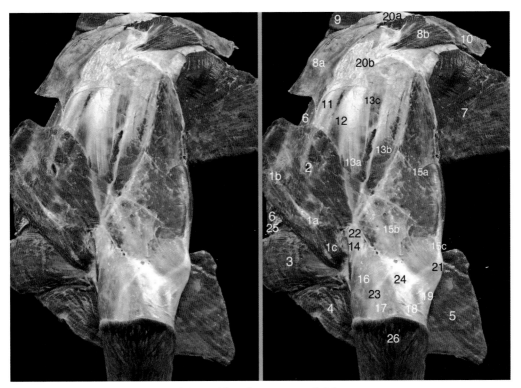

Fig. A.9 Lateral aspect of the shoulder and brachium: superficial structures.

Cervical and thoracic muscles: 1- Brachiocephalicus muscle, 1a- clavicular intersection, 1b- cleidocephalicus muscle, 1c- cleidobrachialis muscle; 2- Omotransversarius muscle; 3- Pectoralis descendens muscle; 4- Pectoralis transversus muscle; 5- Pectoralis profundus (ascendens) muscle; 6- Subclavius muscle; 7- Latissimus dorsi muscle; 8- Trapezius muscle, 8a- cervical part, 8b- thoracic part; 9- Rhomboideus cervicis muscle; 10- Rhomboideus thoracis muscle;

Shoulder muscles: 11- Supraspinatus muscle; 12- Infraspinatus muscle; 13- Deltoideus muscle, 13a- cranial (spinal) head, 13b- caudal (long) head, 13c- aponeurosis (covering the infraspinatus muscle);

Brachial and antebrachial muscles: 14- Brachialis muscle; 15- Triceps brachii muscle; 15a- long head, 15b- lateral head, 15c- tendon; 16- Extensor carpi radialis muscle; 17- Dorsal (common) digital extensor muscle; 18- Ulnaris lateralis muscle; 19- Deep digital flexor muscle (ulnar head).

Other structures: 20- Scapula, 20a- cartilage, 20b- tuberculum of the spine; 21- Olecranon; 22- Brachial fascia; 23- Antebrachial fascia; 24- Lateral collateral ligament of the elbow joint; 25- Cervical superficial artery; 26- Skin.

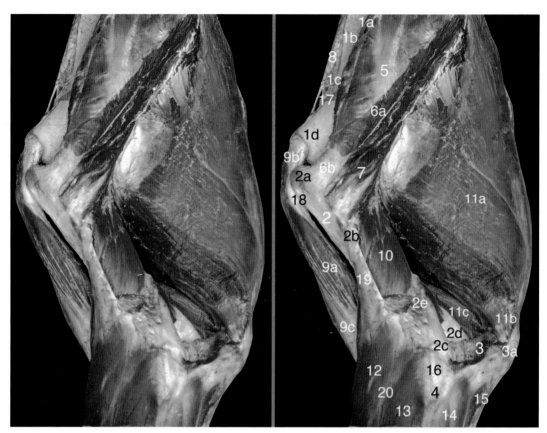

Fig. A.10 Lateral aspect of the shoulder and brachium: intermediate structures.

1- Scapula, 1a- spine, 1b- supraspinatus fossa, 1c- neck, 1d- tuberculum supraglenoidale; 2- Humerus, 2a- major tuberculum, 2b- deltoid tuberosity, 2c- lateral epicondyle, 2d- medial epicondyle and olecranon fossa, 2e- supracondylar crest; 3- Olecranon, 3a- tuber olecrani; 4- Radius (proximolateral tuberosity); 5- Aponeurosis of the deltoid muscle (cut); 6- Infraspinatus muscle, 6a- body, 6b- tendon; 7- Teres minor muscle; 8- Intramuscular aponeurosis of the supraspinatus muscle; 9- Biceps brachii muscle, 9a- body, 9b- proximal tendon, 9c- intramuscular tendon; 10- Brachialis muscle; 11- Triceps brachii muscle, 11a- long head, 11b- tendon, 11c- medial head (lateral head removed); 12- Extensor carpi radialis muscle; 13- Dorsal (common) digital extensor muscle; 14- Ulnaris lateralis muscle; 15- Deep digital flexor muscle (ulnar head); 16- Lateral collateral ligament of the elbow joint; 17- Suprascapular nerve; 18- Bicipital bursa; 19- Brachial fascia; 20- Antebrachial fascia.

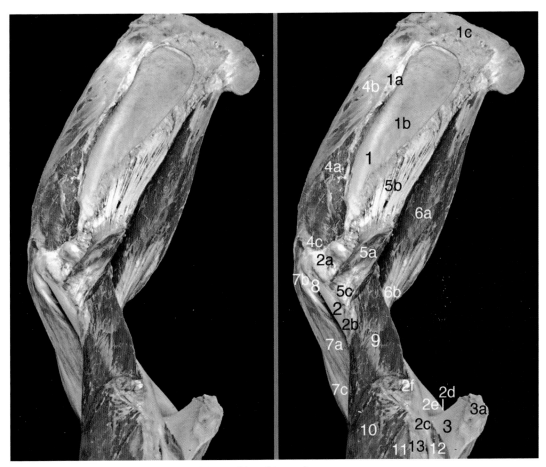

Fig. A.11 **Lateral aspect of the shoulder and brachium: deep structures.**

1- Scapula, 1a- spine, 1b- infraspinatus fossa, 1c- cartilage; 2- Humerus, 2a- major tuberculum, 2b- deltoid tuberosity, 2c- lateral epicondyle, 2d- medial epicondyle, 2e- olecranon fossa, 2f- supracondylar crest; 3- Olecranon, 3a- tuber olecrani; 4- Supraspinatus muscle, 4a- body, 4b- superficial aponeurosis, 4c- lateral tendon; 5- Teres minor muscle, 5a- body, 5b- proximal aponeurosis, 5c- distal insertion; 6- Teres major muscle, 6a- body, 6b- distal tendon; 7- Biceps brachii muscle, 7a- body, 7b- proximal tendon, 7c- intramuscular tendon; 8- Bicipital bursa; 9- Brachialis muscle; 10- Extensor carpi radialis muscle; 11- Dorsal (common) digital extensor muscle; 12- Ulnaris lateralis muscle; 13- Lateral collateral ligament of the elbow joint.

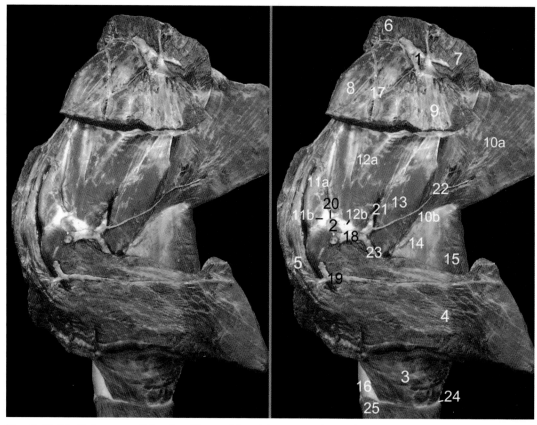

Fig. A.12 Medial aspect of the shoulder and brachium: muscles and arteries.

Bones: 1- Scapula (scapular cartilage); 2- Humerus (minor tuberculum).

Thoracic muscles: 3- Pectoralis transversus muscle; 4- Pectoralis profundus (ascendens); 5- Subclavius muscle; 6- Rhomboideus cervicalis muscle; 7- Rhomboideus thoracis muscle; 8- Serratus ventralis cervicis muscle; 9- Serratus ventralis thoracis muscle; 10- Latissimus dorsi muscle, 10a- muscle body, 10b- tendon;

Shoulder muscles: 11- Supraspinatus muscle, 11a- muscle body, 11b- medial tendon; 12- Subscapular muscle, 12a- muscle body, 12b- distal tendon; 13- Teres major muscle;

Brachial muscles: 14- Triceps brachii muscle (long head); 15- Tensor fasciae antebrachii muscle; **Antebrachial muscle:** 16- Extensor carpi radialis muscle;

Arteries: 17- Dorsal scapular artery; 18- Axillary artery; 19- External thoracic artery; 20- Suprascapular artery; 21- Subscapular artery; 22- Thoracodorsal artery; 23- Brachial artery

Other structures: 24- Antebrachial fascia; 25- Skin.

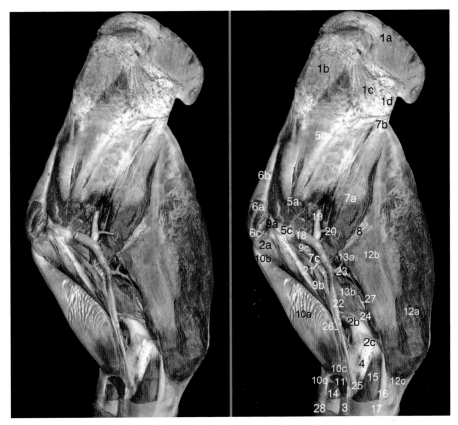

Fig. A.13 **Medial aspect of the shoulder and brachium: muscles and arteries.**

Bones and joints: 1- Scapula (costal face), 1a- scapular cartilage, 1b- cranial serrata face, 1b- caudal serrata face, 1d- caudal angle; 2- Humerus, 2a- minor tuberculum (insertion surface of the pectoralis ascendens); 2b- medial face; 2c- medial epicondyle; 3- Radius; 4- Medial collateral ligament of the elbow joint;

Shoulder muscles: 5- Subscapularis muscle, 5a- body, 5b- aponeurosis, 5c- distal tendon; 6- Supraspinatus muscle, 6a- body, 6b- fascia, 6c- medial tendon; 7- Teres major muscle, 7a- body, 7b- proximal tendon, 7c- distal tendon (fused with the tendon of the latissimus dorsi muscle); 8- Tendon of the latissimus dorsi muscle; 9- Coracobrachialis muscle, 9a- proximal tendon, 9b- long head; 9c- short head;

Brachial muscles: 10- Biceps brachii muscle, 10a- body, 10b- proximal tendon, 10c- distal insertion, 10d- lacertus fibrosus; 11- Brachialis muscle; 12- Tensor fasciae antebrachii muscle (covering the long head of the triceps brachii muscle), 12a- body, 12b- proximal aponeurosis, 12c- musculoaponeurotic junction with the antebrachial fascia; 13- Triceps brachii muscle, 13a- long head, 13b- medial head;

Antebrachial muscles: 14- Extensor carpi radialis muscle; 15- Flexor carpi radialis muscle; 16- Flexor carpi ulnaris muscle (humeral head); 17- Antebrachial fascia;

Arteries and nerves: 18- Axillary artery; 19- Subscapular artery; 20- Thoracodorsal artery (cut); 21- Cranial humeral circumflex artery; 22- Brachial (humeral) artery; 23- Deep brachial artery; 24- Ulnar collateral artery; 25- Median artery; 26- Median nerve; 27- Ulnar nerve; 28- Skin.

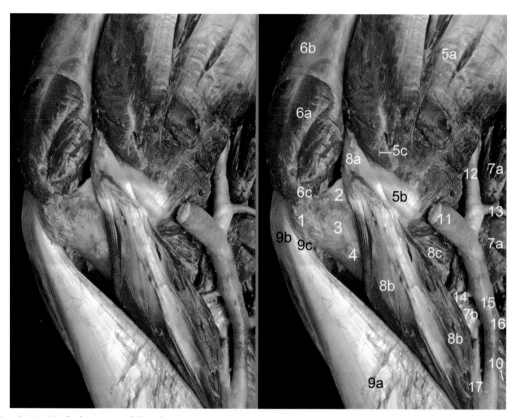

Fig. A.14 **Medial aspect of the shoulder joint area: muscles and arteries.**

Humerus: 1- Cranial part (top) of the minor tuberculum; 2- Caudal part (convexity) of the minor tuberculum; 3- Insertion surface of the pectoralis profundus (ascendens); 4- Proximal metaphysis.

Shoulder muscles: 5- Subscapular muscle, 5a- body, 5b- distal tendon, 5c- motor nerve ramus; 6- Supraspinatus muscle, 6a- body, 6b- fascia, 6c- medial tendon; 7- Teres major muscle, 7a- body, 7b- distal tendon (fused with the latissimus dorsi tendon); 8- Coracobrachialis muscle, 8a- proximal tendon, 8b- long head, 8c- short head;

Brachial muscles: 9- Biceps brachii muscle, 9a- body, 9b- proximal tendon, 9c- bicipital bursa space; 10- Triceps brachii muscle (medial head);

Arteries and nerves: 11- Axillary artery; 12- Subscapular artery; 13- Thoracodorsal artery; 14- Cranial humeral circumflex artery; 15- Brachial (humeral) artery; 16- Deep brachial artery (origin); 17- Median nerve.

A.4 CROSS-SECTIONS

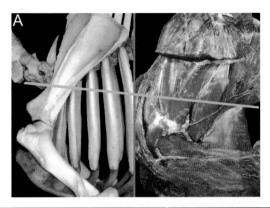

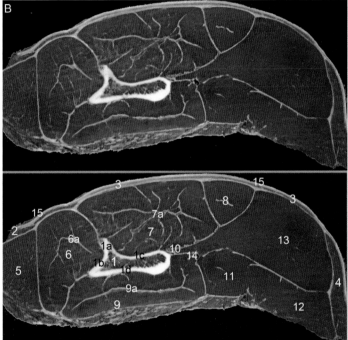

Fig. A.15 **Transverse section of the shoulder. (A) Section level; (B) anatomical structures.**

Scapula: 1- Neck; 1a- spine, 1b- supraspinatus fossa, 1c- infraspinatus fossa, 1d- subscapular fossa;

Muscles: 2- Omotransversarius muscle; 3- Cutaneous omobrachialis muscle; 4- Cutaneous trunci muscle; 5- Subclavius muscle; 6- Supraspinatus muscle, 6a- intramuscular tendon; 7- Infraspinatus muscle, 7a- intramuscular tendon and aponeuroses; 8- Deltoideus muscle; 9- Subscapular muscle, 9a- intramuscular aponeurosis; 10- Teres minor proximal tendon; 11- Teres major muscle; 12- Latissimus dorsi muscle; 13- Triceps brachii muscle (long head);

Vessels and skin: 14- Subscapular artery and vein; 15- Skin.

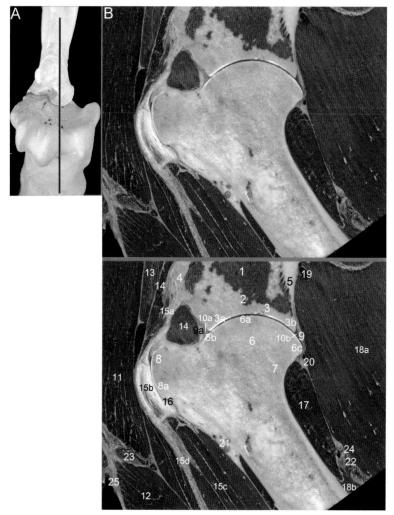

Fig. A.16 Sagittal section of the shoulder joint (A) Section level; (B) anatomical structures.

Scapula: 1- Neck; 2- Ventral angle; 3- Glenoid cavity, articular surface, 3a- articular cartilage, 3b- articular margin; 4- Tuberculum supraglenoidale; 5- Caudal margin of the neck;

Humerus: 6- Head, 6a- articular surface, 6b- articular cartilage, 6c- articular margin; 7- Neck; 8- Intertubercular sulcus, 8a- intermediate tuberculum;

Joint structures: 9- Joint capsule; 9a- glenohumeral fascicules; 10- Joint cavity, 10a- cranial recess, 10b- caudal recess;

Muscles: 11- Brachiocephalicus muscle; 12- Pectoralis descendens muscle; 13- Subclavius muscle; 14- Supraspinatus muscle; 15- Biceps brachii muscle, 15a- proximal tendon, 15b- fibrocartilaginous segment, 15c- body, 15d- intramuscular tendon; 16- Bicipital (intertubercular) bursa; 17- Brachial muscle; 18- Triceps brachii muscle, 18a- long head; 18b- medial head;

Vessels and nerves: 19- Scapular circumflex vein; 20- Caudal humeral circumflex artery and vein; 21- Cranial humeral circumflex artery; 22- Deep brachial artery and veins; 23- Cephalic vein; 24- Radial nerve; 25- Skin.

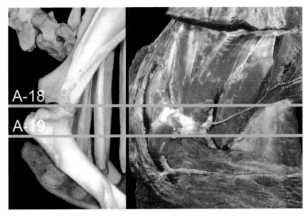

Fig. A.17 Transverse sections of the shoulder joint and proximal brachium: section levels of the following images A.18 and A.19.

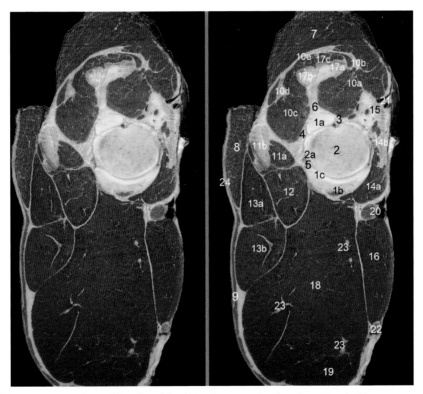

Fig. A.18 Transverse section of the shoulder joint (see section level on Fig. A.17).

Scapula: 1- Glenoid cavity, 1a- dorsal margin, 1b- caudal margin, 1c- articular cartilage;

Humerus: 2- Head, 2a- articular cartilage;

Joint structures: 3- Joint capsule with glenohumeral fascicules; 4- Glenoid labrum; 5- Joint cavity; 6- Fat pad;

Muscles: 7- Subclavius muscle; 8- Omotransversarius muscle; 9- Cutaneous omobrachialis muscle; 10- Supraspinatus muscle, 10a- medial head, 10b- medial tendon, 10c- lateral head, 10d- lateral tendon, 10e- supraspinatus fascia; 11- Infraspinatus muscle, 11a- body, 11b- infraspinatus tendon; 12- Teres minor muscle; 13- Deltoideus muscle, 13a- cranial (spinal) head, 13b- caudal (long) head; 14- Subscapular muscle, 14a- body, 14b- subscapular tendon; 15- Coracobrachialis proximal tendon; 16- Teres major muscle; 17- Proximal tendon of the biceps brachii, 17a- medial lobe, 17b- lateral lobe, 17c- cranial striated muscle fasciculi; 18- Triceps brachii muscle (long head); 19- Tensor fasciae antebrachii muscle;

Vessels and skin: 20- Subscapular artery and vein; 21- Suprascapular rami; 22- Thoracodorsal artery and vein; 23- Muscle rami of the deep brachial artery; 24- Skin.

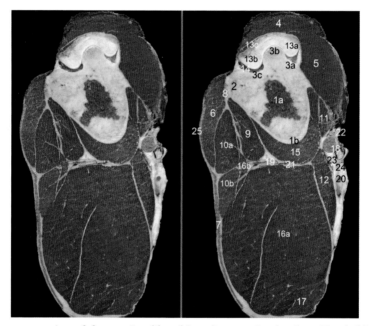

Fig. A.19 **Transverse section of the proximal brachium (see section level on Fig. A.17).**

Humerus: 1- Neck, 1a- spongy bone, 1b- cortex; 2- Base (crest) of the major tuberculum; 3- Sulcus intertubercularis, 3a- medial groove, 3b- intermediate tuberculum, 3c- lateral groove;

Muscles: 4- Subclavius muscle; 5- Pectoralis profundus (ascendens) muscle; 6- Omotransversarius muscle; 7- Cutaneous omobrachialis muscle; 8- Infraspinatus tendon; 9- Teres minor muscle; 10- Deltoideus muscle, 10a- cranial (spinal) head, 10b- caudal (long) head; 11- Coracobrachialis muscle; 12- Teres major muscle; 13- Proximal tendon of the biceps brachii, 13a- medial lobe, 13b- lateral lobe, 13c- cranial striated muscle fasciculi; 14- Bicipital (intertubercular) bursa; 15- Brachialis muscle; 16- Triceps brachii muscle, 16a- long head, 16b- lateral head; 17- Tensor fasciae antebrachii muscle;

Vessels, nerves and skin: 18- Axillary artery and vein; 19- Caudal circumflex artery and vein; 20- Ulnar collateral artery and vein; 21- Axillary nerve; 22- Median nerve; 23- Radial nerve; 24- Ulnar nerve; 25- Skin.

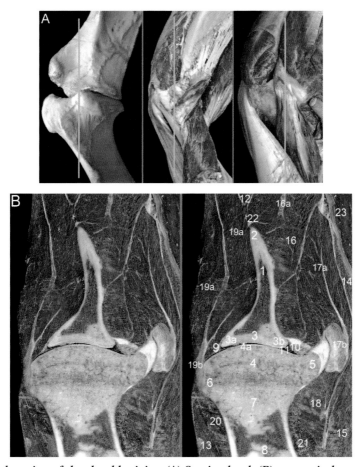

Fig. A.20 **Frontal section of the shoulder joint. (A) Section level; (B) anatomical structures.**

Scapula: 1- Neck; 2- Cranial border; 3- Glenoid cavity, 3a- medial margin, 3b- lateral margin;

Humerus: 4- Head, 4a- articular cartilage; 5- Major tuberculum; 6- Minor tuberculum; 7- Neck; 8- Body;

Joint structures: 9- Joint capsule; 10- Glenoid labrum; 11- Joint cavity;

Muscles: 12- Subclavius muscle; 13- Pectoralis profundus (ascendens) muscle; 14- Omotransversarius muscle; 15- Brachiocephalicus muscle; 16- Supraspinatus muscle, 16a- lateral tendon; 17- Infraspinatus muscle, 17a- body, 17b- infraspinatus tendon; 18- Teres minor muscle; 19- Subscapular muscle, 19a- body, 19b- subscapular tendon; 20- Coracobrachialis muscle; 21- Brachialis muscle;

Vessels, nerves and skin: 22- Suprascapular artery, vein and nerve; 23- Skin.

THE BRACHIUM AND ELBOW

B.1 PHYSICAL ASPECT

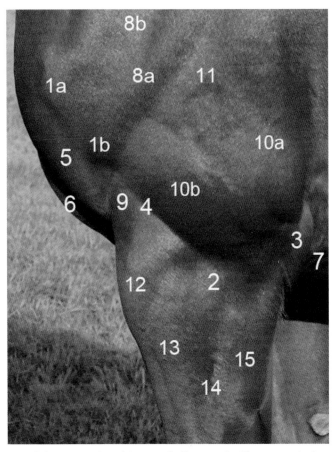

Fig. B.1 **Lateral aspect of the equine brachium and elbow: palpable anatomical structures.**

1- Humerus, 1a- major tuberculum (caudal part or convexity), 1b- deltoid tuberosity; 2- Proximolateral tuberosity of the radius; 3- Point of the elbow (olecranon); 4- Sulcus of the elbow; 5- Brachiocephalicus muscle (covering the biceps brachii muscle); 6- Pectoralis descendens muscle; 7- Pectoralis profundus (ascendens) muscle; 8- Deltoideus muscle, 8a- caudal (long) head, 8b- proximal aponeurosis covering the infraspinatus muscle; 9- Brachial muscle; 10- Triceps brachii muscle, 10a- long head, 10b- lateral head; 11- Cutaneous omobrachialis muscle; 12- Extensor carpi radialis muscle; 13- Dorsal (common) digital extensor muscle; 14- Lateral sulcus of the antebrachium; 15- Ulnaris lateralis muscle.

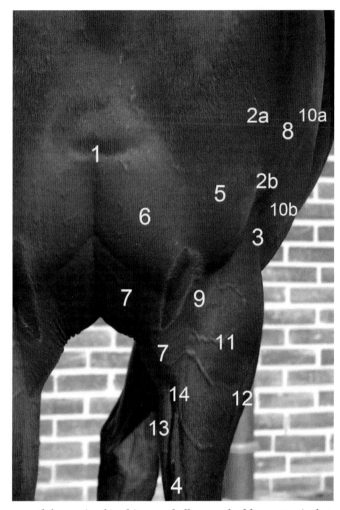

Fig. B.2 **Cranial aspect of the equine brachium and elbow: palpable anatomical structures.**

1- Manubrium of the sternum; 2- Humerus, 2a- major tuberculum (caudal part or convexity), 2b- deltoid tuberosity; 3- Sulcus of the elbow; 4- Radius (medial aspect); 5- Brachiocephalicus muscle (covering the biceps brachii muscle); 6- Pectoralis descendens muscle; 7- Pectoralis transversus muscle; 8- Deltoideus muscle; 9- Brachial muscle (crossed by the lacertus fibrosus of the biceps brachii muscle); 10- Triceps brachii muscle, 10a- long head, 10b- lateral head; 11- Extensor carpi radialis muscle; 12- Dorsal (common) digital extensor muscle; 13- Flexor carpi radialis muscle; 14- Cephalic vein.

B.2 BONES, JOINT AND RADIOGRAPHIC ANATOMY

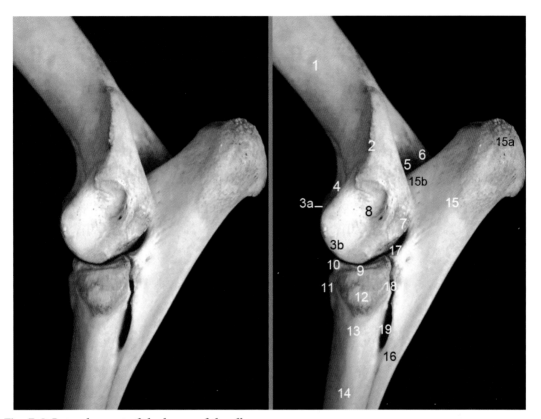

Fig. B.3 **Lateral aspect of the bones of the elbow.**

Humerus: 1- Body; 2- Supracondylar crest; 3- Humeral condyle, 3a- trochlea (medial ridge), 3b- capitulum; 4- Coronoid fossa; 5- Olecranon fossa; 6- Medial epicondyle; 7- Lateral epicondyle; 8- Insertion fossa for the lateral collateral ligament of the elbow;

Radius: 9- Fovea capitis; 10- Coronoid process; 11- Radial tuberosity; 12- Lateral tuberosity; 13- Proximal metaphysis (neck); 14- Body;

Ulna: 15- Olecranon, 15a- olecranon tuberosity, 15b- anconeal process; 16- Body;

Joint and interosseous spaces: 17- Humeroantebrachial joint space; 18- Radioulnar joint; 19- Antebrachial interosseous space.

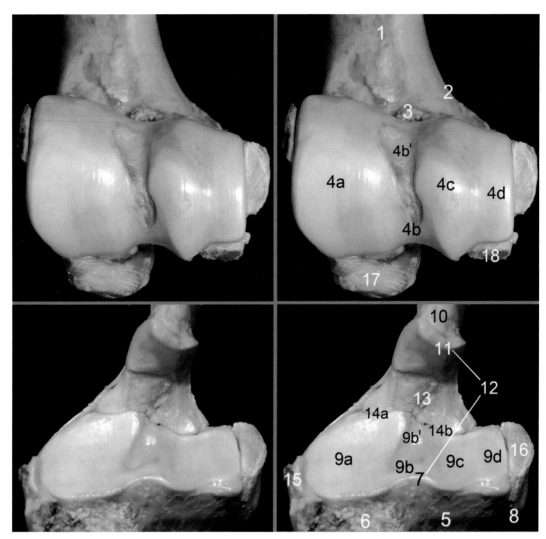

Fig. B.4 **Cranial aspect of the articular surfaces of the elbow.**

Humerus: 1- Body; 2- Supracondylar crest; 3- Coronoid fossa; 4- Humeral condyle, 4a- trochlea (medial ridge), 4b- trochlea (sagittal groove), 4b'- synovial fossa, 4c- trochlea (lateral ridge), 4d- capitulum;

Radius: 5- Proximal epiphysis; 6- Radial tuberosity; 7- Coronoid process; 8- Lateral tuberosity; 9- Fovea capitis, 9a- medial groove, 9b- sagittal ridge, 9b'- synovial fossa, 9c- lateral groove, 9d- lateral glenoid surface for the capitulum;

Ulna: 10- Olecranon; 11- Anconeal process; 12- Trochlear incisura; 13- Synovial fossa;

Joint and tendons: 14- Radioulnar joint space, 14a- medial part, 14b- lateral part; 15- Medial collateral ligament; 16- Lateral collateral ligament; 17- Proximal tendon of the digital flexor muscles; 18- Proximal tendon of the ulnaris lateralis muscle.

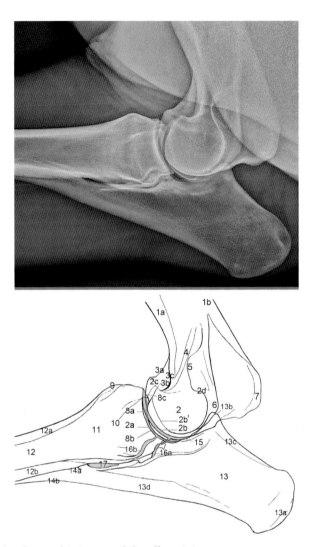

Fig. B.5 **Mediolateral radiographic image of the elbow joint.**

Humerus: 1- Body, 1a- cranial cortex, 1b- caudal cortex; 2- Humeral condyle, 2a- capitulum (lateral part), 2b- trochlea (medial ridge), 2b'- sagittal groove, 2c- proximocranial margin, 2d- proximocaudal margin; 3- Coronoid fossa, 3a- medial margin, 3b- bottom, 3c- lateral margin; 4- Supracondylar crest; 5- Olecranon fossa (bottom); 6- Lateral epicondyle; 7- Medial epicondyle;

Radius: 8- Radial head, 8a- fovea capitis (medial part), 8b- fovea capitis (lateral part), 8c- coronoid process; 9- Radial tuberosity; 10- Lateral tuberosity; 11- Proximal metaphysis (neck); 12- Body, 12a- cranial cortex, 12b- caudal cortex;

Ulna: 13- Olecranon, 13a- olecranon tuberosity, 13b- anconeal process, 13c- cranial cortex, 13d- caudal cortex; 14- Body, 14a- cranial face, 14b- caudal margin;

Radioulnar space: 15- Trochlear incisura; 16- Radioulnar joint, 16a- medial part, 16b- lateral part; 17- Antebrachial interosseous space.

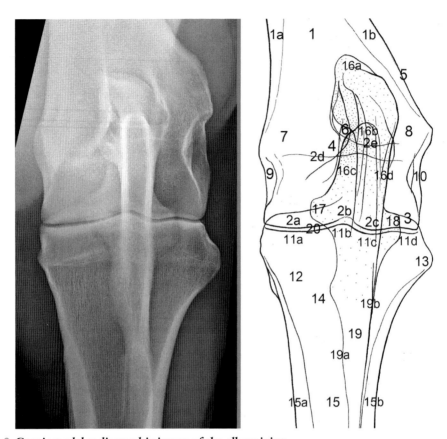

Fig. B.6 **Craniocaudal radiographic image of the elbow joint.**

Humerus: 1- Body, 1a- medial cortex, 1b- lateral cortex; 2- Humeral trochlea, 2a- medial ridge, 2b- sagittal groove, 2c- lateral ridge, 2d- proximocranial margin, 2e- proximocaudal margin; 3- Capitulum; 4- Coronoid fossa; 5- Supracondylar crest; 6- Olecranon fossa; 7- Medial epicondyle; 8- Lateral epicondyle; 9- Insertion fossa of the medial collateral ligament; 10- Insertion fossa of the lateral collateral ligament;

Radius: 11- Radial head: fovea capitis, 11a- medial groove, 11b- sagittal ridge, 11c- lateral groove, 11d- lateral glenoid surface for the capitulum; 12- Radial tuberosity; 13- Lateral tuberosity; 14- Proximal metaphysis; 15- Body, 15a- medial cortex, 15b- lateral cortex;

Ulna: 16- Olecranon, 16a- olecranon tuberosity, 16b- anconeal process, 16c- medial aspect, 16d- lateral aspect; 17- Medial (collateral) coronoid process; 18- Lateral (collateral) coronoid process; 19- Body, 19a- medial margin, 19b- lateral aspect and cortex; 20- Humeroantebrachial joint space.

B.3 DISSECTED SPECIMEN

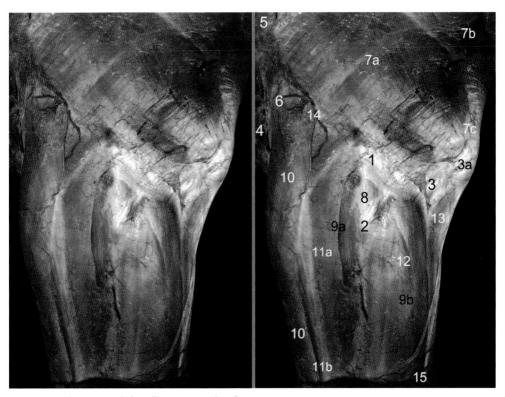

Fig. B.7 **Lateral aspect of the elbow: superficial structures.**

Bones: 1- Humerus (lateral epicondyle); 2- Radius: lateral tuberosity; 3- Ulna (olecranon), 3a- olecranon tuberosity;

Muscles and tendons: 4- Pectoralis descendens muscle; 5- Deltoideus muscle; 6- Brachialis muscle; 7- Triceps brachii muscle, 7a- lateral head, 7b- long head, 7c- distal (olecranon) tendon; 8- Lateral collateral ligament of the elbow joint; 9- Antebrachial fascia, 9a- cranial part, 9b- caudal part; 10- Extensor carpi radialis muscle; 11- Dorsal (common) digital extensor muscle, 11a- muscle body, 11b- tendon; 12- Ulnaris lateralis muscle; 13- Deep digital flexor muscle (ulnar head);

Vessels, nerves and skin: 14- Lateral antebrachial cutaneous nerve (originating from the radial nerve) and satellite arterial ramus; 15- Skin.

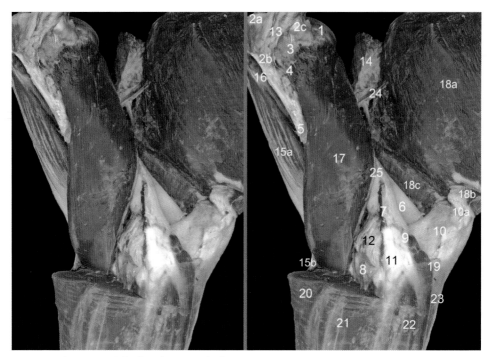

Fig. B.8 **Lateral aspect of the brachium and elbow: intermediate structures.**

Humerus: 1- Head; 2- Major tuberculum, 2a- cranial part (top), 2b- crest, 2c- caudal part (convexity); 3- Neck; 4- Tricipital line; 5- Deltoid tuberosity; 6- Olecranon fossa; 7- Supracondylar crest; 8- Humeral condyle; 9- Lateral epicondyle;

Ulna: 10- Olecranon, 10a- olecranon tuberosity;

Elbow joint structures: 11- Lateral collateral ligament; 12- Dorsal capsule (cut);

Muscles and tendons: 13- Infraspinatus tendon; 14- Teres major muscle; 15- Biceps brachii muscle, 15a- body, 15b- lacertus fibrosus; 16- Bicipital bursa; 17- Brachialis muscle; 18- Triceps brachii muscle, 18a- long head, 18b- distal (olecranon) tendon, 18c- medial head; 19- Antebrachial fascia (cut); 20- Extensor carpi radialis muscle; 21- Dorsal (common) digital extensor muscle; 22- Ulnaris lateralis muscle; 23- Deep digital flexor muscle (ulnar head);

Vessels and nerves: 24- Muscle ramus of the deep brachial artery; 25- Deep ramus of the radial nerve.

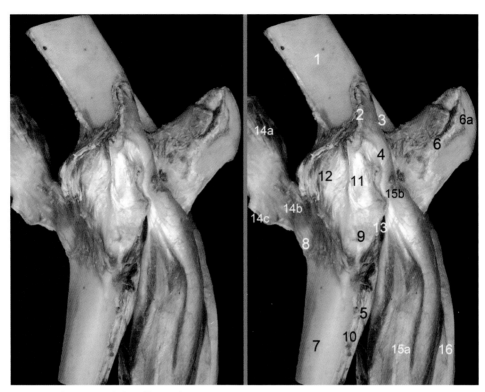

Fig. B.9 **Lateral aspect of the elbow: deep structures.**

Humerus: 1- Body (brachial sulcus); 2- Supracondylar crest; 3- Olecranon fossa; 4- Lateral epicondyle;

Ulna and radius: 5- Body of ulna; 6- Olecranon, 6a- olecranon tuberosity; 7- Body of radius; 8- Radial tuberosity; 9- Lateral tuberosity; 10- Radioulnar syndesmosis;

Elbow joint structures: 11- Lateral collateral ligament; 12- Dorsal capsule; 13- Lateral recess;

Muscles and tendons: 14- Biceps brachii muscle, 14a- body, 14b- distal tendon, 14c- lacertus fibrosus (cut); 15- Ulnaris lateralis, 15a- body, 15b- proximal tendon; 16- Superficial digital flexor muscle (body).

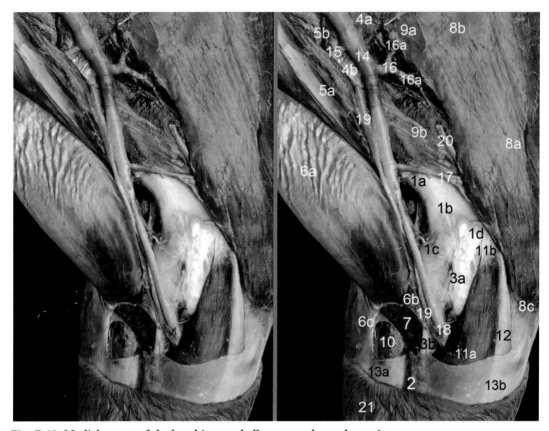

Fig. B.10 **Medial aspect of the brachium and elbow: muscles and arteries.**

Bones and joints: 1- Humerus, 1a- body, 1b- distal metaphysis, 1c- condyle, 1d- medial epicondyle; 2- Radius; 3- Medial collateral ligament of the elbow joint, 3a- caudal fasciculus, 3b- long fasciculus;

Shoulder muscles: 4- Teres major muscle, 4a- body, 4b- distal tendon (fused with the tendon of the latissimus dorsi muscle); 5- Coracobrachialis muscle, 5a- long head; 5b- short head;

Brachial muscles: 6- Biceps brachii muscle, 6a- body, 6b- distal insertion, 6c- lacertus fibrosus (covering partly the extensor carpi radialis muscle body); 7- Brachial muscle; 8- Tensor fasciae antebrachii muscle (covering the long head of the triceps brachii muscle), 8a- body, 8b- proximal aponeurosis, 8c- musculoaponeurotic junction with the antebrachial fascia; 9- Triceps brachii muscle, 9a- long head, 9b- medial head;

Antebrachial muscles: 10- Extensor carpi radialis muscle; 11- Flexor carpi radialis muscle, 11a- body, 11b- proximal tendon; 12- Flexor carpi ulnaris muscle (humeral head); 13- Antebrachial fascia, 13a- cranial part, 13b- caudal part;

Arteries and nerves: 14- Brachial (humeral) artery; 15- Cranial humeral circumflex artery; 16- Deep brachial artery, 16a- muscle rami; 17- Ulnar collateral artery; 18- Median artery; 19- Median nerve; 20- Ulnar nerve; 21- Skin.

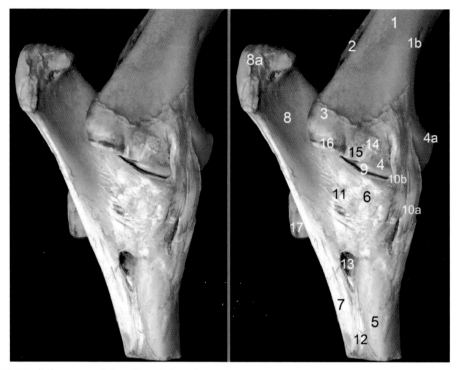

Fig. B.11 **Medial aspect of the elbow joint: deep structures.**

Humerus: 1- Body, 1a- vascular foramen; 2- Olecranon fossa; 3- Medial epicondyle; 4- Humeral condyle (medial aspect of the trochlea), 4a- proximodorsal margin;

Radius and ulna: 5- Body of radius; 6- Proximal epiphysis of radius; 7- Body of ulna; 8- Olecranon, 8a- olecranon tuberosity;

Elbow joint structures: 9- Humeroantebrachial joint space; 10- Medial collateral ligament, 10a- long (cranial) fasciculus, 10b- short (caudal) fasciculus; 11- Medial radioulnar ligament; 12- Antebrachial radioulnar syndesmosis; 13- Antebrachial interosseous space;

Muscles and tendons: 14- Insertion surface for the flexor carpi radialis muscle; 15- Insertion surface for the flexor carpi ulnaris muscle (humeral head); 16- Proximal tendon of the humeral heads of the superficial and deep digital flexor muscles; 17- Ulnaris lateralis muscle body.

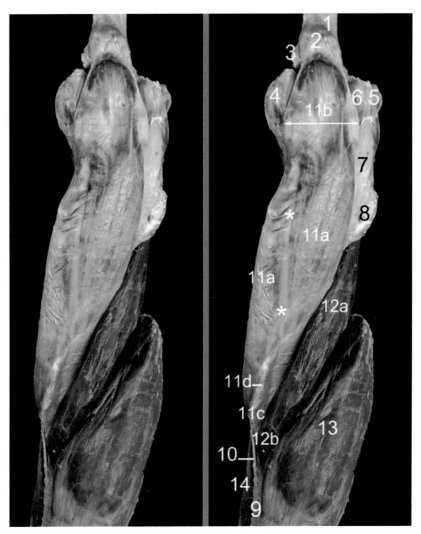

Fig. B.12 **Cranial aspect of the brachium and elbow: intermediate structures.**

Bones: 1- Neck of the scapula; 2- Tuberculum supraglenoidale; 3- Coracoid process; 4- Minor tuberculum of the humerus; 5- Major tuberculum; 6- Intertubercular sulcus; 7- Proximal metaphysis of the humerus; 8- Deltoid tuberosity; 9- Medial aspect of the radius;

Elbow joint structure: 10- Medial collateral ligament;

Muscles: 11- Biceps brachii muscle, 11a- body (*- intramuscular tendon), 11b- proximal tendon (arrow), 11c- distal tendon, 11d- lacertus fibrosus (cut); 12- Brachialis muscle, 12a- body, 12b- distal part; 13- Extensor carpi radialis muscle; 14- Flexor carpi radialis muscle.

B.4 CROSS-SECTIONS

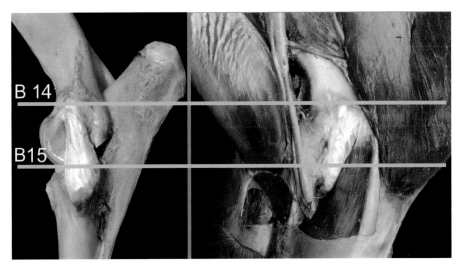

Fig. B.13 Levels of the cross-sections presented on Figures B.14 and B.15.

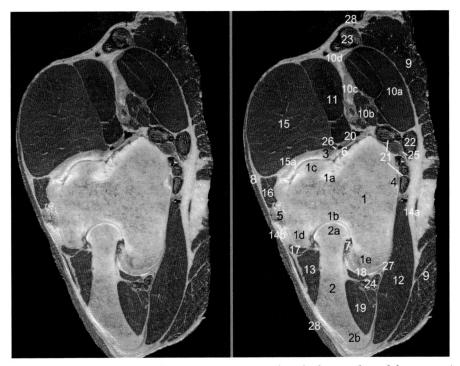

Fig. B.14 Transverse section of the elbow: passing proximal to the humeral condyle: anatomical structures.

Bones: 1- Humerus, 1a- coronoid fossa, 1b- sagittal groove, 1c- lateral trochlear ridge (proximal margin), 1d- lateral epicondyle, 1e- medial epicondyle; 2- Olecranon, 2a- coracoid process and trochlear incisura, 2b- base of the olecranon tuberosity;

Elbow joint structures: 3- Dorsal capsule; 4- Medial collateral ligament (origin); 5- Lateral collateral ligament (origin); 6- Dorsal recess; 7- Olecranon recess;

Cutaneous and pectoral muscles: 8- Cutaneous omobrachialis muscle; 9- Pectoralis transversus muscle;

Brachial muscles: 10- Biceps brachii muscle, 10a- body (medial part), 10b- body (lateral part), 10c- intramuscular tendon (distal part), 10d- lacertus fibrosus (origin); 11- Brachialis muscle; 12- Tensor fasciae antebrachii muscle; 13- Lateral head of the triceps brachii muscle; 14- Brachial and antebrachial fascia, 14a- medial part, 14b- lateral part;

Antebrachial muscles: 15- Extensor carpi radialis muscle, 15a- insertion on the elbow joint capsule; 16- Dorsal digital extensor muscle (origin); 17- Ulnaris lateralis muscle (origin); 18- Superficial digital flexor muscle (origin of proximal tendon); 19- Deep digital flexor muscle (ulnar head);

Arteries and nerves: 20- Transverse cubital artery and vein; 21- Median artery and vein; 22- Median vein of the elbow; 23- Cephalic vein; 24- Collateral ulnar artery and vein; 25- Median nerve; 26- Deep ramus of the radial nerve; 27- Ulnar nerve; 28- Skin.

Bones: 1- Humerus, 1a- medial trochlear ridge, 1b- lateral trochlear ridge; 1c- capitulum; 2- Radius (subchondral bone and articular cartilage of the radial fossa); 3- Ulna (base of olecranon), 3a- medial (collateral) coronoid process, 3b- lateral (collateral) coronoid process;

Elbow joint structures: 4- Dorsal capsule; 5- Medial collateral ligament; 6- Lateral collateral ligament; 7- Humeroantebrachial joint space; 8- Radioulnar joint space; 9- Medial radioulnar ligament;

Cutaneous and pectoral muscles: 10- Cutaneous omobrachialis muscle; 11- Pectoralis transversus muscle;

Brachial muscles: 12- Biceps brachii muscle, 12a- distal part of the muscle body, 12b- distal tendon, 12c- lacertus fibrosus; 13- Brachialis muscle; 14- Tensor fasciae antebrachii muscle; 15- Antebrachial fascia, 15a- medial part, 15b- lateral part;

Antebrachial muscles: 16- Extensor carpi radialis muscle; 17- Dorsal (common) digital extensor muscle; 18- Ulnaris lateralis muscle; 19- Flexor carpi ulnaris, 19a- ulnar head, 19b- humeral head; 20- Flexor carpi radialis origin; 21- Superficial digital flexor muscle; 22- Deep digital flexor muscle, 22a- humeral head, 22b- ulnar head;

Arteries and nerves: 23- Transverse cubital artery and vein; 24- Median artery and vein; 25- Median vein of the elbow; 26- Cephalic vein; 27- Collateral ulnar artery and vein; 28- Median nerve; 29- Deep ramus of the radial nerve; 30- Ulnar nerve; 31- Skin.

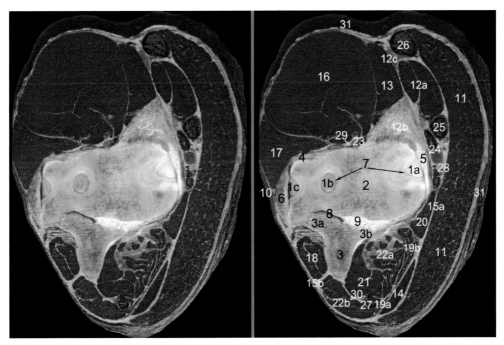

Fig. B.15 Transverse section of the elbow passing through the humeroantebrachial joint space: anatomical structures.

THE ANTEBRACHIUM

C.1 PHYSICAL ASPECT

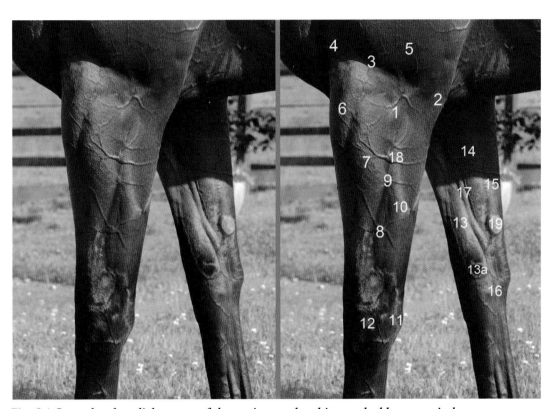

Fig. C.1 **Lateral and medial aspects of the equine antebrachium: palpable anatomical structures.**

1- Proximolateral tuberosity of the radius; 2- Point of the elbow (olecranon); 3- Sulcus of the elbow; 4- Brachialis muscle; 5- Triceps brachii muscle (lateral head); 6- Extensor carpi radialis muscle; 7- Dorsal (common) digital extensor muscle; 8- Lateral digital extensor muscle; 9- Lateral sulcus of the antebrachium; 10- Ulnaris lateralis muscle; 11- Accessory carpal bone; 12- Lateral collateral ligament of the carpus; 13- Radius (medial aspect), 13a- styloid process; 14- Flexor carpi radialis muscle; 15- Flexor carpi ulnaris muscle; 16- Carpal canal; 17- Antebrachial cephalic vein; 18- Cutaneous veins; 19- Chestnut.

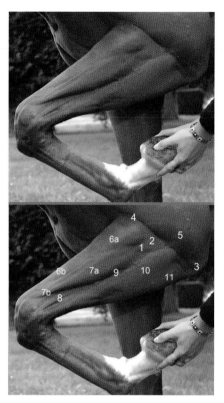

Fig. C.2 **Lateral aspect of the equine antebrachium on the flexed limb: palpable anatomical structures.**

1- Proximolateral tuberosity of the radius; 2- Lateral collateral ligament of the elbow joint; 3- Point of the elbow (olecranon); 4- Sulcus of the elbow; 5- Triceps brachii muscle (lateral head); 6- Extensor carpi radialis muscle, 6a- body, 6b- tendon; 7- Dorsal (common) digital extensor muscle, 7a- body, 7b- tendon; 8- Lateral digital extensor muscle; 9- Lateral sulcus of the antebrachium; 10- Ulnaris lateralis muscle; 11- Deep digital flexor muscle (ulnar head).

C.2 DISSECTED SPECIMEN

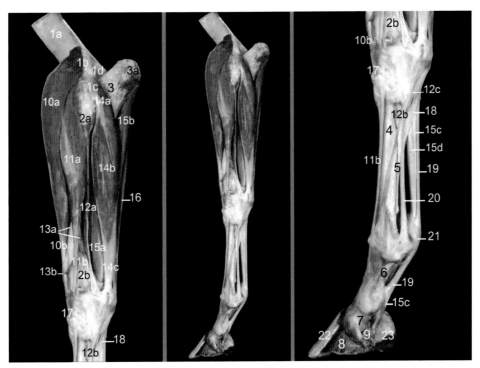

Fig. C.3 **Lateral aspect of the antebrachium and distal thoracic limb.**

Bones: 1- Humerus, 1a- brachial sulcus, 1b- supracondylar crest, 1c- lateral epicondyle, 1d- olecranon fossa; 2- Radius, 2a- lateral tuberosity, 2b- distal metaphysis; 3- Ulna (olecranon), 3a- olecranon tuberosity; 4- Third metacarpal bone; 5- Fourth metacarpal bone; 6- Proximal phalanx; 7- Middle phalanx; 8- Distal phalanx; 9- Distal sesamoid bone;

Muscles and tendons: 10- Extensor carpi radialis muscle, 10a- body, 10b- tendon; 11- Dorsal (common) digital extensor muscle, 11a- body, 11b- tendon; 12- Lateral digital extensor muscle, 12a- body, 12b- tendon, 12c- accessory ligament; 13- Extensor carpi obliquus muscle, 13a- body, 13b- tendon; 14- Ulnaris lateralis muscle, 14a- proximal tendon, 14b- body, 14c- distal tendon; 15- Deep digital flexor muscle, 15a- humeral head, 15b- ulnar head, 15c- tendon, 15d- accessory ligament; 16- Flexor carpi ulnaris muscle (ulnar head); 17- Extensor retinaculum; 18- Flexor retinaculum; 19- Superficial digital flexor tendon; 20- Third interosseous muscle (suspensory ligament); 21- Palmar ligament;

Hoof: 22-Hoof wall; 23- Medial heel.

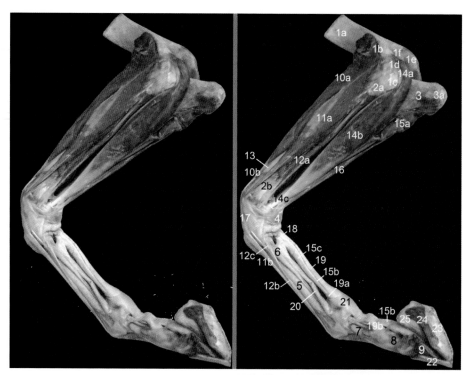

Fig. C.4 **Lateral aspect of the antebrachium and distal thoracic limb in flexion.**

Bones: 1- Humerus, 1a- brachial sulcus, 1b- supracondylar crest, 1c- capitulum, 1d- lateral epicondyle, 1e- medial epicondyle, 1f- olecranon fossa; 2- Radius, 2a- lateral tuberosity, 2b- distal metaphysis; 3- Ulna (olecranon), 3a- olecranon tuberosity; 4- Accessory carpal bone; 5- Third metacarpal bone; 6- Fourth metacarpal bone; 7- Proximal phalanx; 8- Middle phalanx; 9- Distal phalanx;

Muscles and tendons: 10- Extensor carpi radialis muscle, 10a- body, 10b- tendon; 11- Dorsal (common) digital extensor muscle, 11a- body, 11b- tendon; 12- Lateral digital extensor muscle, 12a- body, 12b- tendon, 12c- accessory ligament; 13- Extensor carpi obliquus muscle; 14- Ulnaris lateralis muscle, 14a- proximal tendon, 14b- body, 14c- distal tendon; 15- Deep digital flexor muscle, 15a- ulnar head, 15b- tendon, 15c- accessory ligament; 16- Flexor carpi ulnaris muscle (ulnar head); 17- Extensor retinaculum; 18- Flexor retinaculum; 19- Superficial digital flexor tendon, 19a- manica flexoria, 19b- lateral branch; 20- Third interosseous muscle (suspensory ligament) lateral branch; 21- Palmar ligament;

Hoof: 22-Hoof wall; 23- Sole; 24- Frog; 25- Digital cushion.

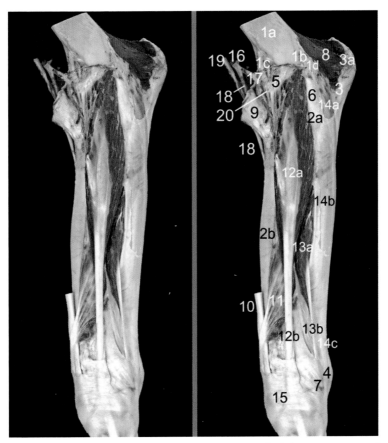

Fig. C.5 **Craniolateral aspect of the antebrachium (after removal of the extensor carpi radialis muscle body).**

Bones and joints: 1- Humerus, 1a- brachial sulcus, 1b- supracondylar crest, 1c- coronoid fossa, 1d- lateral epicondyle; 2- Radius, 2a- lateral tuberosity, 2b- body; 3- Ulna (olecranon), 3a- olecranon tuberosity; 4- Accessory carpal bone; 5- Dorsal capsule of the elbow joint; 6- Lateral collateral ligament of the elbow joint; 7- Lateral collateral ligament of the carpus;

Muscles and tendons: 8- Anconeus muscle; 9- Distal tendon of the biceps brachii muscle; 10- Extensor carpi radialis tendon; 11- Extensor carpi obliquus muscle; 12- Dorsal (common) digital extensor muscle, 12a- body, 12b- tendon; 13- Lateral digital extensor muscle, 13a- body, 13b- tendon; 14- Ulnaris lateralis muscle, 14a- proximal tendon and muscle fibres, 14b- body (covered by the antebrachial fascia), 14c- distal tendon; 15- Extensor retinaculum;

Vessels and nerves: 16- Brachial artery; 17- Transverse cubital artery; 18- Median artery; 19- Median nerve; 20- Deep ramus of the radial nerve.

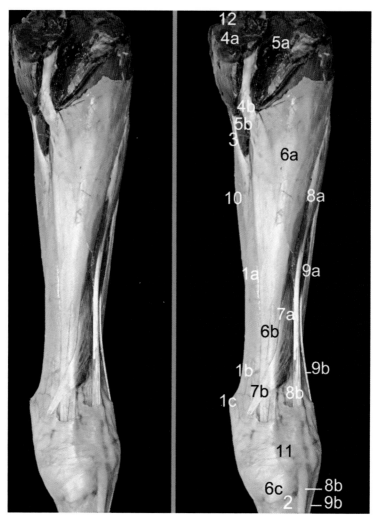

Fig. C.6 **Cranial aspect of the antebrachium.**

Bones and joints: 1- Radius, 1a- body (medial aspect), 1b- distal metaphysis, 1c- styloid process; 2- Third metacarpal bone; 3- Medial collateral ligament of the elbow joint;

Muscles and tendons: 4- Biceps brachii muscle, 4a- distal part of the body, 4b- lacertus fibrosus; 5- Brachialis muscle, 5a- body, 5b- distal part; 6- Extensor carpi radialis muscle, 6a- body (covered by the antebrachial fascia), 6b- tendon, 6c- distal enthesis; 7- Extensor carpi obliquus muscle, 7a- body, 7b- tendon; 8- Dorsal (common) digital extensor muscle, 8a- body, 8b- tendon; 9- Lateral digital extensor muscle, 9a- body, 9b- tendon; 10- Flexor carpi radialis muscle (covered by the antebrachial fascia); 11- Extensor retinaculum;

Vessels and nerves: 12- Median artery and vein.

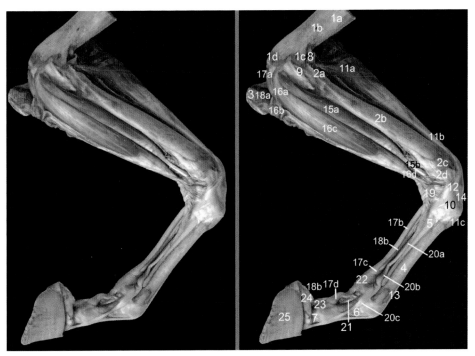

Fig. C.7 Medial aspect of the antebrachium and distal thoracic limb in flexion.

Bones and joints: 1- Humerus, 1a- body, 1b- vascular foramen, 1c- craniomedial crest of the distal metaphysis, 1d- medial epicondyle; 2- Radius, 2a- radial tuberosity, 2b- body, 2c- distal metaphysis, 2d- styloid process; 3- Ulna (olecranon tuberosity); 4- Third metacarpal bone; 5- Second metacarpal bone; 6- Proximal phalanx; 7- Middle phalanx; 8- Dorsal capsule and recess of the elbow joint; 9- Medial collateral ligament of the elbow joint; 10- Medial collateral ligament of the carpus;

Muscles and tendons: 11- Extensor carpi radialis muscle, 11a- body, 11b- tendon, 11c- distal enthesis; 12- Extensor carpi obliquus tendon; 13- Dorsal (common) digital extensor tendon; 14- Extensor retinaculum; 15- Flexor carpi radialis muscle, 15a- body, 15b- distal tendon; 16- Flexor carpi ulnaris muscle, 16a- humeral head, 16b- ulnar head, 16c- body, 16d- distal tendon; 17- Superficial digital flexor muscle, 17a- origin, 17b- tendon, 17c- manica flexoria, 17d- medial branch; 18- Deep digital flexor muscle, 18a- ulnar head, 18b- tendon; 19- Flexor retinaculum; 20- Third interosseous muscle (suspensory ligament), 20a- body, 20b- medial branch, 20c- medial extensor branch; 21- Medial oblique sesamoidean ligament; 22- Palmar ligament; 23- Distal digital annular ligament;

Foot: 24- Medial ungular cartilage; 25- Hoof wall.

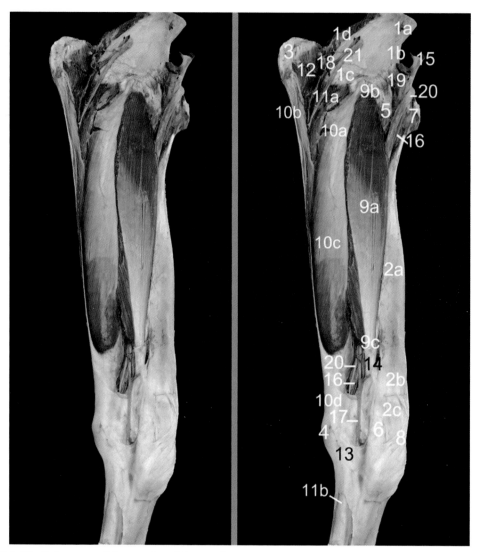

Fig. C.8 **Medial aspect of the antebrachium and carpus.**

Bones and joints: 1- Humerus, 1a- vascular foramen, 1b- craniomedial crest of the distal metaphysis; 1c- medial epicondyle, 1d- olecranon fossa and anconeus muscle; 2- Radius, 2a- body, 2b- distal metaphysis, 2c- styloid process; 3- Ulna (olecranon tuberosity); 4- Accessory carpal bone; 5- Medial collateral ligament of the elbow joint; 6- Medial collateral ligament of the carpus;

Muscles and tendons: 7- Distal tendon of the biceps brachii muscle; 8- Extensor carpi obliquus tendon; 9- Flexor carpi radialis muscle, 9a- body, 9b- proximal tendon, 9c- distal tendon (entering its sheath); 10- Flexor carpi ulnaris muscle, 10a- humeral head, 10b- ulnar head, 10c- body, 10d- distal tendon; 11- Superficial digital flexor muscle, 11a- origin, 11b- tendon; 12- Deep digital flexor muscle (ulnar head); 13- Flexor retinaculum; 14- Tendon sheath of the flexor carpi radialis distal tendon;

Vessels and nerves: 15- Brachial artery; 16- Median artery; 17- Distal radial artery; 18- Collateral ulnar artery; 19- Median vein; 20- Median nerve; 21- Ulnar nerve.

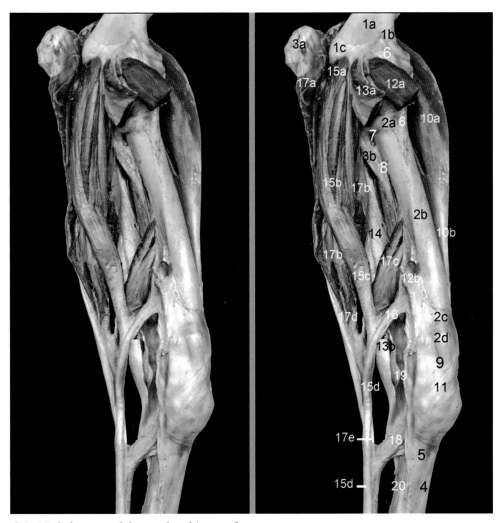

Fig. C.9 **Medial aspect of the antebrachium and carpus.**

Bones and joints: 1- Humerus, 1a- distal metaphysis, 1b- craniomedial crest, 1c- medial epicondyle; 2- Radius, 2a- proximal metaphysis, 2b- body, 2c- distal metaphysis, 2d- styloid process; 3- Ulna, 3a- olecranon tuberosity, 3b- body; 4- Third metacarpal bone; 5- Second metacarpal bone; 6- Medial collateral ligament of the elbow joint; 7- Radioulnar interosseous space; 8- Radioulnar syndesmosis; 9- Medial collateral ligament of the carpus;

Muscles and tendons: 10- Extensor carpi radialis muscle, 10a- body, 10b- tendon; 11- Extensor carpi obliquus tendon; 12- Flexor carpi radialis muscle, 12a- body (cut), 12b- distal tendon (entering its sheath); 13- Flexor carpi ulnaris muscle, 13a- humeral head (cut), 13b- tendon; 14- Ulnaris lateralis muscle; 15- Superficial digital flexor muscle, 15a- origin, 15b- body, 15c- musculotendinous junction, 15d- tendon; 16- Accessory ligament of the superficial digital flexor tendon; 17- Deep digital flexor muscle, 17a- ulnar head, 17b- humeral head, 17c- radial head, 17d- musculotendinous junction, 17e- tendon; 18- Accessory ligament of the deep digital flexor tendon; 19- Flexor retinaculum (cut, the carpal canal is open); 20- Third interosseous muscle (suspensory ligament).

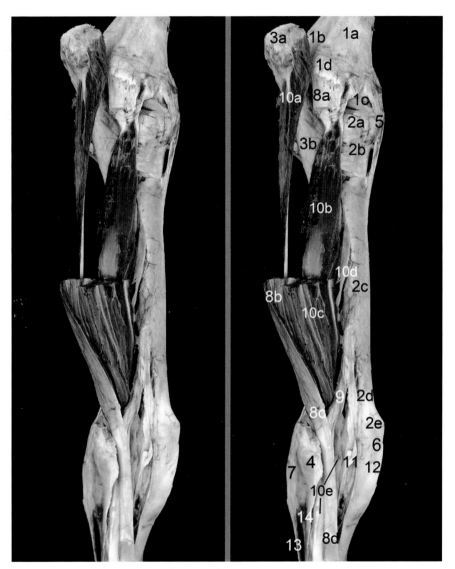

Fig. C.10 **Caudal aspect of the antebrachium and carpus.**

Bones and joints: 1- Humerus, 1a- distal metaphysis, 1b- olecranon fossa, 1c- humeral trochlea, 1d- medial epicondyle; 2- Radius, 2a- proximal epiphysis, 2b- proximal metaphysis, 2c- body, 2d- distal metaphysis, 2e- styloid process; 3- Ulna, 3a-olecranon tuberosity, 3b- body; 4- Accessory carpal bone; 5- Medial collateral ligament of the elbow joint; 6- Medial collateral ligament of the carpus; 7- Lateral collateral ligament of the carpus;

Muscles and tendons: 8- Superficial digital flexor muscle, 8a- origin, 8b- body, 8c- musculo-tendinous junction, 8d- tendon; 9- Accessory ligament of the superficial digital flexor tendon; 10- Deep digital flexor muscle, 10a- ulnar head, 10b- humeral head, cranial part, 10c- humeral head, caudal part, 10d- radial head, 10e- tendon; 11- Flexor carpi radialis tendon in its sheath; 12- Extensor carpi obliquus; 13- Accessory ligament of the lateral digital extensor tendon; 14- Accessoriometacarpal ligament.

C.3 CROSS-SECTIONS

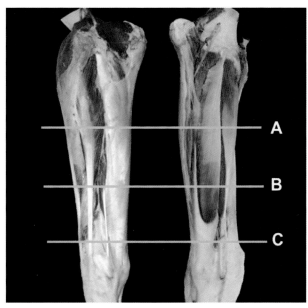

Fig. C.11 Levels of the cross-sections presented on Figs C.12 through C.14.

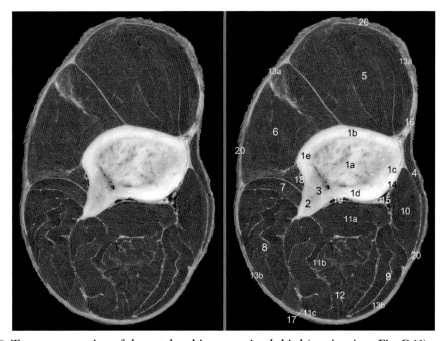

Fig. C.12 Transverse section of the antebrachium: proximal third (section A on Fig. C.11).

Bones: 1- Radius, 1a- medullary cavity, 1b- cranial cortex, 1c- medial cortex, 1d- caudal cortex, 1e- lateral cortex; 2- Ulna (body); 3- Radioulnar synostosis;

Muscles and tendons: 4- Pectoralis transversus muscle; 5- Extensor carpi radialis muscle; 6- Dorsal (common) digital extensor muscle; 7- Lateral digital extensor muscle; 8- Ulnaris lateralis muscle; 9- Flexor carpi ulnaris muscle; 10- Flexor carpi radialis muscle; 11- Deep digital flexor muscle, 11a- cranial part of the humeral head, 11b- caudal part of the humeral head (fused with the superficial digital flexor muscle body), 11c- tendon of the ulnar head; 12- Superficial digital flexor muscle; 13- Antebrachial fascia, 13a- cranial part, 13b- caudal part;

Vessels and nerves: 14- Median nerve; 15- Median artery and veins; 16- Cephalic vein (collapsed); 17- Ulnar nerve and collateral ulnar artery and vein; 18- Cranial antebrachial interosseous artery and vein; 19- Caudal antebrachial interosseous artery and vein; 20- Skin.

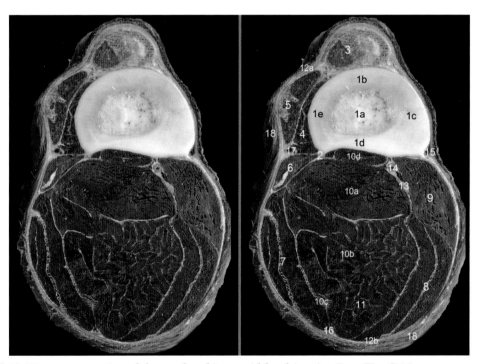

Fig. C.13 **Transverse section of the antebrachium: mid-level (section B on Fig. C.11).**

Bones: 1- Radius, 1a- medullary cavity, 1b- cranial cortex, 1c- medial cortex, 1d- caudal cortex, 1e- lateral cortex; 2- Ulna (fibrous part of the body);

Muscles and tendons: 3- Extensor carpi radialis musculotendinous junction; 4- Extensor carpi obliquus muscle; 5- Dorsal (common) digital extensor muscle; 6- Lateral digital extensor muscle; 7- Ulnaris lateralis muscle; 8- Flexor carpi ulnaris muscle; 9- Flexor carpi radialis muscle; 10- Deep digital flexor muscle, 10a- cranial part of the humeral head, 10b- caudal part of the humeral head (fused with the superficial digital flexor muscle body), 10c- tendon of the ulnar head; 11- Superficial digital flexor muscle; 12- Antebrachial fascia, 12a- cranial part, 12b- caudal part;

Vessels and nerves: 13- Median nerve; 14- Median artery and veins; 15- Cephalic vein (collapsed); 16- Ulnar nerve and collateral ulnar artery and vein; 17- Cranial antebrachial interosseous artery and vein; 18- Skin.

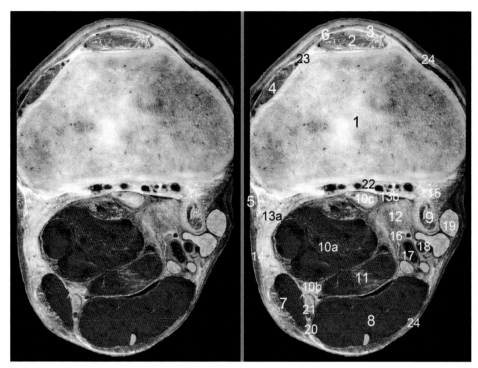

Fig. C.14 **Transverse section of the antebrachium: distal fourth (section C on Fig. C.11).**

Bones: 1- Radius (distal metaphysis);

Muscles and tendons: 2- Extensor carpi radialis tendon; 3- Extensor carpi obliquus tendon; 4- Dorsal (common) digital extensor tendon; 5- Lateral digital extensor tendon; 6- Extensor retinaculum; 7- Ulnaris lateralis musculotendinous junction; 8- Flexor carpi ulnaris muscle; 9- Flexor carpi radialis tendon (in its sheath); 10- Deep digital flexor muscle, 10a- humeral head, 10b- tendon of the ulnar head, 10c- tendon of the radial head; 11- Superficial digital flexor musculotendinous junction; 12- Accessory ligament of the superficial digital flexor tendon; 13- Carpal sheath, 13a- fibrous wall, 13b- cavity; 14- Antebrachial fascia; 15- Proximomedial part of the flexor retinaculum;

Vessels and nerves: 16- Median nerve; 17- Median artery and veins; 18- Distal radial artery; 19- Cephalic vein; 20- Ulnar nerve; 21- Collateral ulnar artery and vein; 22- Palmar network of the carpus; 23- Dorsal network of the carpus; 24- Skin.

THE CARPUS

D.1 PHYSICAL ASPECT

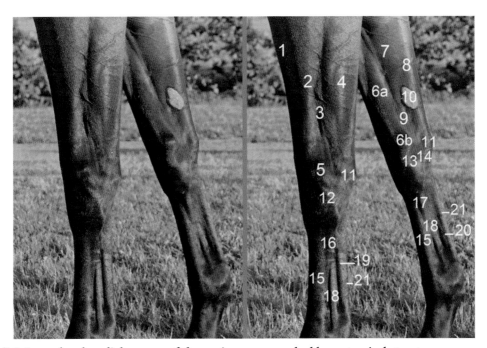

Fig. D.1 **Lateral and medial aspects of the equine carpus: palpable anatomical structures.**

Antebrachium: 1- Extensor carpi radialis muscle; 2- Dorsal (common) digital extensor muscle; 3- Lateral digital extensor muscle; 4- Ulnaris lateralis muscle; 5- Styloid process of the ulna; 6- Radius, 6a- body, 6b- styloid process; 7- Flexor carpi radialis muscle; 8- Flexor carpi ulnaris muscle; 9- Cephalic vein; 10- Chestnut;

Carpus: 11- Accessory carpal bone; 12- Lateral collateral ligament; 13- Medial collateral ligament; 14- Carpal canal;

Metacarpus: 15- Third metacarpal bone; 16- Fourth metacarpal bone; 17- Second metacarpal bone; 18- Third interosseous muscle (suspensory ligament); 19- Accessory ligament of the deep digital flexor tendon; 20- Deep digital flexor tendon; 21- Superficial digital flexor tendon.

D.2 RADIOGRAPHIC ANATOMY

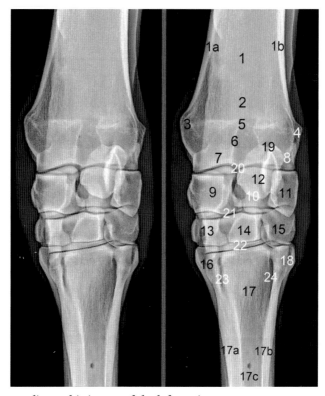

Fig. D.2 **Dorsopalmar radiographic image of the left equine carpus.**

Antebrachial bones: 1- Body (diaphysis) of the radius, 1a- medial cortex, 1b- lateral cortex; 2- Distal metaphysis of the radius; 3- Radial styloid process; 4- Ulnar styloid process; 5- Transverse crest of the radius (insertion of the common palmar ligament); 6- Distal epiphysis of the radius; 7- Radial (antebrachial) condyle; 8- Distal epiphysis of the ulna (fused with the radius);

Proximal row: 9- Radial carpal bone; 10- Intermediate carpal bone; 11- Ulnar carpal bone; 12- Accessory carpal bone;

Distal row: 13- Second carpal bone (no first carpal bone on this carpus); 14- Third carpal bone; 15- Fourth carpal bone;

Metacarpal bones: 16- Second metacarpal bone; 17- Third metacarpal bone, 17a- medial cortex superimposed with the second metacarpal bone, 17b- lateral cortex superimposed with the fourth metacarpal bone, 17c- vascular foramen; 18- Fourth metacarpal bone;

Joints: 19- Radioulnar synostosis; 20- Antebrachiocarpal joint; 21- Mediocarpal joint; 22- Carpometacarpal joint; 23- Second intermetacarpal syndesmosis; 24- Third intermetacarpal syndesmosis.

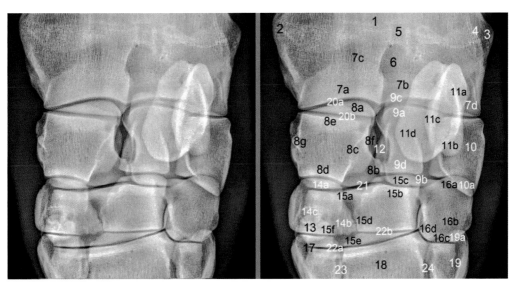

Fig. D.3 **Dorsopalmar radiographic image of the left equine carpus.**

Antebrachial bones: 1- Distal metaphysis of the radius; 2- Radial styloid process; 3- Ulnar styloid process; 4- Sulcus of the lateral digital extensor tendon; 5- Transverse crest of the radius (insertion of the common palmar ligament); 6- Sagittal fossa (palmar aspect); 7- Radial (antebrachial) condyle, 7a- medial part, 7b- intermediate part, 7c- caudal margin, 7d- lateral part (distal part of the ulna);

Proximal row: 8- Radial carpal bone, 8a- dorsal condyle, 8b- distoaxial process for the intermediate carpal bone, 8c- intermediate part, 8d- distal glenoid cavity, 8e- palmar glenoid surface, 8f- palmar tubercle, 8g- medial surface (irregular); 9- Intermediate carpal bone (blue), 9a- dorsal condyle, 9b- dorsodistal angular surface articulating with the dorsal parts of the third and fourth carpal bones, 9c- proximopalmar margin, 9d- palmar tubercle articulating with the palmar tubercle of the third carpal bone; 10- Ulnar carpal bone, 10a- distopalmar part; 11- Accessory carpal bone (yellow), 11a- proximodorsal part articulating with the ulna, 11b- distodorsal part articulating with the ulnar carpal bone, 11c- medial aspect, 11d- palmar part; 12- Radiointermediate interosseous space;

Distal row: 13- First carpal bone; 14- Second carpal bone (green), 14a- head, 14b- palmar part articulating with the third carpal bone, 14c- bed for the first carpal bone; 15- Third carpal bone, 15a- radial fossa, 15b- intermediate fossa, 15c- palmar tubercle, 15d- palmar surface for the second carpal bone, 15e- distodorsal surface for the third metacarpal bone, 15f- distopalmar surface for the second metacarpal bone; 16- Fourth carpal bone, 16a- dorsal part, 16b- palmar tubercle (opacity), 16c- Distal surface for the fourth metacarpal bone, 16d- Distoaxial surface for the third metacarpal bone;

Metacarpal bones: 17- Second metacarpal bone; 18- Third metacarpal bone; 19- Fourth metacarpal bone, 19a- palmar tubercle;

Joints: 20- Antebrachiocarpal joint, 20a- dorsal part, 20b- palmar part; 21- Mediocarpal joint; 22- Carpometacarpal joint, 22a- dorsal part, 22b- palmar part; 23- Second intermetacarpal syndesmosis (palmar part); 24- Third intermetacarpal syndesmosis (palmar part).

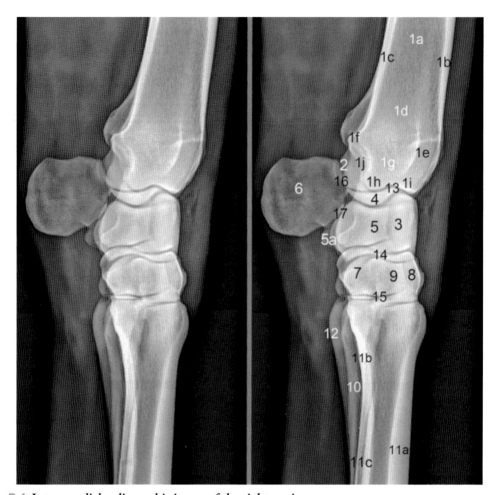

Fig. D.4 **Lateromedial radiographic image of the right equine carpus.**

Antebrachial bones: 1- Radius, 1a- body (diaphysis), 1b- cranial cortex, 1c- caudal cortex, 1d- distal metaphysis, 1e- sulcus of the dorsal digital extensor tendon, 1f- transverse crest (insertion of the common palmar ligament), 1g- distal epiphysis of the radius, 1h- radial (antebrachial) condyle, 1i- dorsal locking surface, 1j- sagittal fossa; 2- Distal epiphysis of the ulna (fused with the radius);

Proximal row: 3- Radial carpal bone; 4- Intermediate carpal bone; 5- Ulnar carpal bone, 5a- distopalmar tubercle; 6- Accessory carpal bone;

Distal row: 7- Second carpal bone (no first carpal bone on this carpus); 8- Third carpal bone; 9- Fourth carpal bone;

Metacarpal bones: 10- Second metacarpal bone; 11- Third metacarpal bone, 11a- dorsal cortex, 11b- palmar cortex (superimposed with the second and fourth metacarpal bones), 11c- vascular foramen; 12- Fourth metacarpal bone;

Joints: 13- Antebrachiocarpal joint; 14- Mediocarpal joint; 15- Carpometacarpal joint; 16- Accessorioulnar joint; 17- accessoriocarpoulnar joint.

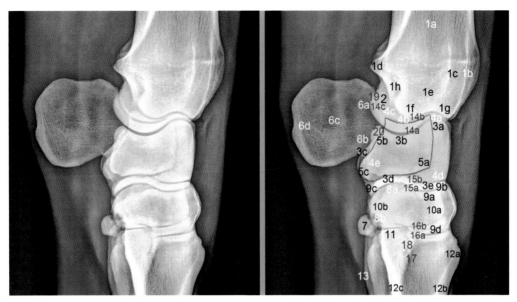

Fig. D.5 Lateromedial radiographic image of the right equine carpus.

Antebrachial bones: 1- Radius, 1a- distal metaphysis, 1b- sulcus of the extensor carpi radialis tendon, 1c- sulcus of the dorsal digital extensor tendon, 1d- transverse crest (insertion of the common palmar ligament), 1e- distal epiphysis of the radius, 1f- radial (antebrachial) condyle, 1g- dorsal locking surface, 1h- sagittal fossa; 2- Distal epiphysis of the ulna (fused with the radius);

Proximal row: 3- Radial carpal bone, 3a- dorsal condyle, 3b- palmar glenoid surface, 3c- palmar tubercle, 3d- distal glenoid cavity, 3e- distodorsal articular surface for the third carpal bone; 4- Intermediate carpal bone (blue), 4a- dorsal condyle, 4b- palmar articular surface, 4c- proximopalmar margin, 4d- dorsodistal angular surface articulating with the dorsal parts of the third and fourth carpal bones, 4e- palmar tubercle; 5- Ulnar carpal bone (red outline), 5a- distodorsal angle, 5b- articular surface for the accessory carpal bone, 5c- distopalmar tubercle; 6- Accessory carpal bone, 6a- proximodorsal part articulating with the ulna, 6b- distodorsal part articulating with the ulnar carpal bone, 6c- intermediate part (crossed by the sulcus of the ulnaris lateralis long tendon), 6d- palmar part;

Distal row: 7- First carpal bone; 8- Second carpal bone (green), 8a- head, 8b- bed for the first carpal bone; 9- Third carpal bone, 9a- radial fossa, 9b- intermediate fossa, 9c- palmar tubercle, 9d- distal surface for the third metacarpal bone; 10- Fourth carpal bone (yellow), 10a- dorsal part, 10b- palmar tubercle;

Metacarpal bones: 11- Second metacarpal bone (head); 12- Third metacarpal bone, 12a- proximal tuberosity (insertion of the extensor carpi radialis tendon), 12b- dorsal cortex, 12c- palmar cortex (superimposed with the second and fourth metacarpal bones); 13- Fourth metacarpal bone;

Joints: 14- Antebrachiocarpal joint, 14a- medial part, 14b- intermediate part, 14c- lateral part; 15- Mediocarpal joint, 15a- medial part, 15b- lateral part; 16- Carpometacarpal joint, 16a- medial part, 16b- lateral part; 17- Second intermetacarpal syndesmosis; 18- Third intermetacarpal syndesmosis; 19- Accessorioulnar joint; 20- Accessoriocarpoulnar joint.

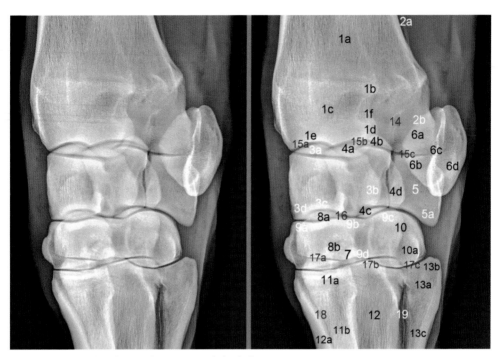

Fig. D.6 **Dorsolateral radiographic image of the left equine carpus.**

Antebrachial bones: 1- Radius, 1a- distal metaphysis, 1b- transverse crest (insertion of the common palmar ligament), 1c- distal epiphysis of the radius, 1d- radial (antebrachial) condyle, 1e- dorsal locking surface, 1f- sagittal fossa; 2- Ulna, 2a- body, 2b- distal epiphysis (fused with the radius);

Proximal row: 3- Radial carpal bone, 3a- dorsal condyle, 3b- palmar tubercle, 3c- distal glenoid cavity, 3d- distodorsal articular surface for the third carpal bone; 4- Intermediate carpal bone, 4a- dorsal condyle, 4b- proximopalmar margin, 4c- dorsodistal angular surface articulating with the dorsal parts of the third and fourth carpal bones, 4d- palmar tubercle; 5- Ulnar carpal bone, 5a- distopalmar tubercle; 6- Accessory carpal bone, 6a- proximodorsal part articulating with the ulna, 6b- distodorsal part articulating with the ulnar carpal bone, 6c- medial aspect, 6d- palmar part;

Distal row: 7- First carpal bone; 8- Second carpal bone, 8a- head, 8b- bed for the first carpal bone; 9- Third carpal bone, 9a- radial fossa, 9b- intermediate fossa, 9c- palmar tubercle, 9d- distal surface for the third metacarpal bone; 10- Fourth carpal bone, 10a- palmar tubercle;

Metacarpal bones: 11- Second metacarpal bone, 11a- base, 11b- body; 12- Third metacarpal bone, 12a- dorsomedial cortex; 13- Fourth metacarpal bone, 13a- base, 13b- palmar tubercle, 13c- body;

Joints: 14- Radioulnar synostosis; 15- Antebrachiocarpal joint, 15a- medial part, 15b- intermediate part, 15c- lateral part; 16- Mediocarpal joint; 17- Carpometacarpal joint, 17a- medial part, 17b- intermediate part, 17c- lateral part; 18- Second intermetacarpal syndesmosis (dorsal aspect); 19- Third intermetacarpal syndesmosis.

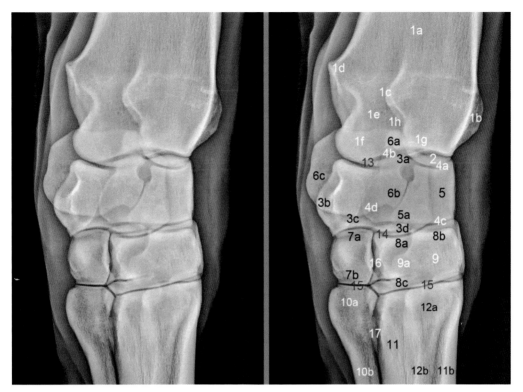

Fig. D.7 **Dorsomedial radiographic image of the left equine carpus.**

Antebrachial bones: 1- Radius, 1a- distal metaphysis, 1b- crest separating the extensor tendon sulci, 1c- transverse crest (insertion of the common palmar ligament), 1d- styloid process, 1e- distal epiphysis of the radius, 1f- radial (antebrachial) condyle, 1g- dorsal locking surface, 1h- sagittal fossa; 2- Ulna (distal epiphysis fused with the radius);

Proximal row: 3- Radial carpal bone, 3a- dorsal condyle, 3b- palmar tubercle, 3c- distal glenoid cavity, 3d- distodorsal articular surface for the third carpal bone; 4- Intermediate carpal bone (violet), 4a- dorsal condyle, 4b- proximopalmar margin, 4c- dorsodistal angular surface articulating with the dorsal parts of the third and fourth carpal bones, 4d- palmar tubercle; 5- Ulnar carpal bone, 5a- distopalmar tubercle; 6- Accessory carpal bone, 6a- proximodorsal part articulating with the ulna, 6b- distodorsal part articulating with the ulnar carpal bone, 6c- palmar part;

Distal row: 7- Second carpal bone, 7a- head, 7b- distal facet for the second metacarpal bone; 8- Third carpal bone, 8a- radial fossa, 8b- intermediate fossa, 8c- distal surface for the third metacarpal bone; 9- Fourth carpal bone, 9a- palmar tubercle;

Metacarpal bones: 10- Second metacarpal bone, 10a- base, 10b- body; 11- Third metacarpal bone, 11a- dorsolateral cortex; 12- Fourth metacarpal bone, 12a- base, 12b- body;

Joints: 13- Antebrachiocarpal joint; 14- Mediocarpal joint; 15- Carpometacarpal joint; 16- Secondotercer interosseous space; 17- Second intermetacarpal syndesmosis.

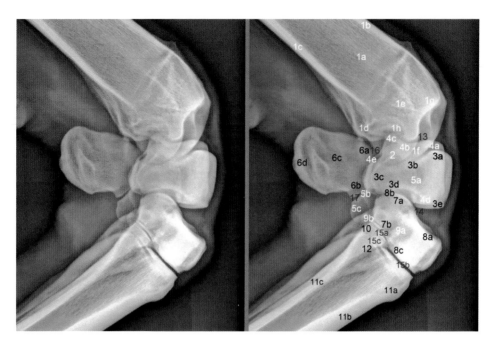

Fig. D.8 **Lateromedial radiographic image of the flexed right carpus.**

Antebrachial bones: 1- Radius, 1a- distal metaphysis, 1b- cranial cortex, 1c- caudal cortex, 1d- transverse crest (insertion of the common palmar ligament), 1e- distal epiphysis of the radius, 1f- radial (antebrachial) condyle, 1g- dorsal locking surface, 1h- sagittal fossa; 2- Distal epiphysis of the ulna (fused with the radius);

Proximal row: 3- Radial carpal bone, 3a- dorsal condyle, 3b- palmar glenoid surface, 3c- palmar tubercle, 3d- distal glenoid cavity, 3e- distodorsal articular surface for the third carpal bone; 4- Intermediate carpal bone, 4a- dorsal condyle, 4b- palmar articular surface, 4c- proximopalmar margin, 4d- distodorsal angular surface articulating with the dorsal parts of the third and fourth carpal bones, 4e- palmar tubercle; 5- Ulnar carpal bone, 5a- dorsal margin, 5b- articular surface for the accessory carpal bone, 5c- distopalmar tubercle; 6- Accessory carpal bone, 6a- proximodorsal part articulating with the ulna, 6b- distodorsal part articulating with the ulnar carpal bone, 6c- intermediate part with the sulcus of the ulnaris lateralis long tendon, 6d- palmar part;

Distal row: 7- Second carpal bone, 7a- head, 7b- distal facet; 8- Third carpal bone, 8a- radial fossa, 8b- palmar tubercle, 8c- distal surface for the third metacarpal bone; 9- Fourth carpal bone, 9a- dorsal part, 9b- palmar tubercle;

Metacarpal bones: 10- Second metacarpal bone (base); 11- Third metacarpal bone, 11a- proximal tuberosity (insertion of the extensor carpi radialis tendon), 11b- dorsal cortex, 11c- palmar cortex (superimposed with the second and fourth metacarpal bones); 12- Fourth metacarpal bone;

Joints: 13- Antebrachiocarpal joint; 14- Mediocarpal joint; 15- Carpometacarpal joint, 15a- medial part, 15b- sagittal part, 15c- lateral part; 16- Accessorioulnar joint; 17- Accessoriocarpoulnar joint.

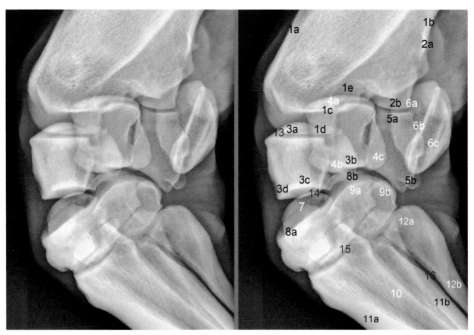

Fig. D.9 **Dorsolaterodistal radiographic image of the flexed left carpus.**

Antebrachial bones: 1- Radius, 1a- craniomedial cortex, 1b- caudolateral cortex, 1c- transverse crest; 1d- radial (antebrachial) condyle, 1e- sagittal fossa; 2- Ulna, 2a- distal part of the body, 2b- distal epiphysis of the ulna (fused with the radius);

Proximal row: 3- Radial carpal bone, 3a- dorsal condyle, 3b- palmar tubercle, 3c- distal glenoid cavity, 3d- distodorsal articular surface for the third carpal bone; 4- Intermediate carpal bone, 4a- dorsal condyle, 4b- distodorsal angular surface articulating with the dorsal parts of the third and fourth carpal bones, 4c- palmar tubercle; 5- Ulnar carpal bone, 5a- proximal articular surface for the ulna, 5b- distopalmar tubercle; 6- Accessory carpal bone, 6a- dorsal part, 6b- medial aspect, 6c- palmar part;

Distal row: 7- Second carpal bone; 8- Third carpal bone, 8a- radial fossa, 8b- palmar tubercle; 9- Fourth carpal bone, 9a- proximal surface, 9b- palmar tubercle;

Metacarpal bones: 10- Second metacarpal bone; 11- Third metacarpal bone, 11a- dorsomedial cortex, 11b- palmarolateral cortex; 12- Fourth metacarpal bone, 12a- base, 12b- body;

Joints: 13- Antebrachiocarpal joint; 14- Mediocarpal joint; 15- Carpometacarpal joint; 16- Third intermetacarpal syndesmosis.

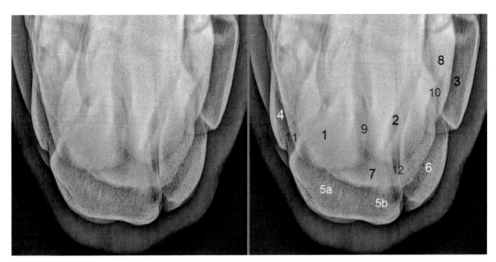

Fig. D.10 **Proximodistal radiographic image of the flexed left carpus.**

Proximal row: 1- Radial carpal bone; 2- Intermediate carpal bone; 3- Ulnar carpal bone;

Distal row: 4- Second carpal bone; 5- Third carpal bone, 5a- radial fossa, 5b- intermediate fossa; 6- Fourth carpal bone;

Metacarpus: 7- Third metacarpal bone; 8- Fourth metacarpal bone;

Joints: 9- Radiointermediate joint; 10- Intermedioulnar joint; 11- Secondotertius joint, 12- Tertioquartal joint.

D.3 DISSECTED SPECIMEN

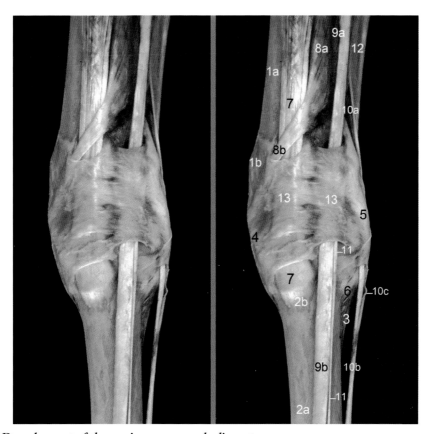

Fig. D.11 **Dorsal aspect of the equine carpus and adjacent areas.**

Bones: 1- Radius, 1a- body (medial aspect), 1b- styloid process; 2- Third metacarpal bone, 2a- body, 2b- proximal tuberosity; 3- Fourth metacarpal bone;

Joints: 4- Medial collateral ligament; 5- Lateral collateral ligament; 6- Third intermetacarpal syndesmosis;

Muscles and tendons: 7- Extensor carpi radialis tendon; 8- Extensor carpi obliquus muscle, 8a- body, 8b- tendon; 9- Dorsal (common) digital extensor muscle, 9a- body, 9b- tendon; 10- Lateral digital extensor muscle, 10a- body, 10b- tendon, 10c- accessory ligament; 11- Accessory digital extensor tendon; 12- Ulnaris lateralis muscle; 13- Extensor retinaculum.

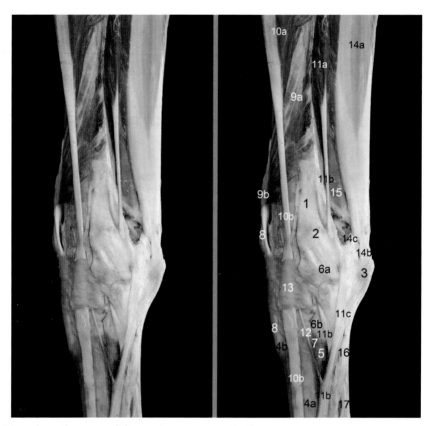

Fig. D.12 **Dorsolateral aspect of the equine carpus and adjacent areas.**

Bones: 1- Radius (distal metaphysis); 2- Lateral styloid process (ulna); 3- Accessory carpal bone; 4- Third metacarpal bone, 4a- body, 4b- proximal tuberosity; 5- Fourth metacarpal bone;

Joints: 6- Lateral collateral ligament, 6a- superficial layer, 6b- deep layer; 7- Third intermetacarpal syndesmosis;

Muscles and tendons: 8- Extensor carpi radialis tendon; 9- Extensor carpi obliquus muscle, 9a- body, 9b- tendon; 10- Dorsal (common) digital extensor muscle, 10a- body, 10b- tendon; 11- Lateral digital extensor muscle, 11a- body, 11b- tendon, 11c- accessory ligament; 12- Accessory digital extensor tendon; 13- Extensor retinaculum; 14- Ulnaris lateralis muscle, 14a- body, 14b- short tendon, 14c- origin of the long tendon; 15- Deep digital flexor muscle; 16- Flexor retinaculum; 17- Superficial digital flexor tendon.

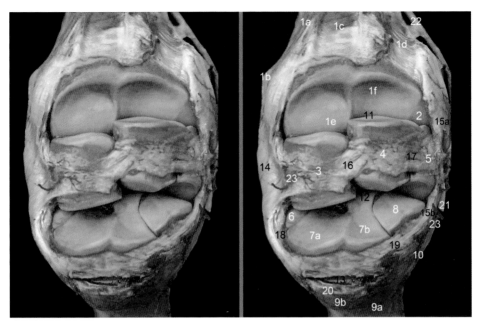

Fig. D.13 **Dorsal aspect of the flexed equine carpus: deep structures.**

Antebrachial bones: 1- Radius, 1a- distal metaphysis, 1b- radial styloid process, 1c- sulcus of the extensor carpi radialis tendon, 1d- sulcus of the dorsal digital extensor tendon, 1e- radial (antebrachial) condyle, 1f- dorsal locking glenoid surface; 2- Ulna (distal condyle);

Carpal bones: 3- Radial carpal bone; 4- Intermediate carpal bone; 5- Ulnar carpal bone; 6- Second carpal bone; 7- Third carpal bone, 7a- radial fossa, 7b- intermediate fossa; 8- Fourth carpal bone;

Metacarpal bones: 9- Third metacarpal bone, 9a- body, 9b- proximal tuberosity; 10- Fourth metacarpal bone;

Joints: 11- Antebrachiocarpal joint; 12- Mediocarpal joint; 13- Carpometacarpal joint; 14- Medial collateral ligament; 15- Lateral collateral ligament, 15a- superficial layer, 15b- deep layer; 16- Dorsal radiointermediate ligament; 17- Dorsal intermedioulnar ligament; 18- Dorsal secondotertius ligament; 19- Dorsal tertioquartal ligament;

Other structures: 20- Extensor carpi radialis distal insertion; 21- Lateral digital extensor tendon; 22- Dorsal antebrachial interosseous artery; 23- Dorsal arterial network of the carpus.

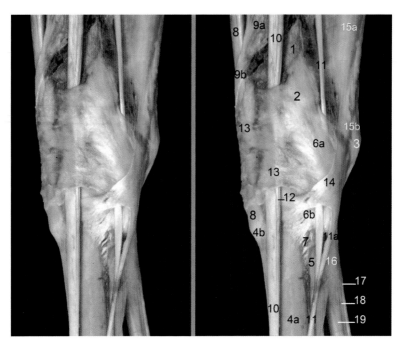

Fig. D.14 **Lateral aspect of the equine carpus.**

Bones: 1- Radius (distal metaphysis); 2- Lateral styloid process (ulna); 3- Accessory carpal bone; 4- Third metacarpal bone, 4a- body, 4b- proximal tuberosity; 5- Fourth metacarpal bone;

Joints: 6- Lateral collateral ligament, 6a- superficial layer, 6b- deep layer; 7- Third intermetacarpal syndesmosis;

Muscles and tendons: 8- Extensor carpi radialis tendon; 9- Extensor carpi obliquus muscle, 9a- body, 9b- tendon; 10- Dorsal (common) digital extensor tendon; 11- Lateral digital extensor tendon, 11a- accessory ligament; 12- Accessory digital extensor tendon; 13- Extensor retinaculum; 14- Dorsolateral carpal fascia; 15- Ulnaris lateralis muscle, 15a- body, 15b- short tendon; 16- Flexor retinaculum and palmar metacarpal fascia; 17- Superficial digital flexor tendon; 18- Deep digital flexor tendon; 19- Accessory ligament of the deep digital flexor tendon.

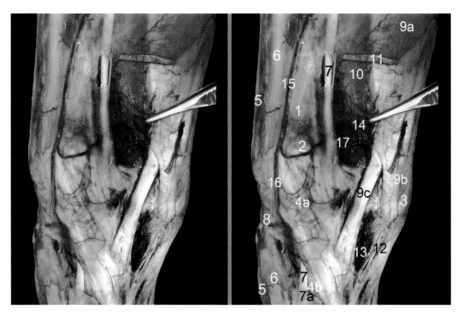

Fig. D.15 **Lateral aspect of the equine carpus.**

1- Radius (distal metaphysis); 2- Lateral styloid process (ulna); 3- Accessory carpal bone; 4- Lateral collateral ligament, 4a- superficial layer, 4b- deep layer; 5- Extensor carpi radialis tendon; 6- Dorsal (common) digital extensor tendon; 7- Lateral digital extensor tendon, 7a- accessory ligament (cut); 8- Extensor retinaculum; 9- Ulnaris lateralis muscle, 9a- body, 9b- short tendon, 9c- long tendon; 10- Deep digital flexor muscle; 11- Antebrachial fascia (cut); 12- Accessoriometacarpal ligament; 13- Palmarolateral recess of the mediocarpal joint; 14- Proximolateral recess of the carpal sheath; 15- Dorsal antebrachial interosseous artery; 16- Dorsal arterial network of the carpus; 17- Palmar arterial network of the carpus.

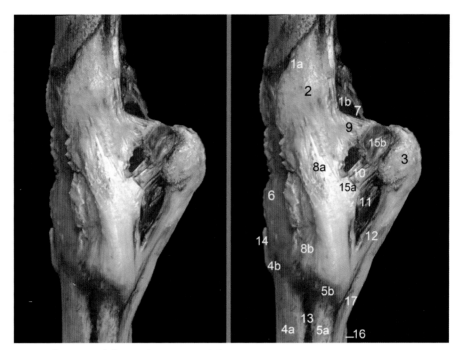

Fig. D.16　Lateral aspect of the equine carpus: joint structures.

Bones: 1- Radius, 1a- distal metaphysis, 1b- transverse crest; 2- Lateral styloid process (ulna); 3- Accessory carpal bone; 4- Third metacarpal bone, 4a- body, 4b- proximal tuberosity; 5- Fourth metacarpal bone, 5a- body, 5b- base;

Joint structures: 6- Dorsal capsule of the carpus; 7- Common palmar ligament of the carpus; 8- Lateral collateral ligament, 8a- superficial layer, 8b- deep layer; 9- Accessorioulnar ligament; 10- Accessoriocarpoulnar ligament; 11- Accessorioquartal ligament (covered by synovial membrane and connective tissue); 12- Accessoriometacarpal ligament; 13- Third intermetacarpal syndesmosis;

Tendons: 14- Extensor carpi radialis tendon; 15- Long tendon of the ulnaris lateralis muscle, 15a- distal part (cut), 15b- subtendinous bursa; 16- Third interosseous muscle (suspensory ligament); 17- Flexor retinaculum (distolateral part).

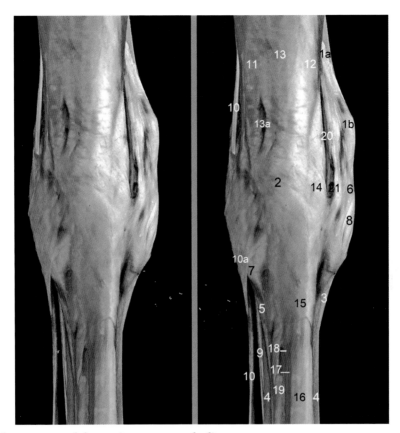

Fig. D.17 **Palmar aspect of the equine carpus and adjacent areas.**

Bones: 1- Radius, 1a- medial aspect, 1b- styloid process; 2- Accessory carpal bone; 3- Second metacarpal bone; 4- Third metacarpal bone; 5- Fourth metacarpal bone;

Joint structures: 6- Medial collateral ligament; 7- Lateral collateral ligament (superficial layer);

Muscles and tendons: 8- Extensor carpi obliquus tendon; 9- Dorsal (common) digital extensor tendon; 10- Lateral digital extensor tendon, 10a- accessory ligament; 11- Ulnaris lateralis muscle; 12- Flexor carpi ulnaris muscle; 13- Antebrachial fascia, 13a- opening for the dorsal ramus of the ulnar nerve; 14- Flexor retinaculum; 15- Palmar metacarpal fascia; 16- Superficial digital flexor tendon; 17- Deep digital flexor tendon; 18- Accessory ligament of the deep digital flexor tendon; 19- Third interosseous muscle (suspensory ligament); 20- Distal radial artery; 21- Cephalic vein (cut).

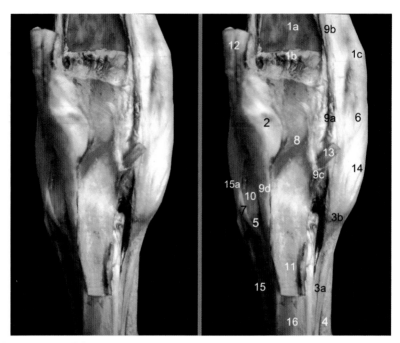

Fig. D.18 **Palmar aspect of the equine carpus: joint structures.**

Bones: 1- Radius, 1a- distal metaphysis, 1b- transverse crest, 1c- styloid process; 2- Accessory carpal bone; 3- Second metacarpal bone, 3a- body, 3b, base; 4- Third metacarpal bone (medial aspect); 5- Fourth metacarpal bone (base);

Joint structures: 6- Medial collateral ligament; 7- Lateral collateral ligament (superficial layer); 8- Common palmar ligament of the carpus; 9- Flexor retinaculum, 9a- medial section plane, 9b- proximomedial part, 9c- tendon sheath for the flexor carpi radialis tendon, 9d- distolateral part; 10- Accessoriometacarpal ligament; 11- Accessory ligament of the deep digital flexor tendon;

Tendons: 12- Ulnaris lateralis distal tendon; 13- Flexor carpi radialis tendon; 14- Extensor carpi obliquus tendon; 15- Lateral digital extensor tendon, 15a- accessory ligament; 16- Third interosseous muscle (suspensory ligament).

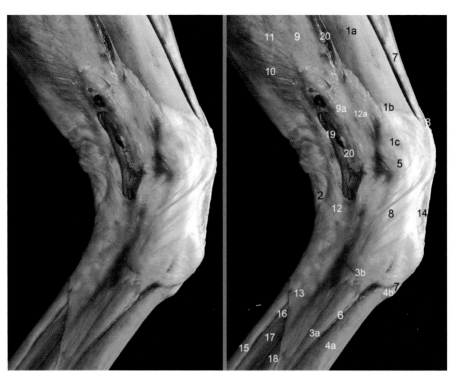

Fig. D.19 **Medial aspect of the equine carpus and adjacent areas.**

Bones: 1- Radius, 1a- body, 1b- distal metaphysis, 1c- styloid process; 2- Accessory carpal bone; 3- Second metacarpal bone, 3a- body, 3b- base; 4- Third metacarpal bone, 4a- body, 4b- proximal tuberosity;

Joint structures: 5- Medial collateral ligament; 6- Second intermetacarpal syndesmosis;

Muscles and tendons: 7- Extensor carpi radialis tendon; 8- Extensor carpi obliquus tendon; 9- Flexor carpi radialis muscle, 9a- tendon sheath within the flexor retinaculum; 10- Flexor carpi ulnaris muscle; 11- Antebrachial fascia; 12- Flexor retinaculum, 12a- proximomedial part; 13- Palmar metacarpal fascia; 14- Extensor retinaculum; 15- Superficial digital flexor tendon; 16- Deep digital flexor tendon; 17- Accessory ligament of the deep digital flexor tendon; 18- Third interosseous muscle (suspensory ligament);

Vessels: 19- Distal radial artery; 20- Cephalic vein pathway.

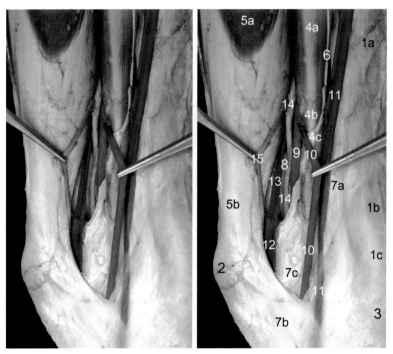

Fig. D.20 **Palmaromedial aspect of the equine carpus: vessels and nerves.**

Bones and joint: 1- Radius, 1a- body, 1b- distal metaphysis, 1c- styloid process; 2- Accessory carpal bone;

Joint structure: 3- Medial collateral ligament;

Muscles and tendons: 4- Flexor carpi radialis muscle, 4a- body, 4b- tendon, 4c- tendon sheath within the flexor retinaculum; 5- Flexor carpi ulnaris muscle, 5a- body, 5b- tendon; 6- Antebrachial fascia (cut); 7- Flexor retinaculum, 7a- proximomedial part, 7b- superficial layer, 7c- deep layer; 8- Accessory ligament of the superficial digital flexor tendon;

Vessels: 9- Median artery; 10- Distal radial artery; 11- Cephalic vein; 12- Ramus communicans coming from the lateral common digital vein; 13- Median vein (empty); 14- Median nerve; 15- Ramus communicans from median to ulnar nerves.

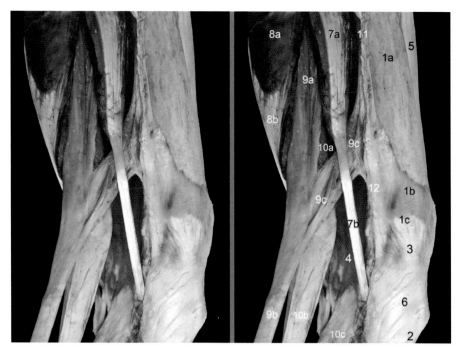

Fig. D.21 Medial aspect of the equine carpus: flexor retinaculum removed, carpal canal open.

Bones and joint: 1- Radius, 1a- body, 1b- distal metaphysis, 1c- styloid process; 2- Third metacarpal bone;

Joint structures: 3- Medial collateral ligament; 4- Common palmar ligament of the carpus;

Muscles and tendons: 5- Extensor carpi radialis tendon; 6- Extensor carpi obliquus tendon; 7- Flexor carpi radialis muscle, 7a- body, 7b- tendon; 8- Flexor carpi ulnaris muscle, 8a- body, 8b- tendon; 9- Superficial digital flexor muscle, 9a- body, 9b- tendon, 9c- accessory ligament of the superficial digital flexor tendon; 10- Deep digital flexor muscle, 10a- body, 10b- tendon, 10c- accessory ligament of the deep digital flexor tendon; 11- Antebrachial fascia (cut); 12- Flexor retinaculum (proximomedial part).

D.4 CROSS-SECTIONS

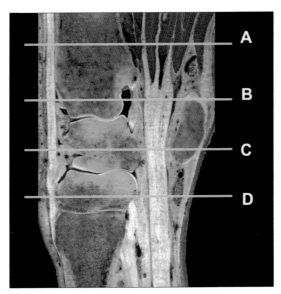

Fig. D.22 **Levels of the cross-sections presented on Figs D.23 through D.26.**

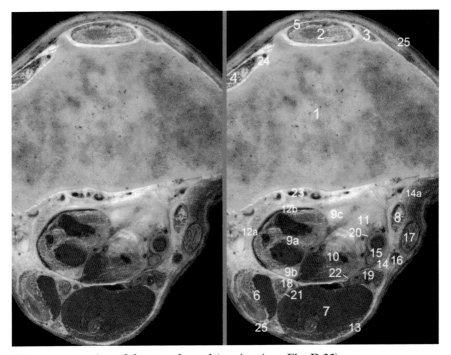

Fig. D.23 **Transverse section of the carpal canal (section A on Fig. D.22).**

Bone: 1- Radius (distal metaphysis);

Muscles and tendons: 2- Extensor carpi radialis tendon; 3- Extensor carpi obliquus tendon; 4- Dorsal (common) digital extensor tendon; 5- Extensor retinaculum; 6- Ulnaris lateralis musculotendinous junction; 7- Flexor carpi ulnaris muscle; 8- Flexor carpi radialis tendon (in its sheath); 9- Deep digital flexor musculotendinous junction, 9a- humeral head, 9b- tendon of the ulnar head, 9c- tendon of the radial head; 10- Superficial digital flexor musculotendinous junction; 11- Accessory ligament of the superficial digital flexor tendon; 12- Carpal canal, 12a- fibrous wall, 12b- cavity; 13- Antebrachial fascia; 14- Flexor retinaculum, 14a- proximomedial part;

Vessels and nerves: 15- Median artery and veins; 16- Distal radial artery; 17- Cephalic vein; 18- Collateral ulnar artery and vein; 19- Rami communicans with the collateral ulnar artery and vein connected to the lateral palmar common digital artery and vein; 20- Median nerve; 21- Ulnar nerve; 22- Ramus communicans from median to ulnar nerves; 23- Palmar network of the carpus; 24- Dorsal network of the carpus; 25- Skin.

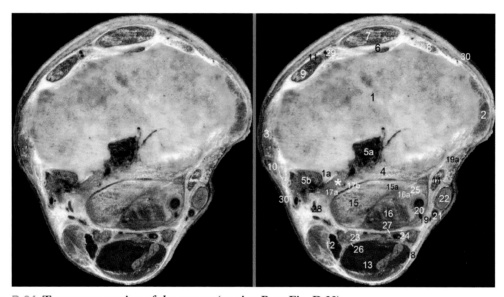

Fig. D.24 **Transverse section of the carpus (section B on Fig. D.22).**

Bone and joint: 1- Radius, 1a- transverse crest; 2- Medial collateral ligament; 3- Lateral collateral ligament; 4- Common palmar ligament of the carpus; 5- Synovial fluid cavity of the antebrachiocarpal joint, 5a- palmarosagittal recess, 5b- proximopalmarolateral recess; 6- Dorsal capsule of the carpus; *- Origin of the antebrachioradial ligament;

Muscles and tendons: 7- Extensor carpi radialis tendon and sheath; 8- Extensor carpi obliquus tendon; 9- Dorsal (common) digital extensor tendon and sheath; 10- Lateral digital extensor tendon; 11- Extensor retinaculum; 12- Ulnaris lateralis musculotendinous junction; 13- Flexor carpi ulnaris muscle; 14- Flexor carpi radialis tendon (in its sheath); 15- Deep digital flexor tendon, 15a- radial head; 16- Superficial digital flexor tendon, 16a- accessory ligament; 17- Carpal canal, 17a- fibrous wall, 17b- cavity; 18- Antebrachial fascia; 19- Flexor retinaculum, 19a- proximomedial part;

Vessels and nerves: 20- Median artery and vein; 21- Distal radial artery; 22- Cephalic vein; 23- Collateral ulnar artery and vein; 24- Rami communicans with the collateral ulnar artery and vein connected to the lateral palmar common digital artery and vein; 25- Median nerve; 26- Ulnar nerve; 27- Ramus communicans from median to ulnar nerves; 28- Palmar network of the carpus; 29- Dorsal network of the carpus; 30- Skin.

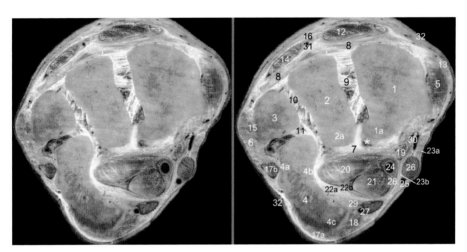

Fig. D.25 **Transverse section of the carpus: proximal row (section C on Fig. D.22).**

Bone and joints: 1- Radial carpal bone, 1a- palmar tubercle; 2- Intermediate carpal bone, 2a- palmar tubercle; 3- Ulnar carpal bone; 4- Accessory carpal bone, 4a- lateral sulcus, 4b- medial aspect, 4c- palmar part; 5- Medial collateral ligament; 6- Lateral collateral ligament; 7- Common palmar ligament of the carpus; 8- Dorsal capsule of the carpus; 9- Radiointermediate interosseous ligaments; 10- Intermedioulnar interosseous ligaments; 11- Accessoriocarpoulnar interosseous ligament; *- Distal insertion of the antebrachioradial ligament;

Muscles and tendons: 12- Extensor carpi radialis tendon and sheath; 13- Extensor carpi obliquus tendon; 14- Dorsal (common) digital extensor tendon and sheath; 15- Lateral digital extensor tendon; 16- Extensor retinaculum; 17- Ulnaris lateralis tendons, 17a- short, 17b- long; 18- Flexor carpi ulnaris tendon insertion; 19- Flexor carpi radialis tendon (in its sheath); 20- Deep digital flexor tendon; 21- Superficial digital flexor tendon; 22- Carpal canal, 22a- fibrous wall, 22b- cavity; 23- Flexor retinaculum, 23a- superficial layer, 23b- deep layer;

Vessels and nerves: 24- Median artery; 25- Distal radial artery; 26- Cephalic vein; 27- Collateral ulnar artery and vein connected to the lateral palmar common digital artery and vein; 28- Median nerve; 29- Ulnar nerve; 30- Palmar network of the carpus; 31- Dorsal network of the carpus; 32- Skin.

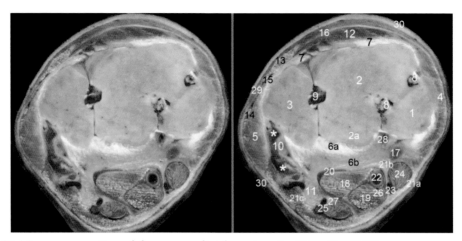

Fig. D.26 **Transverse section of the carpus: distal row (section D on Fig. D.22).**

Bone and joints: 1- Second carpal bone; 2- Third carpal bone, 2a- palmar tubercle; 3- Fourth carpal bone; 4- Medial collateral ligament; 5- Lateral collateral ligament; 6- Common palmar ligament of the carpus, 6a- proximal fibers of the third interosseous muscle, 6b- origin of the accessory ligament of the deep digital flexor tendon; 7- Dorsal capsule of the carpus; 8- Secondotertius interosseous ligaments and spaces; 9- Tertioquartal interosseous ligament and space; 10- Accessorioquartal interosseous ligament; 11- Accessoriometacarpal ligament; *- Palmarolateral recess of the mediocarpal joint;

Muscles and tendons: 12- Extensor carpi radialis tendon and sheath; 13- Dorsal (common) digital extensor tendon and sheath; 14- Lateral digital extensor tendon; 15- Accessory digital extensor tendon; 16- Extensor retinaculum; 17- Flexor carpi radialis tendon; 18- Deep digital flexor tendon; 19- Superficial digital flexor tendon; 20- Carpal canal; 21- Flexor retinaculum, 21a- superficial layer, 21b- deep layer, 21c- distolateral part;

Vessels and nerves: 22- Median artery; 23- Distal radial artery; 24- Cephalic vein; 25- Collateral ulnar artery and vein connected to the lateral palmar common digital artery and vein; 26- Median nerve; 27- Ulnar nerve; 28- Palmar network of the carpus; 29- Dorsal network of the carpus; 30- Skin.

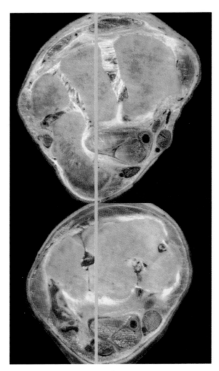

Fig. D.27a Sagittal section of the carpus: section plane.

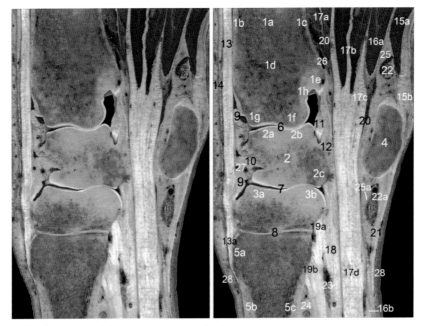

Fig. D.27b Sagittal section of the carpus: anatomical structures.

Bones and joints: 1- Radius, 1a- body, 1b- cranial cortex, 1c- caudal cortex, 1d- distal metaphysis, 1e- transverse crest, 1f- distal condyle, 1g- dorsal locking glenoid cavity, 1h- sagittal fossa; 2- Intermediate carpal bone, 2a- dorsal condyle, 2b- palmar glenoid surface, 2c- palmar tubercle; 3- Third carpal bone, 3a- intermediate fossa, 3b- palmar tubercle; 4- Accessory carpal bone (palmar part); 5- Third metacarpal bone, 5a- proximal tuberosity, 5b- dorsal cortex, 5c- palmar cortex; 6- Antebrachiocarpal joint; 7- Mediocarpal joint; 8- Carpometacarpal joint; 9- Dorsal capsule of the carpus; 10- Radiointermediate interosseous ligament; 11- Antebrachioradial ligament; 12- Common palmar ligament of the carpus;

Muscles and tendons: 13- Extensor carpi radialis tendon, 13a- distal enthesis; 14- Extensor retinaculum; 15- Ulnaris lateralis muscle, 15a- body, 15b- short tendon; 16- Superficial digital flexor muscle, 16a- body, 16b- superficial digital flexor tendon (lateral margin); 17- Deep digital flexor muscle, 17a- muscle body of the radial head, 17b- muscle body of the humeral head, 17c- tendon of the ulnar head, 17d- deep digital flexor tendon; 18- Accessory ligament of the deep digital flexor tendon; 19- Third interosseous muscle (suspensory ligament), 19a- carpal origin, 19b- metacarpal origin; 20- Carpal canal sheath cavity; 21- Flexor retinaculum;

Vessels and nerves: 22- Collateral ulnar artery and vein, 22a- connection to the lateral palmar common digital artery and vein; 23- Proximal deep palmar arch; 24- Palmar metacarpal artery and vein in fat; 25- Ulnar nerve, 25a- palmar ramus; 26- Palmar network of the carpus; 27- Dorsal network of the carpus; 28- Skin.

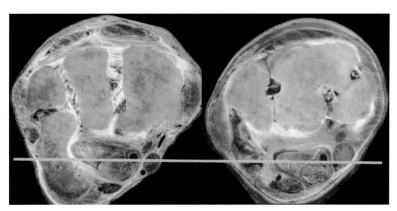

Fig. D.28a **Frontal section of the carpus: section plane.**

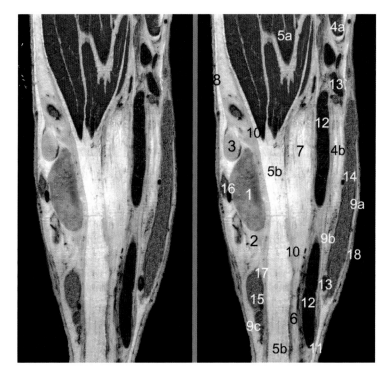

Fig. D.28b **Frontal section of the carpus: anatomical structures.**

Bone, muscles and tendons: 1- Accessory carpal bone; 2- Accessoriometacarpal ligament; 3- Ulnaris lateralis long tendon; 4- Flexor carpi radialis muscle, 4a- muscle body, 4b- tendon sheath (opened); 5- Deep digital flexor muscle, 5a- muscle body of the humeral head, 5b- deep digital flexor tendon; 6- Superficial digital flexor tendon, 7- Accessory ligament of the superficial digital flexor tendon; 8- Antebrachial fascia; 9- Flexor retinaculum, 9a- superficial layer, 9b- deep layer, 9c- distolateral part; 10- Carpal canal sheath cavity; 11- Palmar metacarpal fascia;

Vessels and nerves: 12- Median artery; 13- Distal radial artery; 14- Cephalic vein; 15- Connection to the lateral palmar common digital artery and vein; 16- Rami of the collateral ulnar artery and vein and dorsal ramus of the ulnar nerve; 17- Palmar ramus of the ulnar nerve; 18- Skin.

THE METACARPUS

E.1 PHYSICAL ASPECT

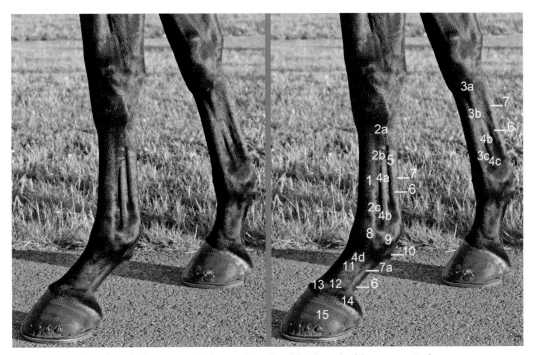

Fig. E.1 **Lateral and medial aspects of the equine distal limb: palpable anatomical structures.**

1- Third metacarpal bone; 2- Fourth metacarpal bone, 2a- base, 2b- body, 2c- distal end; 3- Second metacarpal bone, 3a- base, 3b- body, 3c- distal end; 4- Third interosseous muscle (suspensory ligament), 4a- body, 4b- lateral branch, 4c- medial branch, 4d- lateral extensor branch; 5- Accessory ligament of the deep digital flexor tendon; 6- Deep digital flexor tendon; 7- Superficial digital flexor tendon, 7a- lateral branch; 8- Lateral collateral ligament of the fetlock; 9- Base of the proximal sesamoid bone; 10- Ergot; 11- Proximal phalanx; 12- Middle phalanx; 13- Coronet; 14- Ungular cartilage; 15- Hoof wall.

E.2 RADIOGRAPHIC ANATOMY

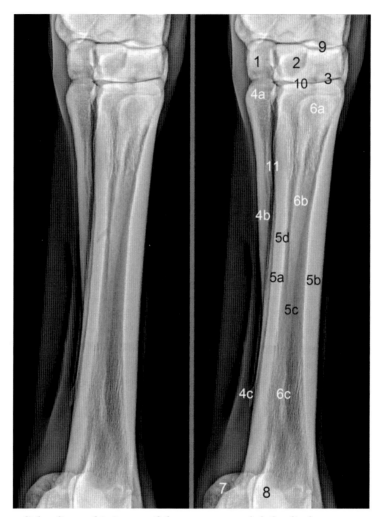

Fig. E.2 **Dorsomedial radiographic image of the metacarpus: left forelimb.**

Carpus: distal row: 1- Second carpal bone; 2- Third carpal bone; 3- Fourth carpal bone;

Metacarpus: 4- Second metacarpal bone, 4a- head, 4b- body, 4c- end; 5- Third metacarpal bone, 5a- palmaromedial cortex, 5b- dorsolateral cortex, 5c- medullary cavity superimposed with the fourth metacarpal bone, 5d- vascular foramen; 6- Fourth metacarpal bone, 6a- head, 6b- body, 6c- end;

Proximal sesamoid bones: 7- Medial proximal sesamoid bone; 8- Lateral proximal sesamoid bone;

Joints: 9- Mediocarpal joint; 10- Carpometacarpal joint; 11- Second intermetacarpal syndesmosis.

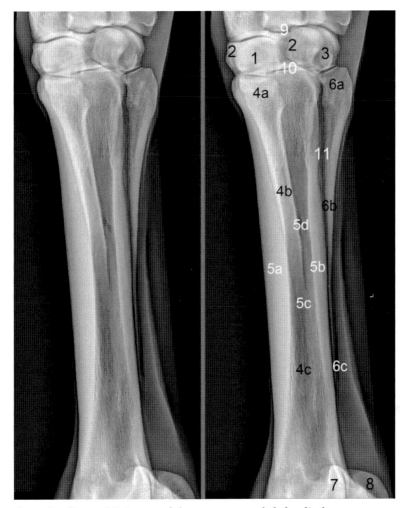

Fig. E.3 **Dorsolateral radiographic image of the metacarpus: left forelimb.**

Carpus: distal row: 1- Second carpal bone; 2- Third carpal bone; 3- Fourth carpal bone;

Metacarpus: 4- Second metacarpal bone, 4a- head, 4b- body, 4c- end; 5- Third metacarpal bone, 5a- dorsomedial cortex, 5b- palmarolateral cortex, 5c- medullary cavity superimposed with the second metacarpal bone, 5d- vascular foramen; 6- Fourth metacarpal bone, 6a- head, 6b- body, 6c- end;

Proximal sesamoid bones: 7- Medial proximal sesamoid bone; 8- Lateral proximal sesamoid bone;

Joints: 9- Mediocarpal joint; 10- Carpometacarpal joint; 11- Fourth intermetacarpal syndesmosis.

E.3 DISSECTED SPECIMEN

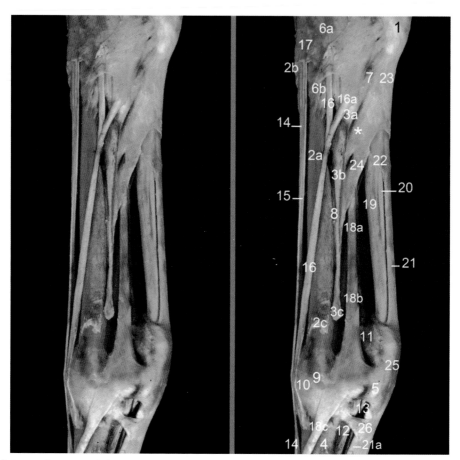

Fig. E.4 **Lateral aspect of the metacarpus: left forelimb.**

Bones: 1- Accessory carpal bone; 2- Third metacarpal bone, 2a- body, 2b- proximal tuberosity (covered by the extensor carpi radialis tendon), 2c- distal metaphysis; 3- Fourth metacarpal bone, 3a- base, 3b- body, 3c- distal end; 4- Proximal phalanx; 5- Base of the proximal sesamoid bone;

Joints: 6- Lateral collateral ligament of the carpus, 6a- superficial layer, 6b- deep layer; 7- Accessoriometacarpal ligament; 8- Third intermetacarpal syndesmosis; 9- Lateral collateral ligament of the fetlock joint (superficial layer); 10- Dorsal capsule of the fetlock joint; 11- Palmar (intersesamoidean) ligament (suprasesamoidean part); 12- Lateral oblique sesamoidean ligament; 13- Straight sesamoidean ligament;

Tendons: 14- Dorsal (common) digital extensor tendon; 15- Accessory digital extensor tendon; 16- Lateral digital extensor tendon, 16a- accessory ligament; 17- Extensor retinaculum; 18- Third interosseous muscle (suspensory ligament), 18a- body, 18b- lateral branch, 18c- lateral extensor branch; 19- Accessory ligament of the deep digital flexor tendon; 20- Deep digital flexor tendon; 21- Superficial digital flexor tendon, 21a- lateral branch; 22- Accessoriosuperficial fibers; 23- Flexor retinaculum, *- distolateral part; 24- Palmar metacarpal fascia; 25- Palmar annular ligament; 26- Proximal digital annular ligament (proximolateral attachment).

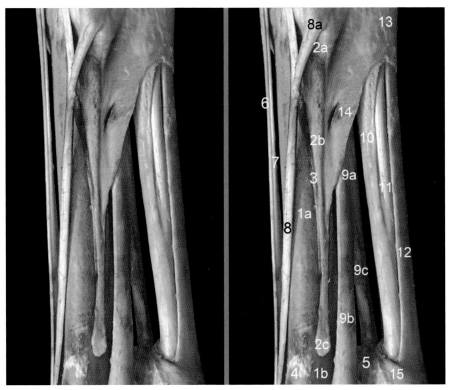

Fig. E.5 **Lateral aspect of the metacarpus: left forelimb.**

Bones: 1- Third metacarpal bone, 1a- body, 1b- distal metaphysis; 2- Fourth metacarpal bone, 2a- base, 2b- body, 2c- distal end;

Joints: 3- Third intermetacarpal syndesmosis; 4- Lateral collateral ligament of the fetlock joint (superficial layer); 5- Palmar (intersesamoidean) ligament (suprasesamoidean part);

Tendons: 6- Dorsal (common) digital extensor tendon; 7- Accessory digital extensor tendon; 8- Lateral digital extensor tendon, 8a- accessory ligament; 9- Third interosseous muscle (suspensory ligament), 9a- body, 9b- lateral branch, 9c- medial branch; 10- Accessory ligament of the deep digital flexor tendon; 11- Deep digital flexor tendon; 12- Superficial digital flexor tendon; 13- Flexor retinaculum; 14- Palmar metacarpal fascia; 15- Palmar annular ligament.

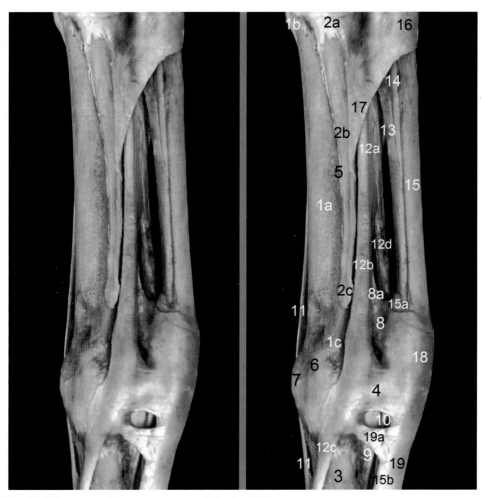

Fig. E.6 **Medial aspect of the metacarpus: right forelimb.**

Bones: 1- Third metacarpal bone, 1a- body, 1b- proximal tuberosity (covered by the extensor carpi radialis tendon), 1c- distal metaphysis; 2- Second metacarpal bone, 2a- base, 2b- body, 2c- distal end; 3- Proximal phalanx; 4- Base of the proximal sesamoid bone;

Joints: 5- Second intermetacarpal syndesmosis; 6- Medial collateral ligament of the fetlock joint (superficial layer); 7- Dorsal capsule of the fetlock joint; 8- Palmar (intersesamoidean) ligament (suprasesamoidean part), 8a- metacarpopalmar ligament; 9- Medial oblique sesamoidean ligament; 10- Straight sesamoidean ligament;

Tendons: 11- Dorsal (common) digital extensor tendon; 12- Third interosseous muscle (suspensory ligament), 12a- body, 12b- medial branch, 12c- medial extensor branch, 12d- lateral branch; 13- Accessory ligament of the deep digital flexor tendon; 14- Deep digital flexor tendon; 15- Superficial digital flexor tendon, 15a- manica flexoria, 15b- medial branch; 16- Flexor retinaculum; 17- Palmar metacarpal fascia; 18- Palmar annular ligament; 19- Proximal digital annular ligament, 19a- proximomedial attachment.

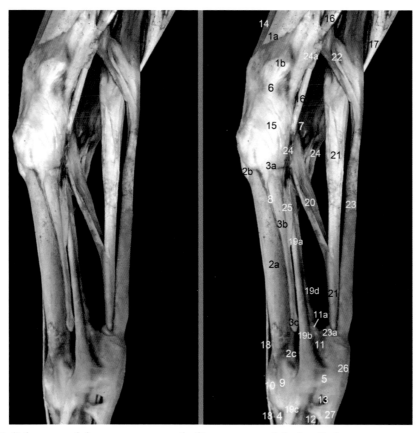

Fig. E.7 **Medial aspect of the metacarpus and adjacent areas: right forelimb.**

Bones: 1- Radius, 1a- distal metaphysis, 1b- styloid process; 2- Third metacarpal bone, 2a- body, 2b- proximal tuberosity (covered by the extensor carpi radialis tendon), 2c- distal metaphysis; 3- Second metacarpal bone, 3a- base, 3b- body, 3c- distal end; 4- Proximal phalanx; 5- Base of the medial proximal sesamoid bone;

Joints: 6- Medial collateral ligament of the carpus; 7- Common palmar ligament of the carpus; 8- Second intermetacarpal syndesmosis; 9- Medial collateral ligament of the fetlock joint (superficial layer); 10- Dorsal capsule of the fetlock joint; 11- Palmar (intersesamoidean) ligament (suprasesamoidean part), 11a- metacarpopalmar ligament; 12- Medial oblique sesamoidean ligament; 13- Straight sesamoidean ligament;

Tendons: 14- Extensor carpi radialis tendon; 15- Extensor carpi obliquus tendon; 16- Flexor carpi radialis tendon; 17- Flexor carpi ulnaris tendon; 18- Dorsal (common) digital extensor tendon; 19- Third interosseous muscle (suspensory ligament), 19a- body, 19b- medial branch, 19c- medial extensor branch, 19d- lateral branch; 20- Accessory ligament of the deep digital flexor tendon; 21- Deep digital flexor tendon; 22- Accessory ligament of the superficial digital flexor tendon; 23- Superficial digital flexor tendon, 23a- manica flexoria; 24- Flexor retinaculum (cut), 24a- sheath of the flexor carpi radialis tendon; 25- Palmar metacarpal fascia; 26- Palmar annular ligament; 27- Proximal digital annular ligament.

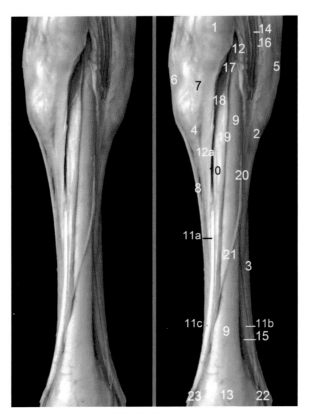

Fig. E.8 **Palmar aspect of the metacarpus: left forelimb.**

Bones: 1- Accessory carpal bone; 2- Second metacarpal bone; 3- Third metacarpal bone; 4-Fourth metacarpal bone;

Joints: 5- Medial collateral ligament of the carpus; 6- Lateral collateral ligament of the carpus; 7- Accessoriometacarpal ligament;

Tendons: 8- Lateral digital extensor tendon; 9- Superficial digital flexor tendon; 10- Accessory ligament of the deep digital flexor tendon; 11- Third interosseous muscle, 11a- body, 11b- medial branch, 11c- lateral branch; 12- Flexor retinaculum (open), 12a- Distolateral part; 13- Palmar annular ligament; 14- Distal radial artery; 15- Medial palmar common digital artery; 16- Cephalic vein; 17- Palmar ramus of the ulnar nerve (having incorporated the proximal ramus communicans of the median nerve); 18- Deep ramus of the ulnar nerve; 19- Superficial ramus providing the lateral palmar common digital nerve; 20- Medial palmar common digital nerve; 21- Distal ramus communicans; 22- Medial proper digital artery and nerve; 23- Lateral proper digital artery and nerve.

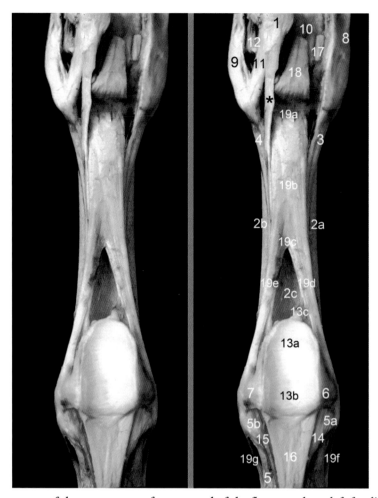

Fig. E.9 **Palmar aspect of the metacarpus after removal of the flexor tendons: left forelimb.**

Bones: 1- Accessory carpal bone; 2- Third metacarpal bone, 2a- medial aspect, 2b- lateral aspect, 2c- palmar aspect; 3- Second metacarpal bone; 4- Fourth metacarpal bone; 5- Proximal phalanx, 5a- medial palmar eminence, 5b- lateral palmar eminence; 6- Base of the medial proximal sesamoid bone; 7- Base of the lateral proximal sesamoid bone;

Joints: 8- Medial collateral ligament of the carpus; 9- Lateral collateral ligament of the carpus; 10- Common palmar ligament of the carpus; 11- Accessoriometacarpal ligament; 12- Accessoriocarpoulnar ligament; *- Flexor retinaculum (distolateral part); 13- Palmar (intersesamoidean) ligament, 13a- suprasesamoidean part, 13b- sesamoidean part, 13c- interosseopalmar ligament; 14- Medial oblique sesamoidean ligament; 15- Lateral oblique sesamoidean ligament; 16- Straight sesamoidean ligament;

Tendons: 17- Flexor carpi radialis tendon (distal part); 18- Accessory ligament of the deep digital flexor tendon (reclined proximally); 19 - Third interosseous muscle (suspensory ligament), 19a- origin, 19b- body, 19c- bifurcation, 19d- medial branch, 19e- lateral branch, 19f- medial extensor branch, 19g- lateral extensor branch.

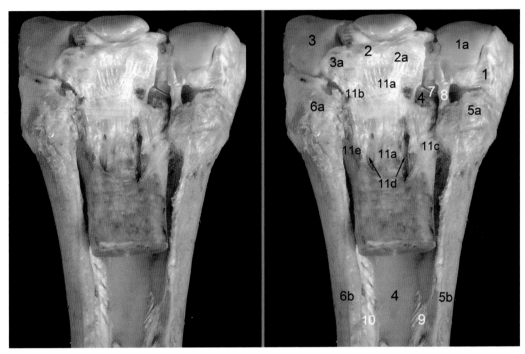

Fig. E.10 Palmar aspect of the proximal metacarpus after removal of the flexor tendons: left forelimb.

Bones: 1- Second carpal bone, 1a- head; 2- Third carpal bone, 2a- palmar tubercle; 3- Fourth carpal bone, 3a- palmar tubercle; 4- Third metacarpal bone; 5- Second metacarpal bone, 5a- base, 5b- body; 6- Fourth metacarpal bone, 6a- base, 6b- body;

Joints: 7- Carpometacarpal joint; 8- Secondometacarpal ligament; 9- Second intermetacarpal syndesmosis; 10- Third intermetacarpal syndesmosis;

Tendons: 11- Third interosseous muscle (suspensory ligament), 11a- third carpal bone origin, 11b- fourth carpal bone origin, 11c- second metacarpal bone origin, 11d- third metacarpal bone origin (seen through the neurovascular pathways), 11e- fourth metacarpal bone origin.

E.4 CROSS-SECTIONS

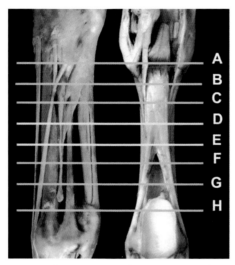

Fig. E.11 Levels of the transverse sections presented on Figs E.12 through E.20.

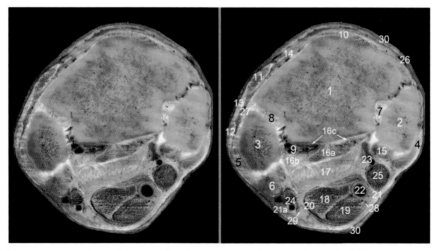

Fig. E.12 Transverse section of the proximal metacarpus (section A on Fig. E.11).

Bones and joints: 1- Third metacarpal bone; 2- Second metacarpal bone; 3- Fourth metacarpal bone; 4- Medial collateral ligament of the carpus; 5- Lateral collateral ligament of the carpus; 6- Accessoriometacarpal ligament; 7- Second intermetacarpal syndesmosis; 8- Third intermetacarpal syndesmosis; 9- Palmarolateral recess of the carpometacarpal joint;

Muscles and tendons: 10- Extensor carpi radialis enthesis; 11- Dorsal (common) digital extensor tendon and sheath; 12- Lateral digital extensor tendon; 13- Accessory digital extensor tendon; 14- Extensor retinaculum; 15- Flexor carpi radialis tendon (distal enthesis); 16-Third interosseous muscle, 16a- third carpal bone origin, 16b- fourth carpal bone origin, 16c- third metacarpal bone origin; 17- Accessory ligament of the deep digital flexor tendon; 18- Deep digital flexor tendon;

19- Superficial digital flexor tendon; 20- Carpal canal sheath cavity; 21- Flexor retinaculum, 21a- distolateral part;

Vessels and nerves: 22- Medial palmar common digital artery; 23- Distal radial artery; 24- Lateral palmar common digital artery and vein; 25- Medial palmar common digital vein; 26- Medial dorsal metacarpal artery; 27- Lateral dorsal metacarpal artery; 28- Medial palmar common digital nerve; 29- Lateral palmar common digital nerve; 30- Skin.

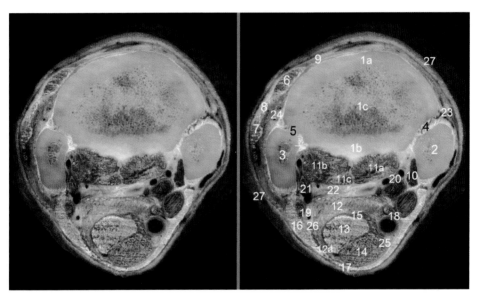

Fig. E.13 **Transverse section of the proximal metacarpus (section B on Fig. E.11).**

Bones and joints: 1- Third metacarpal bone, 1a- dorsal cortex, 1b- palmar cortex, 1c- spongy bone; 2- Second metacarpal bone; 3- Fourth metacarpal bone; 4- Second intermetacarpal syndesmosis; 5- Third intermetacarpal syndesmosis;

Muscles and tendons: 6- Dorsal (common) digital extensor tendon; 7- Lateral digital extensor tendon and its accessory ligament; 8- Accessory digital extensor tendon; 9- Dorsal metacarpal fascia; 10- Second interosseous muscle (vestigial); 11- Third interosseous muscle, 11a- medial lobe, 11b- lateral lobe, 11c- third carpal bone origin; 12- Accessory ligament of the deep digital flexor tendon, 12a- accessoriosuperficial fibers; 13- Deep digital flexor tendon; 14- Superficial digital flexor tendon; 15- Distal recess of the carpal canal; 16- Flexor retinaculum (distolateral part); 17- Palmar metacarpal fascia;

Vessels and nerves: 18- Medial palmar common digital artery and vein; 19- Lateral palmar common digital artery and vein; 20- Medial palmar metacarpal artery and vein; 21- Lateral palmar metacarpal artery and vein; 22- Deep palmar arch; 23- Medial dorsal metacarpal artery; 24- Lateral dorsal metacarpal artery; 25- Medial palmar common digital nerve; 26- Lateral palmar common digital nerve; 27- Skin.

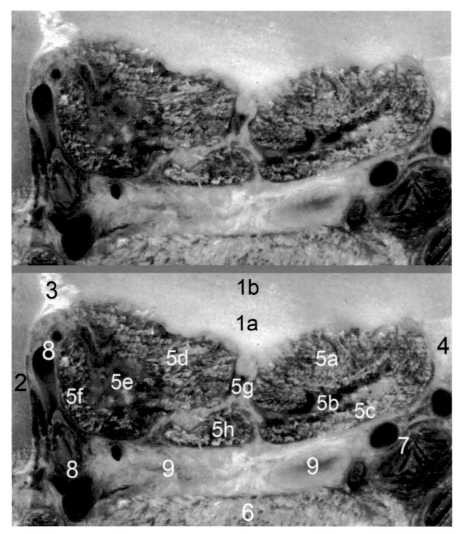

Fig. E.14 **Transverse section of the proximal third interosseous metacarpal enthesis (section B on Fig. E.11).**

Bones and joint: 1- Third metacarpal bone, 1a- palmar cortex, 1b- spongy bone; 2- Fourth metacarpal bone; 3- Third intermetacarpal syndesmosis; 4- Fat;

Muscles and tendons: 5-Third interosseous muscle, 5a- dorsal tendinous part of the medial lobe, 5b- fat and striated muscle fibers, 5c- palmar tendinous part of the medial lobe, 5d- dorsal tendinous part of the lateral lobe, 5e- fat and striated muscle fibers, 5f- palmar tendinous part of the lateral lobe, 5g- sagittal connective tissue, 5h- third carpal bone origin; 6- Accessory ligament of the deep digital flexor tendon;

Vessels and nerves: 7- Medial palmar metacarpal artery and vein; 8- Lateral palmar metacarpal artery and vein; 9- Deep palmar arch.

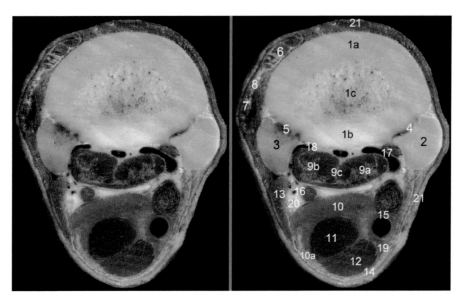

Fig. E.15 **Transverse section of the proximal metacarpus (section C on Fig. E.11).**

Bones and joints: 1- Third metacarpal bone, 1a- dorsal cortex, 1b- palmar cortex, 1c- spongy bone; 2- Second metacarpal bone; 3- Fourth metacarpal bone; 4- Second intermetacarpal syndesmosis; 5- Third intermetacarpal syndesmosis;

Muscles and tendons: 6- Dorsal (common) digital extensor tendon; 7- Lateral digital extensor tendon and its accessory ligament; 8- Accessory digital extensor tendon; 9- Third interosseous muscle, 9a- medial lobe, 9b- lateral lobe, 9c- sagittal connective tissue; 10- Accessory ligament of the deep digital flexor tendon, 10a- accessoriosuperficial fibers; 11- Deep digital flexor tendon; 12- Superficial digital flexor tendon; 13- Flexor retinaculum (distolateral part); 14- Palmar metacarpal fascia;

Vessels and nerves: 15- Medial palmar common digital artery and vein; 16- Lateral palmar common digital artery and vein; 17- Medial palmar metacarpal artery and vein; 18- Lateral palmar metacarpal artery; 19- Medial palmar common digital nerve; 20- Lateral palmar common digital nerve; 21- Skin.

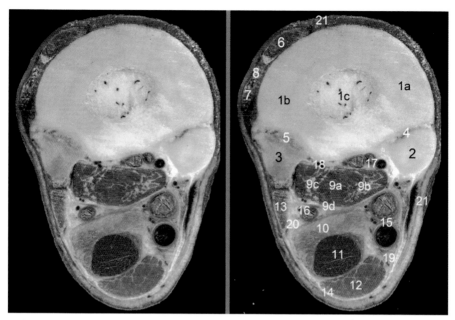

Fig. E.16 **Transverse section of the metacarpus: middle third (section D on Fig. E.11).**

Bones and joints: 1- Third metacarpal bone, 1a- medial cortex, 1b- lateral cortex, 1c- medullary cavity; 2- Second metacarpal bone; 3- Fourth metacarpal bone; 4- Second intermetacarpal syndesmosis; 5- Third intermetacarpal syndesmosis;

Muscles and tendons: 6- Dorsal (common) digital extensor tendon; 7- Lateral digital extensor tendon; 8- Accessory digital extensor tendon; 9- Third interosseous muscle body, 9a- sagittal tendon part, 9b- medial part, 9c- lateral part, 9d- interosseous fascia; 10- Accessory ligament of the deep digital flexor tendon; 11- Deep digital flexor tendon; 12- Superficial digital flexor tendon; 13- Flexor retinaculum (distolateral part); 14- Palmar metacarpal fascia;

Vessels and nerves: 15- Medial palmar common digital artery and vein; 16- Lateral palmar common digital artery and vein; 17- Medial palmar metacarpal artery and vein; 18- Lateral palmar metacarpal artery; 19- Medial palmar common digital nerve; 20- Lateral palmar common digital nerve; 21- Skin.

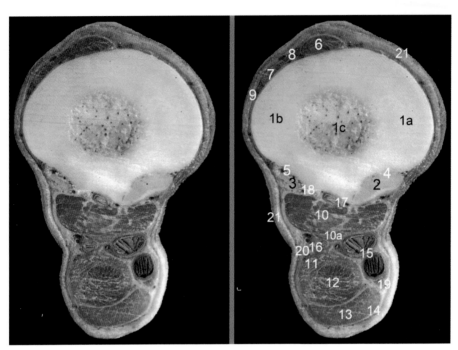

Fig. E.17 **Transverse section of the metacarpus: middle third (section E on Fig. E.11).**

Bones and joints: 1- Third metacarpal bone, 1a- medial cortex, 1b- lateral cortex, 1c- medullary cavity; 2- Second metacarpal bone; 3- Fourth metacarpal bone (distal end); 4- Second intermetacarpal syndesmosis; 5- Third intermetacarpal syndesmosis;

Muscles and tendons: 6- Dorsal (common) digital extensor tendon; 7- Lateral digital extensor tendon; 8- Accessory digital extensor tendon; 9- Dorsal metacarpal fascia; 10- Third interosseous muscle body, 10a- interosseous fascia; 11- Accessory ligament of the deep digital flexor tendon (fused with the tendon); 12- Deep digital flexor tendon; 13- Superficial digital flexor tendon; 14- Palmar metacarpal fascia;

Vessels and nerves: 15- Medial palmar common digital artery and vein; 16- Lateral palmar common digital artery and vein; 17- Medial palmar metacarpal artery and vein; 18- Lateral palmar metacarpal artery; 19- Medial palmar common digital nerve; 20- Lateral palmar common digital nerve; 21- Skin.

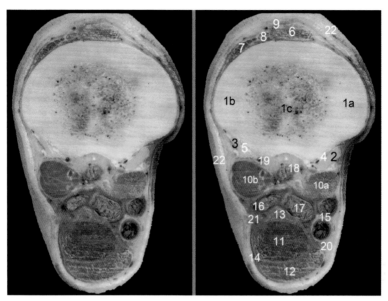

Fig. E.18 **Transverse section of the metacarpus: distal third (section F on Fig. E.11).**

Bones and joints: 1- Third metacarpal bone, 1a- medial cortex, 1b- lateral cortex, 1c- medullary cavity; 2- Second metacarpal bone; 3- Fourth metacarpal bone; 4- Second intermetacarpal syndesmosis; 5- Third intermetacarpal syndesmosis;

Muscles and tendons: 6- Dorsal (common) digital extensor tendon; 7- Lateral digital extensor tendon; 8- Accessory digital extensor tendon; 9- Dorsal metacarpal fascia; 10- Third interosseous muscle, 10a- medial branch, 10b- lateral branch; 11- Deep digital flexor tendon; 12- Superficial digital flexor tendon; 13- Synovial membrane of the proximodorsal recess of the digital flexor tendon sheath; 14- Palmar metacarpal fascia;

Vessels and nerves: 15- Medial palmar common digital artery and vein; 16- Lateral palmar common digital artery and vein; 17- Distal palmar anastomosis; 18- Medial palmar metacarpal artery and vein; 19- Lateral palmar metacarpal artery; 20- Medial palmar common digital nerve; 21- Lateral palmar common digital nerve; 22- Skin.

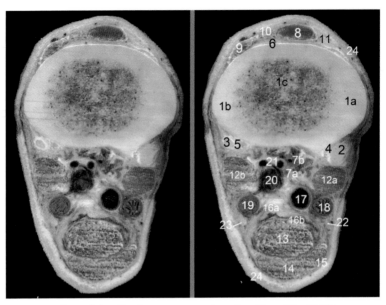

Fig. E.19 **Transverse section of the distal metacarpus (section G on Fig. E.11).**

Bones and joints: 1- Third metacarpal bone, 1a- medial cortex, 1b- lateral cortex, 1c- spongy bone; 2- Second metacarpal bone (distal end); 3- Fourth metacarpal bone (distal end); 4- Second intermetacarpal syndesmosis; 5- Third intermetacarpal syndesmosis and metacarposesamoidean ligament; 6- Proximal attachment of the dorsal capsule of the metacarpophalangeal joint; 7- Proximopalmar recess of the metacarpophalangeal joint, 7a- wall, 7b- cavity and synovial plica;

Muscles and tendons: 8- Dorsal (common) digital extensor tendon; 9- Lateral digital extensor tendon; 10- Accessory digital extensor tendon; 11- Dorsal metacarpophalangeal fascia; 12- Third interosseous muscle, 12a- medial branch, 12b- lateral branch; 13- Deep digital flexor tendon; 14- Superficial digital flexor tendon; 15- Palmar metacarpal fascia; 16- Digital flexor tendon sheath, 16a- wall and synovial membrane, 16b- cavity;

Vessels and nerves: 17- Medial palmar common digital artery; 18- Medial palmar common digital vein; 19- Lateral palmar common digital vein; 20- Palmar metacarpal vein; 21- Palmar metacarpal arteries; 22- Medial palmar common digital nerve; 23- Lateral palmar common digital nerve; 24- Skin.

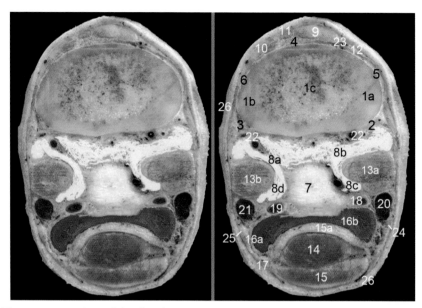

Fig. E.20 **Transverse section of the distal metacarpus (section H on Fig. E.11).**

Bones and joints: 1- Third metacarpal bone distal metaphysis, 1a- medial cortex, 1b- lateral cortex, 1c- spongy bone; 2- Medial metacarposesamoidean ligament; 3- Lateral metacarposesamoidean ligament; 4- Proximal attachment of the dorsal capsule of the metacarpophalangeal joint; 5- Medial collateral ligament of the metacarpophalangeal joint (proximal fibers of the superficial layer); 6- Lateral collateral ligament of the metacarpophalangeal joint (proximal fibers of the superficial layer); 7- Palmar (intersesamoidean) ligament (suprasesamoidean part); 8- Proximopalmar recess of the metacarpophalangeal joint, 8a- synovial membrane, 8b- synovial cavity, 8c- medial interosseopalmar recess, 8d- lateral interosseopalmar recess;

Muscles and tendons: 9- Dorsal (common) digital extensor tendon; 10- Lateral digital extensor tendon; 11- Accessory digital extensor tendon; 12- Dorsal metacarpophalangeal fascia; 13- Third interosseous muscle, 13a- medial branch, 13b- lateral branch; 14- Deep digital flexor tendon; 15- Superficial digital flexor tendon, 15a- manica flexoria (proximal part); 16- Digital flexor tendon sheath, 16a- wall and synovial membrane, 16b- cavity (proximodorsal recess); 17- Palmar metacarpal fascia;

Vessels and nerves: 18- Medial proper palmar digital artery; 19- Lateral proper palmar digital artery; 20- Medial proper palmar digital vein; 21- Lateral proper palmar digital vein; 22- Palmar network of the metacarpophalangeal joint; 23- Dorsal network of the metacarpophalangeal joint; 24- Medial proper palmar digital nerve; 25- Lateral proper palmar digital nerve; 26- Skin.

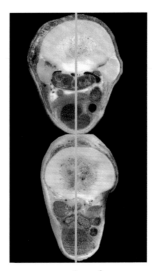

Fig. E.21 **Sagittal section of the metacarpus: section plane.**

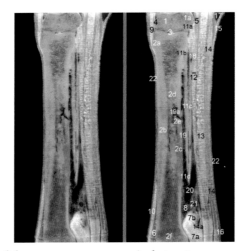

Fig. E.22 **Sagittal section of the metacarpus: anatomical structures.**

Bones and joints: 1- Third carpal bone, 1a- palmar tubercle; 2- Third metacarpal bone, 2a- proximal tuberosity, 2b- dorsal cortex, 2c- palmar cortex, 2d- medullary cavity, 2e- nutrient foramen, 2f- metacarpal condyle; 3- Carpometacarpal joint; 4- Dorsal capsule of the carpus; 5- Common palmar ligament of the carpus; 6- Dorsal capsule of the metacarpophalangeal joint; 7- Palmar (intersesamoidean) ligament, 7a- sesamoidean part, 7b- suprasesamoidean part; 8- Proximopalmar recess of the metacarpophalangeal joint;

Muscles and tendons: 9- Extensor carpi radialis tendon (distal enthesis); 10- Dorsal (common) digital extensor tendon; 11- Third interosseous muscle (suspensory ligament), 11a- third carpal bone origin, 11b- third metacarpal bone origin, 11c- body, 11d- bifurcation; 12- Accessory ligament of the deep digital flexor tendon; 13- Deep digital flexor tendon; 14- Superficial digital flexor tendon, 14a- manica flexoria; 15- Flexor retinaculum; 16- Palmar annular ligament;

Vessels and nerves: 17- Collateral ulnar vein; 18- Deep palmar arch; 19- Palmar metacarpal arteries and veins in adipose connective tissue, 19a- nutrient vessels of the third metacarpal bone; 20- Distal palmar anastomosis; 21- Lateral proper palmar digital artery; 22- Skin.

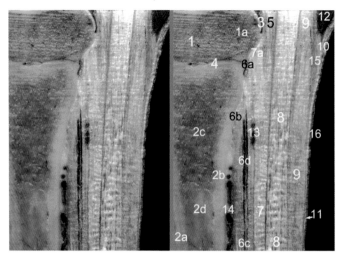

Fig. E.23 **Sagittal section of the proximal metacarpus (see Fig. E.21, image at the top).**

Bones and joint: 1- Third carpal bone, 1a- palmar tubercle; 2- Third metacarpal bone, 2a- dorsal cortex, 2b- palmar cortex, 2c- spongy bone, 2d- medullary cavity; 3- Palmar recess of the medio-carpal joint; 4- Carpometacarpal joint; 5- Common palmar ligament of the carpus;

Muscles and tendons: 6- Third interosseous muscle (suspensory ligament), 6a- third carpal bone origin (palmar wall of the palmar recess of the carpometacarpal joint), 6b- third metacarpal bone origin, 6c- body, 6d- striated muscles fibers; 7- Accessory ligament of the deep digital flexor tendon, 7a- third carpal bone origin; 8- Deep digital flexor tendon; 9- Superficial digital flexor tendon; 10- Flexor retinaculum; 11- Palmar metacarpal fascia;

Vessels and nerves: 12- Collateral ulnar vein; 13- Deep palmar arch; 14- Palmar metacarpal arteries and veins in adipose connective tissue; 15- Palmar ramus of the ulnar nerve; 16- Skin.

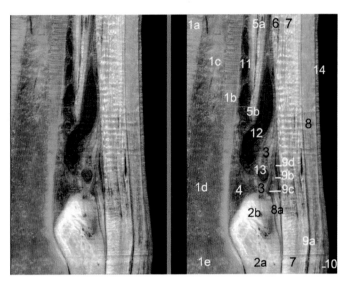

Fig. E.24 **Sagittal section of the distal metacarpus (see Fig. E.21, image at the bottom).**

Bones and joint: 1- Third metacarpal bone, 1a- dorsal cortex, 1b- palmar cortex, 1c- medullary cavity, 1d- spongy bone, 1e- metacarpal condyle; 2- Palmar (intersesamoidean) ligament, 2a- sesamoidean part, 2b- suprasesamoidean part; 3- Interosseopalmar ligament; 4- Proximopalmar recess of the metacarpophalangeal joint;

Muscles and tendons: 5- Third interosseous muscle (suspensory ligament), 5a- body, 5b- bifurcation; 6- Accessory ligament of the deep digital flexor tendon; 7- Deep digital flexor tendon; 8- Superficial digital flexor tendon, 8a- manica flexoria; 9- Digital flexor tendon sheath, 9a- synovial cavity, 9b- synovial membrane attaching on the manica flexoria, 9c- dorsal recess, 9d- proximal recess; 10- Palmar annular ligament;

Vessels and nerves: 11- Palmar metacarpal arteries and veins in adipose connective tissue; 12- Distal palmar anastomosis (between proper digital, metacarpal and common digital veins); 13- Lateral proper palmar digital artery (origin); 14- Skin.

THE DIGITAL AREA

F.1 PHYSICAL ASPECT

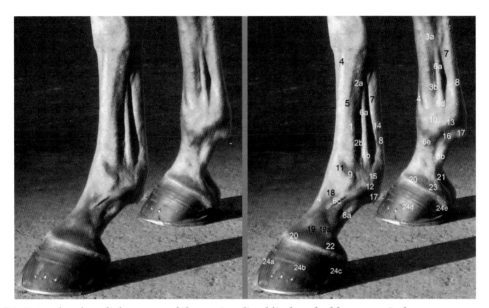

Fig. F.1 **Lateral and medial aspects of the equine distal limb: palpable anatomical structures.**

1- Third metacarpal bone; 2- Fourth metacarpal bone, 2a- body, 2b- distal end; 3- Second metacarpal bone, 3a- body, 3b- distal end; 4- Dorsal digital extensor tendon; 5- Lateral digital extensor tendon; 6- Third interosseous muscle (suspensory ligament), 6a- body, 6b- lateral branch, 6c- lateral extensor branch, 6d- medial branch, 6e- medial extensor branch; 7- Deep digital flexor tendon and accessory ligament; 8- Superficial digital flexor tendon, 8a- lateral branch, 8b- medial branch; 9- Lateral collateral ligament of the fetlock; 10- Medial collateral ligament of the fetlock; 11- Dorsal capsule of the fetlock; 12- Base of the lateral proximal sesamoid bone; 13- Base of the medial proximal sesamoid bone; 14- Neurovascular anastomosis; 15- Lateral proper palmar digital vessels; 16- Medial proper palmar digital vessels; 17- Ergot; 18- Proximal phalanx; 19- Middle phalanx, 19a- lateral tubercle of the flexor tuberosity; 20- Coronet; 21- Distal pastern fossa; 22- Lateral ungular cartilage; 23- Medial ungular cartilage; 24- Hoof wall, 24a- toe, 24b- lateral quarter, 24c- lateral heel, 24d- medial quarter, 24e- medial heel.

F.2 RADIOGRAPHIC ANATOMY

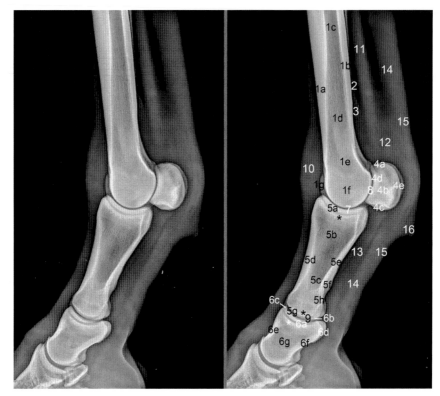

Fig. F.2 Lateromedial radiographic image of the left fetlock and pastern.

Metacarpus: 1- Third metacarpal bone, 1a- dorsal cortex, 1b- palmar cortex, 1c- medullary cavity, 1d- spongy bone, 1e- distal metaphysis, 1f- metacarpal condyle, 1g- sagittal ridge; 2- Second metacarpal bone (distal end); 3- Fourth metacarpal bone (distal end);

Proximal sesamoid bones: 4a- apex, 4b- body, 4c- base, 4d- articular surface, 4e- palmar margin;

Proximal phalanx: 5a- glenoid cavity, *- subchondral bone of the sagittal groove, 5b- spongy bone, 5c- medullary cavity, 5d- dorsal cortex, 5e- palmar cortex, 5f- trigonum (insertion of the oblique sesamoidean ligaments), 5g- condyle, *- subchondral bone of the sagittal groove, 5h- supracondylar fossa for insertion of the scutocompedal ligament (attachment of the scutum medium and through it, superficial digital flexor tendon);

Middle phalanx: 6a- glenoid cavity, *- subchondral bone, 6b- sagittal ridge (palmar part), 6c- extensor process, 6d- flexor tuberosity, 6e- dorsal compact bone, 6f- palmar compact bone, 6g- spongy bone;

Joints: 7- Metacarpophalangeal joint (MPJ); 8- Metacarposesamoidean joint; 9- Proximal interphalangeal joint;

Soft tissues: 10- Dorsal capsule of the fetlock joint and extensor tendons; 11- Third interosseous muscle (suspensory ligament); 12- Palmar (intersesamoidean) ligament (suprasesamoidean part); 13-Sesamoidean ligaments; 14- Deep digital flexor tendon; 15- Superficial digital flexor tendon; 16- Ergot.

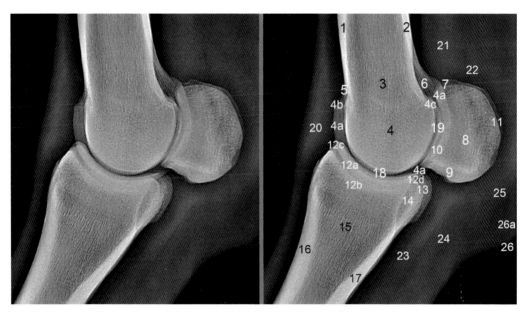

Fig. F.3 **Lateromedial radiographic image of the left metacarpophalangeal joint.**

Third metacarpal bone: 1- Dorsal cortex; 2- Palmar cortex; 3- Spongy bone of the metaphysis; 4- Metacarpal condyle, 4a- sagittal ridge, 4b- proximodorsal margin, 4c- proximopalmar margin; 5- Dorsal supracondylar fossa; 6- Palmar supracondylar fossa;

Proximal sesamoid bones: 7- Apex; 8- Body; 9- Base; 10- Articular surface; 11- Palmar margin;

Proximal phalanx: 12- glenoid cavity, 12a- sagittal groove, 12b- subchondral bone of the sagittal groove, 12c- dorsal margin, 12d- palmar margin; 13- Palmar eminence; 14- Sagittal fossa between palmar eminences; 15- Spongy bone; 16- Dorsal cortex; 17- Palmar cortex;

Joints: 18- Metacarpophalangeal joint (cartilaginous space); 19- Metacarposesamoidean joint (cartilaginous space);

Soft tissues: 20- Dorsal capsule of the fetlock joint and extensor tendons; 21- Third interosseous muscle (suspensory ligament) branches; 22- Palmar (intersesamoidean) ligament (suprasesamoidean part); 23-Sesamoidean ligaments; 24- Deep digital flexor tendon; 25- Superficial digital flexor tendon; 26- Ergot, 26a- pulvinus.

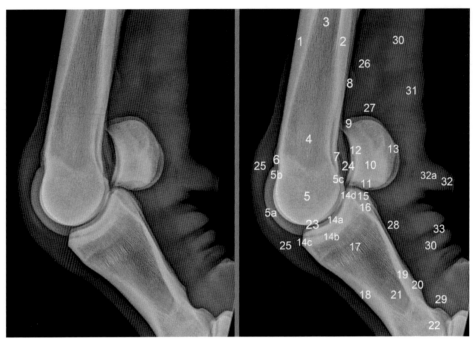

Fig. F.4 **Lateromedial radiographic image of the flexed metacarpophalangeal joint.**

Third metacarpal bone: 1- Dorsal cortex; 2- Palmar cortex; 3- Medullary cavity, 4- Spongy bone of the metaphysis; 5- Metacarpal condyle, 5a- sagittal ridge, 5b- proximodorsal margin, 5c- proximopalmar margin; 6- Dorsal supracondylar fossa; 7- Palmar supracondylar fossa;

Fourth metacarpal bone: 8- Distal end;

Proximal sesamoid bones: 9- Apex; 10- Body; 11- Base; 12- Articular surface; 13- Palmar margin;

Proximal phalanx: 14- glenoid cavity, 14a- sagittal groove, 14b- subchondral bone of the sagittal groove, 14c- dorsal margin, 14d- palmar margin; 15- Palmar eminence; 16- Sagittal fossa between palmar eminences; 17- Spongy bone; 18- Dorsal cortex; 19- Palmar cortex; 20- Trigonum (insertion of the oblique sesamoidean ligaments) distal end; 21- Medullary cavity; 22- Condyle;

Joints: 23- Metacarpophalangeal joint; 24- Metacarposesamoidean joint;

Soft tissues: 25- Dorsal capsule of the fetlock joint and extensor tendons; 26- Third interosseous muscle (suspensory ligament) branches; 27- Palmar (intersesamoidean) ligament (suprasesamoidean part); 28- Sesamoidean ligaments; 29- Middle scutum; 30- Deep digital flexor tendon; 31- Superficial digital flexor tendon; 32- Ergot, 32a- pulvinus; 33- Skin folds.

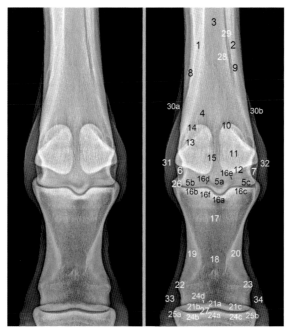

Fig. F.5 **Dorsopalmar radiographic image of the left fetlock and pastern regions.**

Third metacarpal bone: 1- Medial cortex; 2- Lateral cortex; 3- Medullary cavity; 4- Spongy bone; 5- Metacarpal condyle, 5a- sagittal ridge, 5b- medial part, 5c- lateral part; 6- Medial collateral fossa; 7- Lateral collateral fossa;

Second and fourth metacarpal bones: 8- Second metacarpal bone (distal end); 9- Fourth metacarpal bone (distal end);

Proximal sesamoid bones: 10- Apex; 11- Body; 12- Base; 13- Interosseous face; 14- Palmar margin; 15- Axial margin;

Proximal phalanx: 16- Glenoid cavity, 16a- sagittal groove, 16b- medial part, 16c- lateral part, 16d- dorsal margin, 16e- palmar margin, 16f- subchondral bone; 17- Spongy bone; 18- Medullary cavity; 19- Medial cortex; 20- Lateral cortex; 21- Condyle, 21a- sagittal groove, 21b- medial part, 21c- lateral part; 22- Medial epicondyle; 23- Lateral epicondyle;

Middle phalanx: 24- Glenoid cavity, 24a- sagittal ridge, 24b- medial part, 24c- lateral part, 24d- palmar margin; 25- Flexor tuberosity, 25a- medial tubercle, 25b- lateral tubercle;

Joints: 26- Metacarpophalangeal joint; 27- Proximal interphalangeal joint.

Soft tissues: 28- Flexor tendons; 29- Radiolucent space between flexor tendons and lateral cortex of the metacarpal bone; 30- Third interosseous muscle (suspensory ligament), 30a- medial branch, 30b- lateral branch; 31- Medial collateral ligament of the metacarpophalangeal joint; 32- Lateral collateral ligament of the metacarpophalangeal joint; 33- Medial collateral ligament of the proximal interphalangeal joint; 34- Lateral collateral ligament of the proximal interphalangeal joint.

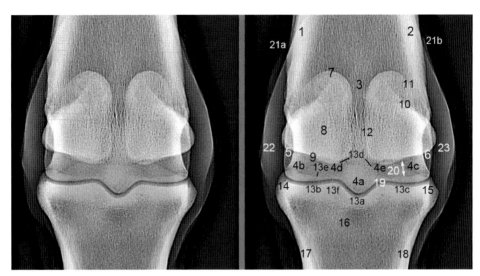

Fig. F.6 **Dorsopalmar radiographic image of the left fetlock.**

Third metacarpal bone: 1- Medial cortex; 2- Lateral cortex; 3- Spongy bone of the metaphysis; 4- Metacarpal condyle, 4a- sagittal ridge, 4b- medial part, 4c- lateral part, 4d- medial parasagittal sulcus, 4e- lateral parasagittal sulcus; 5- Medial collateral fossa; 6- Lateral collateral fossa;

Medial proximal sesamoid bone: 7- Apex; 8- Body; 9- Base;

Lateral proximal sesamoid bone: 10- Interosseous face; 11- Palmar margin; 12- Axial margin;

Proximal phalanx: 13- Glenoid cavity, 13a- sagittal groove, 13b- medial part, 13c- lateral part, 13d- dorsal margin, 13e- palmar margin, 13f- subchondral bone; 14- Medial palmar eminence; 15- Lateral palmar eminence; 16- Spongy bone; 17- Medial cortex; 18- Lateral cortex;

Joints: 19- Metacarpophalangeal joint (cartilaginous space); 20- Sesamoidophalangeal space;

Soft tissues: 21- Third interosseous muscle (suspensory ligament), 21a- medial branch, 21b- lateral branch; 22- Medial collateral ligament of the metacarpophalangeal joint; 23- Lateral collateral ligament of the metacarpophalangeal joint.

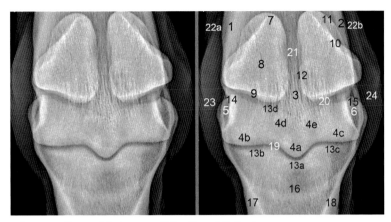

Fig. F.7 **Dorsopalmar radiographic image of the flexed fetlock.**

Third metacarpal bone: 1- Medial cortex; 2- Lateral cortex; 3- Spongy bone; 4- Metacarpal condyle (palmarodistal profile), 4a- sagittal ridge, 4b- medial part, 4c- lateral part, 4d- medial parasagittal sulcus, 4e- lateral parasagittal sulcus; 5- Medial collateral fossa; 6- Lateral collateral fossa;

Medial proximal sesamoid bone: 7- Apex; 8- Body; 9- Base;

Lateral proximal sesamoid bone: 10- Interosseous face; 11- Palmar margin; 12- Axial margin;

Proximal phalanx: 13- Glenoid cavity (dorsal profile), 13a- sagittal groove, 13b- medial part, 13c- lateral part, 13d- palmar margin; 14- Medial palmar eminence; 15- Lateral palmar eminence; 16- Spongy bone; 17- Medial cortex; 18- Lateral cortex;

Joints: 19- Metacarpophalangeal joint (cartilaginous space); 20- Sesamoidophalangeal space; 21- Intersesamoidean space;

Soft tissues: 22- Third interosseous muscle (suspensory ligament), 22a- medial branch, 22b- lateral branch; 23- Medial collateral ligament of the metacarpophalangeal joint; 24- Lateral collateral ligament of the metacarpophalangeal joint.

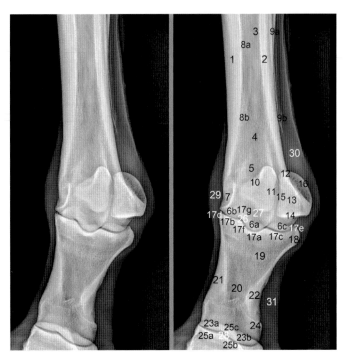

Fig. F.8 **Dorsolateral radiographic image of the left fetlock and pastern.**

Third metacarpal bone: 1- Dorsomedial cortex; 2- Palmarolateral cortex; 3- Medullary cavity; 4- Spongy bone; 5- Distal metaphysis and palmar supracondylar fossa; 6- Metacarpal condyle, 6a- sagittal ridge, 6b- medial part, 6c- lateral part; 7- Medial collateral fossa;

Second and fourth metacarpal bones: 8- Second metacarpal bone, 8a- body, 8b- distal end; 9- Fourth metacarpal bone, 9a- body, 9b- distal end;

Medial proximal sesamoid bone: 10- Interosseous face; 11- Flexor surface;

Lateral proximal sesamoid bone: 12- Apex; 13- Body; 14- Base; 15- Axial margin; 16-Palmar margin;

Proximal phalanx: 17- Glenoid cavity, 17a- sagittal groove, 17b- medial part, 17c- lateral part, 17d- dorsomedial margin, 17e- palmarolateral margin, 17f- subchondral bone, 17g- palmaromedial margin; 18- Lateral palmar eminence; 19- Spongy bone; 20- Medullary cavity; 21- Dorsomedial cortex; 22- Palmarolateral cortex; 23- Condyle, 23a- medial part, 23b- lateral part; 24- Lateral epicondyle;

Middle phalanx: 25- Glenoid cavity, 25a- medial part, 25b- lateral part, 25c- palmar margin;

Joints: 26- Metacarpophalangeal joint; 27- Sesamoidophalangeal space; 28- Proximal interphalangeal joint;

Soft tissues: 29- Joint capsule of the metacarpophalangeal joint; 30- Flexor tendons and lateral branch of the third interosseous muscle (suspensory ligament); 31- Lateral branch of the superficial digital flexor tendon.

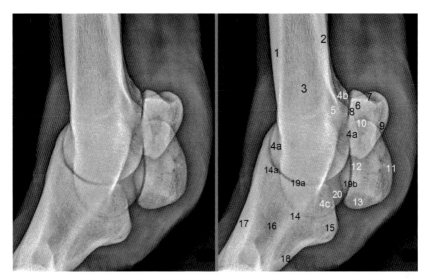

Fig. F.9 Frontal proximolateral radiographic image of the left fetlock.

Third metacarpal bone: 1- Dorsal cortex; 2- Palmar cortex; 3- Spongy bone; 4- Metacarpal condyle, 4a- sagittal ridge, 4b- medial part, 4c- lateral part; 5- Palmar supracondylar fossa;

Medial proximal sesamoid bone: 6- Apex; 7- Interosseous face; 8- Articular surface; 9- Flexor surface;

Lateral proximal sesamoid bone: 10- Apex; 11- Palmar margin; 12- Articular surface; 13- Base;

Proximal phalanx: 14- Glenoid cavity (lateral part), 14a- sagittal groove; 15- Lateral palmar eminence; 16- Spongy bone; 17- Dorsal cortex; 18- Palmar cortex;

Joints: 19- Metacarpophalangeal joint (cartilaginous space); 20- Sesamoidophalangeal space.

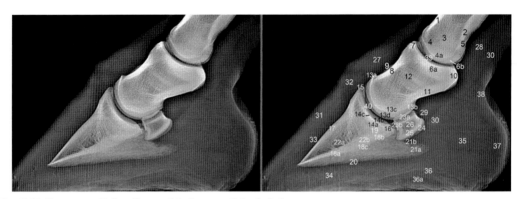

Fig. F.10 **Lateromedial radiographic image of the left foot.**

Proximal phalanx: 1- Dorsal cortex; 2- Palmar cortex; 3- Spongy bone; 4- Condyle, 4a- Subchondral bone of the sagittal groove; 5- Supracondylar fossa for insertion of the scuto-compedal ligament (attachment of the scutum medium and through it, superficial digital flexor tendon);

Middle phalanx: 6- Glenoid cavity, 6a- subchondral bone, 6b- sagittal ridge (palmar end); 7- Extensor process; 8- Dorsal compact bone; 9- Dorsal margin of the insertion fossae of the collateral ligaments of the distal interphalangeal joint; 10- Flexor tuberosity; 11- Palmar compact bone; 12- Spongy bone; 13- Condyle, 13a- dorsal margin of the articular surface, 13b- palmar margin of the articular surface, 13c- subchondral bone of the sagittal groove, 13d- medial and lateral parts;

Distal phalanx: 14- Glenoid cavity, 14a- subchondral bone, 14b- sagittal ridge; 14c- medial and lateral parts; 15- Extensor process; 16- Articular surface for the distal sesamoid bone; 17- Parietal surface; 18- Solar surface, 18a- cutaneous plane, 18b- flexor surface; 18c- semilunar line; 19- Insertion fossa of the collateral ligament of the distal interphalangeal joint; 20- Solar margin; 21- Palmar process, 21a- distal part, 21b- palmar incisura (or foramen); 22- Body of the distal phalanx, 22a- semilunar sinus; 22b- solar canal;

Distal sesamoid bone: 23- Articular surface, 23a- proximal part in contact with the middle phalanx, 23b- distal part in contact with the distal phalanx; 24- Flexor surface; 25- Palmar compact bone; 26- Spongy bone;

Soft tissues: 27- Dorsal recess of the distal interphalangeal joint; 28- Straight sesamoidean ligament and scutum medium; 29- Proximal sesamoid ligament; 30- Deep digital flexor tendon; 31- Dorsal hoof wall; 32- Coronal corium; 33- Parietal corium; 34- Sole; 35- Digital cushion; 36- Frog, 36a- sulci; 37- Heel; 38- Distal pastern fossa;

Joints: 39- Proximal interphalangeal joint; 40- Distal interphalangeal joint.

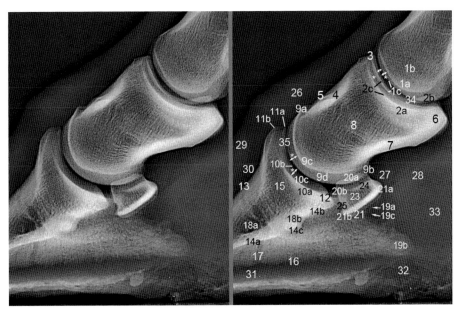

Fig. F.11 **Lateromedial radiographic image of the left foot: interphalangeal joints.**

Proximal phalanx: 1- Condyle, 1a- subchondral bone of the sagittal groove, 1b- spongy bone, 1c- medial and lateral parts;

Middle phalanx: 2- Glenoid cavity, 2a- subchondral bone, 2b- sagittal ridge, 2c- medial and lateral parts; 3- Extensor process; 4- Dorsal compact bone; 5- Dorsal margin of the insertion fossae of the collateral ligaments of the distal interphalangeal joint; 6- Flexor tuberosity; 7- Palmar compact bone; 8- Spongy bone; 9- Condyle, 9a- dorsal margin of the articular surface, 9b- palmar margin of the articular surface, 9c- subchondral bone of the sagittal groove, 9d- medial and lateral parts (superimposed);

Distal phalanx: 10- Glenoid cavity, 10a- subchondral bone, 10b- sagittal ridge, 10c- medial and lateral parts; 11- Extensor process, 11a- periarticular margin, 11b- tubercle of insertion of the dorsal digital extensor tendon; 12- Articular surface of the distal sesamoid bone; 13- Parietal surface; 14- Solar surface, 14a- cutaneous plane, 14b- flexor surface, 14c- semilunar line; 15- Spongy bone; 16- Solar margin; 17- Vascular channel; 18- Body of the distal phalanx, 18a- semilunar sinus; 18b- solar canal; 19- Palmar process, 19a- proximal part, 19b- distal part, 19c- palmar incisura (or foramen);

Distal sesamoid bone: 20- Articular surface, 20a- proximal part in contact with the middle phalanx, 20b- distal part in contact with the distal phalanx; 21- Flexor surface, 21a- proximal margin, 21b- distal margin; 22- Palmar compact bone; 23- Spongy bone; 24- Subchondral bone; 25- Synovial fossae;

Soft tissues: 26- Dorsal recess of the distal interphalangeal joint; 27- Proximal sesamoidean ligament; 28- Deep digital flexor tendon; 29- Dorsal hoof wall; 30- Parietal corium; 31- Sole; 32- Sulcus of the frog; 33- Digital cushion;

Joints: 34- Proximal interphalangeal joint, *- cartilaginous space; 35- Distal interphalangeal joint, *- cartilaginous space.

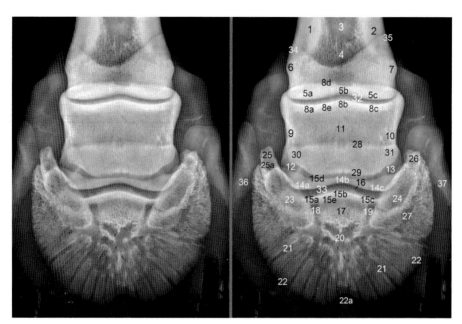

Fig. F.12 **Dorsopalmar radiographic image of the left foot.**

Proximal phalanx: 1- Medial cortex; 2- Lateral cortex; 3- Medullary cavity; 4- Spongy bone; 5- Condyle, 5a- medial part, 5b- sagittal groove, 5c- lateral part; 6- Medial epicondyle; 7- Lateral epicondyle;

Middle phalanx: 8- Glenoid cavity, 8a- medial part, 8b- sagittal ridge, 8c- lateral part; 8d- palmar margin, 8e- subchondral bone; 9- Medial compact bone; 10- Lateral compact bone; 11- Spongy bone; 12- Insertion fossa of the medial collateral ligament of the distal interphalangeal joint; 13- Insertion fossa of the lateral collateral ligament of the distal interphalangeal joint; 14- Condyle, 14a- medial part, 14b- sagittal groove, 14c- lateral part;

Distal phalanx: 15- Glenoid cavity, 15a- medial part; 15b- sagittal ridge, 15c- lateral part, 15d- palmar margin, 15e- subchondral bone; 16- Extensor process; 17- Body of the distal phalanx (spongy bone); 18- Medial solar canal; 19- Lateral solar canal; 20- Semilunar sinus; 21- Vascular channel; 22- Solar margin, 22a- crena; 23- Medial collateral fossa (insertion of the medial collateral ligament of the distal interphalangeal joint (DIPJ)); 24- Lateral collateral fossa (insertion of the lateral collateral ligament of the DIPJ); 25- Medial palmar process, 25a- palmar incisura (or foramen); 26- Lateral palmar process; 27- Parietal sulcus;

Distal sesamoid bone: 28- Proximal margin; 29- Distal articular margin in contact with the distal phalanx; 30- Medial angle; 31- Lateral angle;

Joints and soft tissues: 32- Proximal interphalangeal joint; 33- Distal interphalangeal joint; 34- Shadow of the medial heel bulb; 35- Shadow of the lateral heel bulb; 36- Hoof wall (medial heel); 37- Hoof wall (lateral heel).

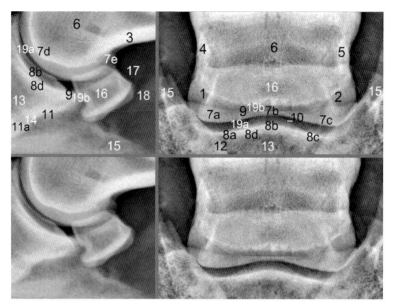

Fig. F.13 **Lateromedial and dorsopalmar radiographic images of the left distal interphalangeal joint.**

Middle phalanx: 1- Insertion fossa of the medial collateral ligament of the DIPJ; 2- Insertion fossa of the lateral collateral ligament of the DIPJ; 3- Palmar compact bone; 4- Medial compact bone; 5- Lateral compact bone; 6- Spongy bone; 7- Condyle, 7a- medial part, 7b- sagittal groove, 7c- lateral part, 7d- subchondral bone of the sagittal groove, 7e- palmar margin;

Distal phalanx: 8- Glenoid cavity, 8a- medial part, 8b- sagittal ridge, 8c- lateral part, 8d- subchondral bone; 9- Articular surface for the distal sesamoid bone (superimposed on the dorsopalmar image with the distal margin of the flexor surface of the distal sesamoid bone); 10- Extensor process; 11- Flexor surface, 11a- compact bone; 12- Semilunar line; 13- Spongy bone (body of the distal phalanx); 14- Solar canal; 15- Palmar process;

Distal sesamoid bone: 16

Soft tissues: 17- Proximal sesamoidean ligament; 18- Deep digital flexor tendon;

Joints: 19- Distal interphalangeal joint, 19a- interphalangeal part, 19b- sesamoidophalangeal part.

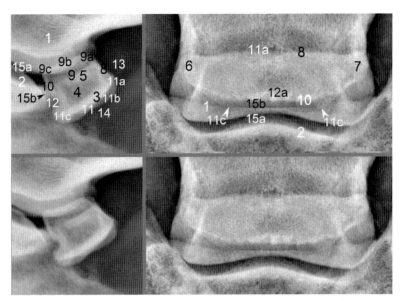

Fig. F.14 Lateromedial and dorsopalmar radiographic images of the left distal sesamoid bone.

Middle phalanx: 1- Condyle;

Distal phalanx: 2- Glenoid cavity;

Distal sesamoid bone: 3- Palmar compact bone; 4- Spongy bone; 5- Subchondral bone; 6- Medial angle; 7- Lateral angle; 8- Proximal border; 9- Articular surface for the middle phalanx, 9a- proximal margin, 9b- sagittal ridge, 9c- dorsal angle; 10- Articular surface for the distal phalanx; 11- Flexor surface, 11a- proximal margin, 11b- sagittal ridge, 11c- distal margin; 12- Synovial sulcus, 12a- synovial fossae;

Soft tissues: 13- Proximal sesamoidean ligament; 14- Deep digital flexor tendon;

Joints: 15- Distal interphalangeal joint, 15a- interphalangeal part, 15b- sesamoidophalangeal part.

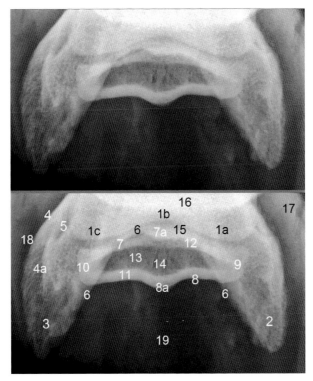

Fig. F.15 **Proximodistal radiographic image of the left distal sesamoid bone.**

Middle phalanx: 1- Condyle, 1a- medial part, 1b- sagittal groove, 1c- lateral part;

Distal phalanx: 2- Medial palmar process; 3- Lateral palmar process; 4- Parietal surface, 4a- parietal sulcus; 5- Insertion fossa of the lateral collateral ligament; 6- Flexor surface;

Distal sesamoid bone: 7- Articular surface for the middle phalanx, 7a- sagittal ridge; 8- Flexor surface, 8a- sagittal ridge; 9- Medial angle; 10- Lateral angle; 11- Palmar compact bone; 12- Subchondral bone; 13- Spongy bone; 14- synovial fossae;

Joints: 15- Distal interphalangeal joint (sesamoidophalangeal part);

Soft tissues and hoof: 16- Shadow of the palmar fetlock; 17- Hoof wall; 18- Parietal corium; 19- Digital cushion and frog.

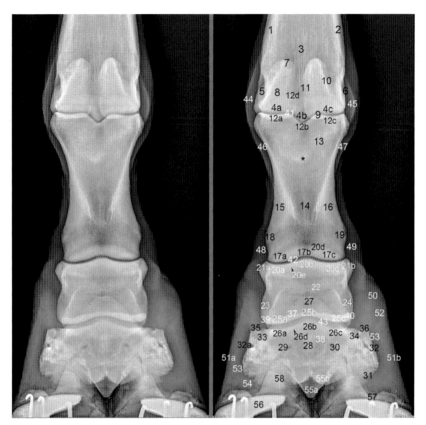

Fig. F.16 Dorsopalmar radiographic image of the weight-bearing left distal limb (fetlock, pastern and foot).

Third metacarpal bone: 1- Medial cortex; 2- Lateral cortex; 3- Spongy bone; 4- Metacarpal condyle, 4a- medial part, 4b- sagittal ridge, 4c- lateral part; 5- Medial collateral fossa; 6- Lateral collateral fossa;

Proximal sesamoid bones: 7- Apex; 8- Body; 9- Base; 10- Interosseous face; 11- Axial margin;

Proximal phalanx: 12- Glenoid cavity, 12a- medial part, 12b- sagittal groove, 12c- lateral part, 12d- dorsal margin; 13- Spongy bone; 14- Medullary cavity; 15- Medial cortex; 16- Lateral cortex; 17- Condyle, 17a- medial part, 17b- sagittal groove, 17c- lateral part; 18- Medial epicondyle; 19- Lateral epicondyle;

Middle phalanx: 20- Glenoid cavity, 20a- medial part, 20b- sagittal ridge, 20c- lateral part, 20d- dorsal margin, 20e- subchondral bone; 21- Flexor tuberosity, 21a- medial tubercle, 21b- lateral tubercle; 22- Spongy bone; 23- Insertion fossa of the medial collateral ligament of the DIPJ; 24- Insertion fossa of the lateral collateral ligament of the DIPJ; 25- Condyle, 25a- medial part, 25b- sagittal groove, 25c- lateral part;

Distal phalanx: 26- Glenoid cavity, 26a- medial part; 26b- sagittal ridge, 26c- lateral part, 26d- subchondral bone; 27- Extensor process; 28- Body of the distal phalanx (spongy bone); 29- Medial solar canal; 30- Lateral solar canal; 31- Solar margin; 32- Parietal surface, 32a- parietal sulcus; 33- Medial collateral fossa (insertion of the medial collateral ligament of the DIPJ);

34- Lateral collateral fossa (insertion of the lateral collateral ligament of the DIPJ); 35- Medial palmar process; 36- Lateral palmar process;

Distal sesamoid bone: 37- Proximal (articular) margin; 38- Distal (flexor surface) margin; 39- Medial angle; 40- Lateral angle;

Joints: 41- Metacarpophalangeal joint; 42- Proximal interphalangeal joint; 43- Distal interphalangeal joint;

Soft tissues and hoof: 44- Medial collateral ligament of the metacarpophalangeal joint (MPJ); 45- Lateral collateral ligament of the MPJ; 46- Medial extensor branch of the third interosseous muscle; 47- Lateral extensor branch of the third interosseous muscle; *- Ergot; 48- Medial collateral ligament of the proximal interphalangeal joint (PIPJ); 49- Lateral collateral ligament of the PIPJ; 50- Coronet; 51- Hoof wall, 51a- medial quarter, 51b- lateral quarter; 52- Coronal corium; 53- Parietal corium; 54- Sole; 55- Frog, 55a- apex, 55b- base;

Shoe and pad: 56- Shoe; 57- Pad; 58- Silicone in the frog sulcus.

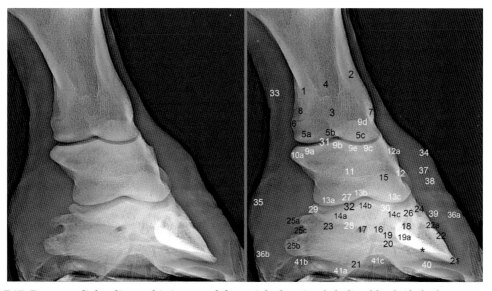

Fig. F.17 **Dorsomedial radiographic image of the weight-bearing left distal limb (fetlock, pastern and foot) (cassette at the palmarolateral aspect of the distal limb).**

Proximal phalanx: 1- Palmaromedial cortex; 2- Dorsolateral cortex; 3- Spongy bone; 4- Medullary cavity; 5- Condyle, 5a- medial part, 5b- sagittal groove, 5c- lateral part; 6- Medial epicondyle; 7- Lateral epicondyle; 8- Insertion fossa of the scutocompedal ligament;

Middle phalanx: 9- Glenoid cavity, 9a- medial part, 9b- sagittal ridge, 9c- lateral part, 9d- dorsal margin, 9e- subchondral bone; 10- Flexor tuberosity, 10a- medial tubercle; 11- Spongy bone; 12- Insertion fossa of the lateral collateral ligament of the DIPJ, 12a- proximal edge; 13- Condyle, 13a- medial part, 13b- sagittal groove, 13c- lateral part;

Distal phalanx: 14- Glenoid cavity, 14a- medial part, 14b- sagittal ridge, 14c- lateral part; 15- Extensor process; 16- Body of the distal phalanx (spongy bone); 17- Medial solar foramen and canal; 18- Lateral solar canal; 19- Flexor surface, 19a- compact bone; 20- Semilunar line;

*- Cutaneous plane; 21- Solar margin; 22- Parietal surface, 22a- parietal sulcus; 23- Medial collateral fossa (insertion of the medial collateral ligament of the DIPJ); 24- Lateral collateral fossa (insertion of the lateral collateral ligament of the DIPJ); 25- Medial palmar process, 25a- proximal part, 25b- distal part, 25c- palmar incisura; 26- Lateral palmar process;

Distal sesamoid bone: 27- Proximal margin; 28- Distal (flexor surface) margin; 29- Medial angle; 30- Lateral angle;

Joints: 31- Proximal interphalangeal joint; 32- Distal interphalangeal joint;

Soft tissues and hoof: 33- Medial branch of the superficial digital flexor tendon; 34- Coronet; 35- Bulb of the medial heel; 36- Hoof wall, 36a- dorsolateral part, 36b- medial heel; 37- Coronal cushion; 38- Coronal corium; 39- Parietal corium; 40- Sole (lateral branch); 41- Frog, 41a- body, 41b- medial sulcus, 41c- lateral sulcus.

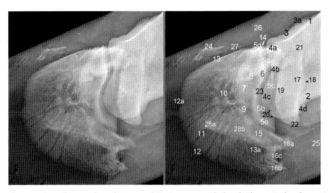

Fig. F.18 **Dorsolateral-proximolateral radiographic image of the left weight-bearing foot (cassette under the foot).**

Middle phalanx: 1- Dorsomedial cortex; 2- Palmarolateral cortex; 3- Insertion fossa of the medial collateral ligament of the DIPJ, 3a- proximal edge; 4- Condyle, 4a- medial part, 4b- sagittal groove, 4c- lateral part, 4d- palmar margin;

Distal phalanx: 5- Glenoid cavity, 5a- medial part, 5b- lateral part, 5c- palmar margin and articular surface for the distal sesamoid bone, 5d- dorsomedial margin, 5e- dorsolateral margin; 6- Extensor process; 7- Body of the distal phalanx (spongy bone); 8- Medial solar canal; 9- Lateral solar canal; 10- Semilunar sinus; 11- Vascular channel; 12- Solar margin, 12a- crena; 13- Parietal surface, 13a- parietal sulcus; 14- Medial collateral fossa (insertion of the medial collateral ligament of the DIPJ); 15- Lateral collateral fossa (insertion of the lateral collateral ligament of the DIPJ); 16- Lateral palmar process, 16a- proximal part, 16b- distal part, 16c- palmar incisura;

Distal sesamoid bone: 17- Proximal articular margin; 18- Proximal margin of the flexor surface; 19- Distal articular margin; 20- Distal margin of the flexor surface; 21- Medial angle; 22- Lateral angle;

Joints: 23- Distal interphalangeal joint;

Soft tissues and hoof: 24- Hoof wall (dorsomedial part); 25- Lateral heel; 26- Coronal corium; 27- Parietal corium; 28- Frog, 28a- apex, 28b- body.

F.3 DISSECTED SPECIMEN

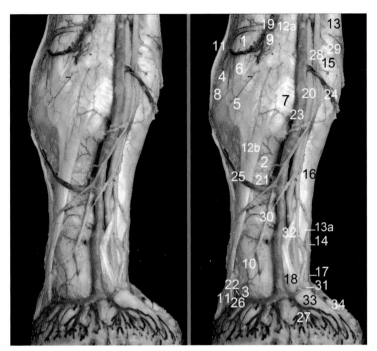

Fig. F.19 **Medial aspect of the right thoracic limb digital area.**

Bones and joints: 1- Third metacarpal bone (distal metaphysis); 2- Proximal phalanx; 3- Middle phalanx; 4- Dorsal capsule of the metacarpophalangeal joint; 5- Metacarpophalangeal fascia; 6- Collateral ligament of the metacarpophalangeal joint (superficial layer); 7- Collateral sesamoidean ligament; 8- Dorsal recess of the metacarpophalangeal joint; 9- Proximopalmar recess of the metacarpophalangeal joint; 10- Collateral ligament of the proximal interphalangeal joint;

Tendons and associated structures: 11- Dorsal digital extensor tendon; 12- Third interosseous muscle (TIOM, suspensory ligament), 12a- medial branch, 12b- medial extensor branch; 13- Superficial digital flexor tendon, 13a- medial branch; 14- Deep digital flexor tendon (covered by the digital sheath wall); 15- Palmar annular ligament; 16- Proximal digital annular ligament; 17- Distal digital annular ligament (proximal part); 18- Chondrocompedal ligament;

Vessels and nerves: 19- Palmar metacarpal artery (endings) and vein; 20- Medial proper digital artery; 21- Dorsal ramus of the proximal phalanx; 22- Dorsal ramus of the middle phalanx; 23- Medial proper digital vein; 24- Ergot ramus; 25- Dorsal ramus of the proximal phalanx; 26- Dorsal ramus of the middle phalanx; 27- Superficial ungular plexus; 28- Medial proper digital nerve; 29- Ergot ramus; 30- Dorsal ramus; 31- Ramus of the digital torus;

Other structures: 32- Ergot ligament; 33- Medial ungular cartilage; 34- Lateral ungular cartilage.

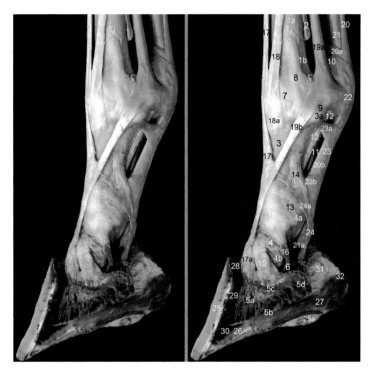

Fig. F.20 **Lateral aspect of the left distal thoracic limb.**

Bones and joints: 1- Third metacarpal bone, 1a- body, 1b- distal metaphysis; 2- Fourth metacarpal bone (end); 3- Proximal phalanx, 3a- palmar eminence; 4- Middle phalanx, 4a- flexor tuberosity, 4b- condyle; 5- Distal phalanx, 5a- Parietal surface, 5b- solar margin, 5c- collateral fossa, 5d-lateral palmar process; 6- Distal sesamoid bone (lateral angle); 7- Dorsal capsule of the MPJ; 8- Lateral collateral ligament of the MPJ (superficial layer); 9- Lateral collateral sesamoidean ligament of the MPJ; 10- Palmar (intersesamoidean) ligament (suprasesamoidean part); 11- Straight sesamoidean ligament; 12- Lateral oblique sesamoidean ligament; 13- Lateral collateral ligament of the proximal interphalangeal joint (PIPJ); 14- Abaxial palmar ligament of the PIPJ (covered by the proximal attachment of the distal digital annular ligament); 15- Collateral ligament of the distal interphalangeal joint; 16- Lateral collateral sesamoidean ligament;

Tendons and associated structures: 17- Dorsal digital extensor tendon, 17a- distal enthesis; 18- Lateral digital extensor tendon, 18a- distal enthesis; 19- Third interosseous muscle (TIOM, suspensory ligament), 19a- lateral branch, 19b- lateral extensor branch; 20- Superficial digital flexor tendon, 20a- manica flexoria, 20b- lateral branch; 21- Deep digital flexor tendon, 21a- fibrocartilaginous pad; 22- Palmar annular ligament; 23- Proximal digital annular ligament, 23a- proximal attachment, 23b- distal attachment; 24- Distal digital annular ligament, 24a- proximal attachment;

Superficial structures: 25- Hoof wall, 25a- bar; 26- Sole; 27- Frog; 28- Coronal corium and cushion; 29- Parietal corium; 30- Corium of the sole; 31- Digital cushion; 32- Bulb of the medial heel.

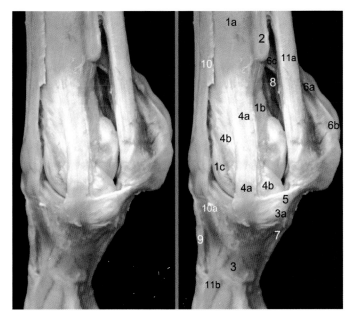

Fig. F.21 **Lateral aspect of the left metacarpophalangeal joint.**

Bones and joints: 1- Third metacarpal bone, 1a- body, 1b- distal metaphysis, 1c- condyle; 2- Fourth metacarpal bone (end); 3- Proximal phalanx, 3a- palmar eminence; 4- Lateral collateral ligament of the metacarpophalangeal joint, 4a- superficial layer, 4b- deep layer; 5- Collateral sesamoidean ligament of the metacarpophalangeal joint; 6- Palmar (intersesamoidean) ligament, 6a- suprasesamoidean part, 6b- sesamoidean part, 6c- metacarpointersesamoidean ligament; 7- Lateral oblique sesamoidean ligament; 8- Proximopalmar recess of the metacarpophalangeal joint;

Tendons: 9- Dorsal digital extensor tendon; 10- Lateral digital extensor tendon (cut longitudinally), 10a- distal enthesis; 11- Third interosseous muscle (suspensory ligament), 11a- lateral branch, 11b- lateral extensor branch (cut).

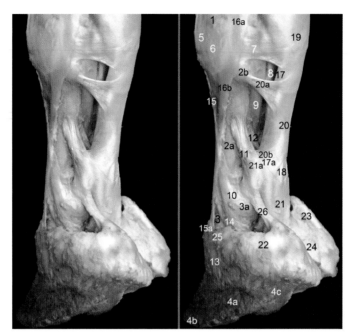

Fig. F.22 **Medial aspect of the right thoracic limb digital area.**

Bones and joints: 1- Third metacarpal bone; 2- Proximal phalanx, 2a- body, 2b- medial palmar eminence; 3- Middle phalanx, 3a- flexor tuberosity; 4- Distal phalanx, 4a- parietal surface, 4b- solar margin, 4c- medial palmar process; 5- Dorsal capsule of the metacarpophalangeal joint; 6- Medial collateral ligament (superficial layer) of the MPJ; 7- Medial collateral sesamoidean ligament of the MPJ; 8- Straight sesamoidean ligament; 9- Medial oblique sesamoidean ligament; 10- Collateral ligament of the PIPJ; 11- Abaxial palmar ligament of the PIPJ (covered by the proximal attachments of the distal digital annular ligament and chondrocompedal ligament); 12- Axial palmar ligament of the PIPJ; 13- Collateral ligament of the distal interphalangeal joint; 14- Collateral sesamoidean ligament;

Tendons and associated structures: 15- Dorsal digital extensor tendon, 15a- distal enthesis; 16- Third interosseous muscle (suspensory ligament), 16a- medial branch (enthesis), 16b- medial extensor branch; 17- Superficial digital flexor tendon, 17a- medial branch (covered by the proximal digital annular ligament); 18- Deep digital flexor tendon; 19- Palmar annular ligament; 20- Proximal digital annular ligament, 20a- proximal attachment, 20b- distal attachment; 21- Distal digital annular ligament, 21a- proximal attachment;

Other foot structures: 22- Medial ungular cartilage; 23- Lateral ungular cartilage; 24- Digital cushion; 25- Chondrocoronal ligament; 26- Chondrocompedal ligament.

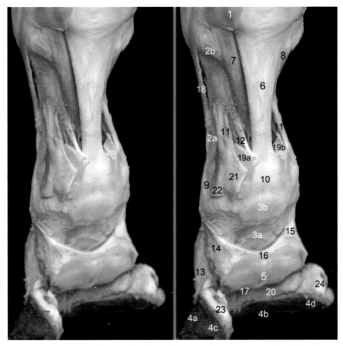

Fig. F.23 **Palmaromedial aspect of the right digital area after removal of the flexor tendons.**

Bones and joints: 1- Medial proximal sesamoid bone (palmar margin); 2- Proximal phalanx, 2a- body, 2b- medial palmar eminence; 3- Middle phalanx, 3a- body, 3b- flexor tuberosity; 4- Distal phalanx, 4a- parietal surface, 4b- solar margin, 4c- medial palmar process, 4d- lateral palmar process; 5- Distal sesamoid bone; 6- Straight sesamoidean ligament; 7- Medial oblique sesamoidean ligament; 8- Lateral oblique sesamoidean ligament; 9- Collateral ligament of the PIPJ; 10- Middle scutum; 11- Abaxial palmar ligament of the PIPJ; 12- Axial palmar ligament of the PIPJ; 13- Collateral ligament of the distal interphalangeal joint; 14- Medial collateral sesamoidean ligament; 15- Lateral collateral sesamoidean ligament; 16- Proximal sesamoidean ligament; 17- Distal sesamoidean ligament;

Tendons and associated structures: 18- Third interosseous muscle (suspensory ligament), medial extensor branch; 19- Superficial digital flexor tendon, 19a- medial branch (cut), 19b- lateral branch (cut); 20- Deep digital flexor tendon (infrasesamoidean part); 21- Proximal attachment of the distal digital annular ligament;

Ungular cartilages: 22- Proximal attachment of the chondrocompedal ligament; 23- Medial ungular cartilage (cut); 24- Lateral ungular cartilage (cut).

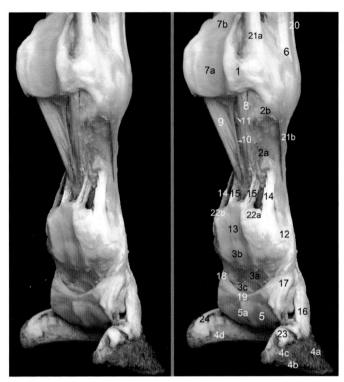

Fig. F.24 **Palmarolateral aspect of the right digital area after removal of the flexor tendons and straight sesamoidean ligament.**

Bones and joints: 1- Lateral proximal sesamoid bone (body); 2- Proximal phalanx, 2a- body, 2b- lateral palmar eminence; 3- Middle phalanx, 3a- body, 3b- flexor tuberosity, 3c- condyle (palmar margin); 4- Distal phalanx, 4a- parietal surface, 4b- solar margin, 4c- lateral palmar process, 4d- medial palmar process; 5- Distal sesamoid bone (flexor surface), 5a- sagittal crest; 6- Lateral collateral ligament of the metacarpophalangeal joint (superficial layer); 7- Palmar (intersesamoidean) ligament, 7a- sesamoidean part, 7b- suprasesamoidean part; 8- Lateral oblique sesamoidean ligament; 9- Medial oblique sesamoidean ligament; 10- Intermediate sesamoidean ligament; 11- Cruciate sesamoidean ligament; 12- Collateral ligament of the PIPJ; 13- Middle scutum; 14- Abaxial palmar ligament of the PIPJ; 15- Axial palmar ligament of the PIPJ; 16- Lateral collateral ligament of the distal interphalangeal joint; 17- Lateral collateral sesamoidean ligament; 18- Medial collateral sesamoidean ligament; 19- Proximal sesamoidean ligament;

Tendons and associated structures: 20- Lateral digital extensor tendon; 21- Third interosseous muscle (suspensory ligament), 21a- lateral branch, 21b- lateral extensor branch; 22- Superficial digital flexor tendon, 22a- lateral branch (cut), 22b- medial branch (cut);

Ungular cartilages: 23- Lateral ungular cartilage (cut); 24- Medial ungular cartilage (cut).

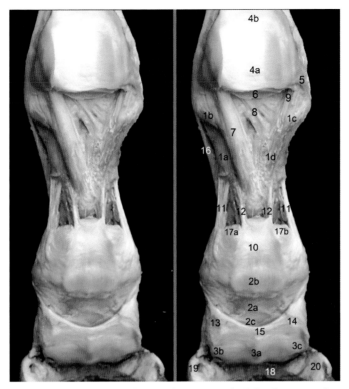

Fig. F.25 **Palmar aspect of the right digital area after removal of the flexor tendons as well as straight and lateral oblique sesamoidean ligaments.**

Bones and joints: 1- Proximal phalanx, 1a- body, 1b- medial palmar eminence, 1c- lateral palmar eminence, 1d- trigonum; 2- Middle phalanx, 2a- body, 2b- flexor tuberosity, 2c- condyle (palmar margin); 3- Distal sesamoid bone (flexor surface), 3a- sagittal crest, 3b- medial angle, 3c- lateral angle; 4- Palmar (intersesamoidean) ligament, 4a- sesamoidean part, 4b- suprasesamoidean part; 5- Collateral sesamoidean ligament; 6- Straight sesamoidean ligament (origin, cut); 7- Medial oblique sesamoidean ligament; 8- Cruciate sesamoidean ligament; 9- Short sesamoidean ligament; 10- Middle scutum; 11- Abaxial palmar ligament of the PIPJ; 12- Axial palmar ligament of the PIPJ; 13- Medial collateral sesamoidean ligament; 14- Lateral collateral sesamoidean ligament; 15- Proximal sesamoidean ligament;

Tendons and associated structures: 16- Third interosseous muscle (suspensory ligament), medial extensor branch; 17- Superficial digital flexor tendon, 17a- medial branch (cut), 17b- lateral branch (cut); 18- Deep digital flexor tendon (distal enthesis, cut);

Ungular cartilages: 19- Medial ungular cartilage (cut); 20- Lateral ungular cartilage (cut).

F.4 CROSS-SECTIONS

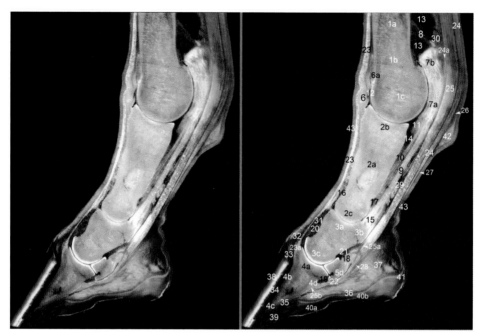

Fig. F.26 **Sagittal section of the thoracic limb digital area.**

Bones and joints: 1- Third metacarpal bone, 1a- body, 1b- distal metaphysis, 1c- condyle; 2- Proximal phalanx, 2a- body, 2b- glenoid cavity, 2c- condyle; 3- Middle phalanx, 3a- glenoid cavity, 3b- flexor tuberosity, 3c- condyle; 4- Distal phalanx, 4a- glenoid cavity, 4b- parietal surface, 4c- solar margin, 4d- flexor surface; 5- Distal sesamoid bone, 5a- flexor surface; 6- Dorsal capsule of the MPJ, 6a- proximodorsal fibrosynovial plica; 7- Palmar (intersesamoidean) ligament (proximal scutum), 7a- sesamoidean part, 7b- suprasesamoidean part; 8- Metacarpointersesamoidean ligament; 9- Straight sesamoidean ligament; 10- Intermediate sesamoidean ligament; 11- Cruciate sesamoidean ligament; 12- Dorsal recess of the MPJ; 13- Proximopalmar recess of the MPJ; 14- Distopalmar recess of the MPJ; 15- Middle scutum; 16- Dorsal recess of the PIPJ; 17- Palmar recess of the PIPJ; 18- Proximal sesamoidean ligament; 19- Distal sesamoidean ligament; 20- Dorsal recess of the DIPJ; 21- Proximopalmar recess of the DIPJ; 22- Distopalmar recess of the DIPJ;

Tendons and associated structures: 23- Dorsal digital extensor tendon, 23a- distal enthesis on the extensor process of the distal phalanx; 24- Superficial digital flexor tendon, 24a- manica flexoria; 25- Deep digital flexor tendon, 25a- fibrocartilaginous pad, 25b- distal enthesis; 26- Palmar annular ligament; 27- Proximal digital annular ligament; 28- Distal digital annular ligament; 29- Digital sheath cavity;

Vessels and nerves: 30- Distal palmar anastomosis between the palmar metacarpal and digital arteries); 31- Dorsal rami (artery and vein) of the middle phalanx; 32- Coronal vein and artery;

Superficial structures and skin: 33- Coronal corium and cushion; 34- Parietal corium; 35- Solar corium; 36- Corium of the frog; 37- Digital cushion; 38- Hoof wall; 39- Sole; 40- Frog, 40a- body, 40b- branch; 41- Heel; 42- Ergot; 43- Skin.

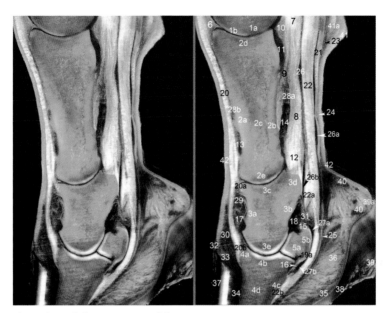

Fig. F.27 **Sagittal section of the pastern and foot.**

Bones and joints: 1- Third metacarpal condyle, 1a- subchondral bone of the sagittal ridge, 1b- articular cartilage; 2- Proximal phalanx, 2a- dorsal cortex, 2b- palmar cortex, 2c- medullary cavity, 2d- subchondral bone of the sagittal groove, 2e- subchondral bone of the condyle; 3- Middle phalanx, 3a- dorsal compact bone, 3b- palmar compact bone, 3c- subchondral bone of the glenoid cavity, 3d- compact bone of the flexor tuberosity, 3e- subchondral bone of the condyle; 4- Distal phalanx, 4a- extensor process, 4b- subchondral bone of the glenoid cavity, 4c- compact bone of the flexor surface, 4d- spongy bone of the body; 5- Distal sesamoid bone, 5a- spongy bone, 5b- compact bone of the flexor surface; 6- Dorsal capsule of the MPJ; 7- Palmar (intersesamoidean) ligament (sesamoidean part); 8- Straight sesamoidean ligament; 9- Intermediate sesamoidean ligament; 10- Cruciate sesamoidean ligament; 11- Distopalmar recess of the MPJ; 12- Middle scutum; 13- Dorsal recess of the PIPJ; 14- Palmar recess of the PIPJ; 15- Proximal sesamoidean ligament; 16- Distal sesamoidean ligament; 17- Dorsal recess of the DIPJ; 18- Proximopalmar recess of the DIPJ; 19- Distopalmar recess of the DIPJ, 19a- synovial fossa;

Tendons and associated structures: 20- Dorsal digital extensor tendon, 20a- enthesis on the extensor process of the middle phalanx, 20b- distal enthesis on the extensor process of the distal phalanx; 21- Superficial digital flexor tendon; 22- Deep digital flexor tendon, 22a- fibrocartilaginous pad, 22b- distal enthesis; 23- Palmar annular ligament; 24- Proximal digital annular ligament; 25- Distal digital annular ligament; 26- Digital sheath cavity, 26a- distopalmar recess, 26b- distodorsal recess; 27- Podotrochlear bursa, 27a- proximal recess, 27b- distal recess;

Vessels and nerves: 28- Rami (artery and vein) of the proximal phalanx, 28a- palmar rami, 28b- dorsal rami; 29- Dorsal rami (artery and vein) of the middle phalanx; 30- Coronal vein and artery; 31- Arteries of the transverse ligament;

Superficial structures and skin: 32- Perioplic and limbic corium; 33- Coronal corium and cushion; 34- Parietal corium; 35- Corium of the frog; 36- Digital cushion; 37- Hoof wall, 38- Frog (body and central sulcus); 39- Heel, 39a- bulb; 40- Rami (artery and vein) of the digital torus; 41- Ergot, 41a- ergot cushion; 42-Skin.

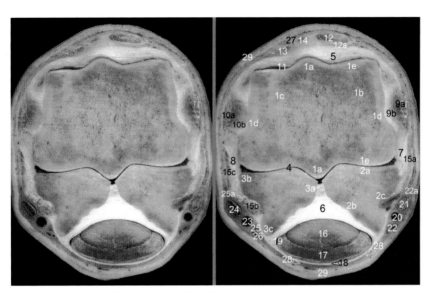

Fig. F.28 **Transverse section of the thoracic limb fetlock.**

Bones and joints: 1- Metacarpal condyle, 1a- sagittal ridge, 1b-medial part (medial condyle), 1c- lateral part (lateral condyle), 1d- collateral fossa, 1e- subchondral bone and articular cartilage; 2- Medial proximal sesamoid bone (body), 2a- articular surface, 2b- flexor surface, 2c- interosseous surface; 3- Lateral proximal sesamoid bone (body), 3a- axial margin, 3b- abaxial margin, 3c- palmar margin; 4- Metacarposesamoidean joint space; 5- Dorsal capsule of MPJ; 6- Palmar (intersesamoidean) ligament (sesamoidean part); 7- Medial collateral sesamoidean ligament; 8- Lateral collateral sesamoidean ligament; 9- Medial collateral ligament, 9a- superficial layer, 9b- deep layer; 10- Lateral collateral ligament, 10a- superficial layer, 10b- deep layer; 11- Dorsal recess of the MPJ;

Tendons and associated structures: 12- Dorsal digital extensor tendon, 12a- subtendinous bursa; 13- Lateral digital extensor tendon; 14- Accessory digital extensor tendon; 15- Third interosseous muscle (suspensory ligament), 15a- medial extensor branch, 15b- lateral branch, 15c- lateral extensor branch; 16- Deep digital flexor tendon; 17- Superficial digital flexor tendon; 18- Palmar annular ligament; 19- Digital sheath cavity;

Vessels and nerves: 20- Medial proper digital artery; 21- Medial proper digital vein; 22- Medial proper digital nerve, 22a- dorsal ramus; 23- Lateral proper digital artery; 24- Lateral proper digital vein; 25- Lateral proper digital nerve, 25a- dorsal ramus; 26- Lymphatic vessels;

Superficial structures and skin: 27- Dorsal metacarpophalangeal fascia; 28- Subcutaneous tissue; 29- Skin.

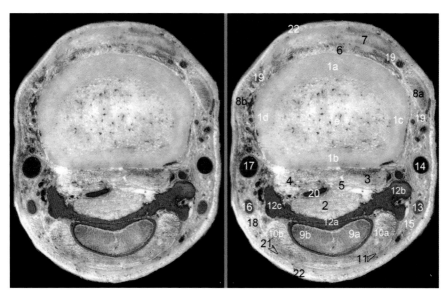

Fig. F.29 **Transverse section of the thoracic limb pastern.**

Bones and joints: 1- Proximal phalanx, 1a- dorsal cortex, 1b- palmar cortex, 1c- medial cortex, 1d- lateral cortex, 1e- spongy bone; 2- Straight sesamoidean ligament; 3- Medial oblique sesamoidean ligament; 4- Lateral oblique sesamoidean ligament; 5- Intermediate sesamoidean ligament; 6- Dorsal recess of the proximal interphalangeal joint (injected with orange latex);

Tendons and associated structures: 7- Dorsal digital extensor tendon; 8- Third interosseous muscle (suspensory ligament), 8a- medial extensor branch, 8b- lateral extensor branch; 9- Deep digital flexor tendon, 9a- origin of the medial lobe, 9b- origin of the lateral lobe; 10- Superficial digital flexor tendon, 10a- origin of the medial branch, 10b- origin of the lateral branch; 11- Proximal digital annular ligament; 12- Digital sheath cavity (injected with green latex), 12a- synovial plica, 12b- medial collateral digital recess, 12c- lateral collateral digital recess;

Vessels and nerves: 13- Medial proper digital artery; 14- Medial proper digital vein; 15- Medial proper digital nerve; 16- Lateral proper digital artery; 17- Lateral proper digital vein; 18- Lateral proper digital nerve; 19- Dorsal ramus (artery) of the proximal phalanx; 20- Palmar ramus (vein) of the proximal phalanx;

Superficial structure and skin: 21- Subcutaneous tissue; 22- Skin.

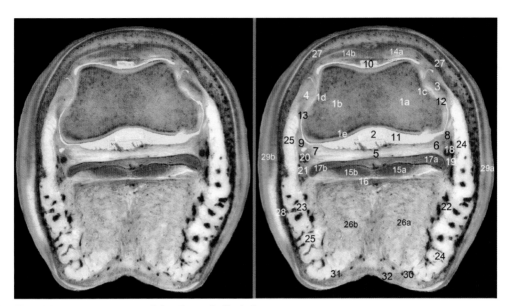

Fig. F.30 **Transverse section of the thoracic limb foot.**

Bones and joints: 1- Condyle of the middle phalanx, 1a- medial part; 1b- lateral part, 1c- medial collateral fossa, 1d- lateral collateral fossa, 1e- subchondral bone and articular cartilage; 2- Proximal articular margin of the distal sesamoid bone; 3- Medial collateral ligament of the DIPJ; 4- Lateral collateral ligament of the DIPJ; 5- Proximal sesamoidean ligament; 6- Origin of the medial collateral sesamoidean ligament; 7- Origin of the lateral collateral sesamoidean ligament; 8- Medial chondrosesamoidean ligament; 9- Lateral chondrosesamoidean ligament; 10- Dorsal recess of the DIPJ; 11- Proximopalmar recess of the DIPJ; 12- Medial collateral recess of the DIPJ; 13- Lateral collateral recess of the DIPJ;

Tendons and associated structures: 14- Dorsal digital extensor tendon, 14a- medial lobe, 14b- lateral lobe; 15- Deep digital flexor tendon, 15a- medial lobe, 15b- lateral lobe; 16- Distal digital annular ligament; 17- Podotrochlear bursa, 17a- medial recess, 17b- lateral recess;

Vessels and nerves: 18- Medial proper digital artery; 19- Medial proper digital nerve; 20- Lateral proper digital artery; 21- Lateral proper digital nerve; 22- Medial (venous) ungular plexus; 23- Lateral (venous) ungular plexus;

Ungular cartilages and superficial structures: 24- Medial ungular cartilage; 25- Lateral ungular cartilage; 26- Digital cushion, 26a- medial lobe, 26b- lateral lobe; 27- Coronal cushion and corium; 28- Parietal corium; 29- Hoof wall, 29a- medial quarter, 29b- lateral quarter; 30- Bulb of the medial heel; 31- Bulb of the lateral heel; 32- Skin.

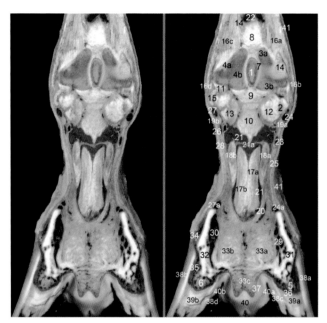

Fig. F.31 **Frontal section of the thoracic limb digital area.**

Bones and joints: 1- Third metacarpal condyle (sagittal ridge); 2- Proximal phalanx (medial palmar eminence); 3-Medial proximal sesamoid bone, 3a- apex, 3b- base; 4- Lateral proximal sesamoid bone, 4a- interosseous surface, 4b- articular surface; 5- Medial palmar process of the distal phalanx; 6- Lateral palmar process of the distal phalanx; 7- Metacarposesamoidean joint space; 8- Palmar (intersesamoidean) ligament (suprasesamoidean part); 9- Cruciate sesamoidean ligaments; 10- Straight sesamoidean ligament; 11- Lateral short sesamoidean ligament; 12- Medial oblique sesamoidean ligament; 13- Lateral oblique sesamoidean ligament; 14- Proximopalmar recess of the metacarpophalangeal joint; 15- Lateral collateropalmar recess of the MPJ;

Tendons and associated structures: 16- Third interosseous muscle (suspensory ligament), 16a- medial branch, 16b- medial extensor branch, 16c- lateral branch, 16d- lateral extensor branch; 17- Deep digital flexor tendon, 17a- medial lobe, 17b- lateral lobe; 18- Superficial digital flexor tendon, 18a- medial branch, 18b- lateral branch; 19- Proximal digital annular ligament, 19a- medial proximal attachment, 19b- lateral proximal attachment; 20- Distal digital annular ligament; 21- Digital sheath cavity, 21a- transverse synovial plica;

Vessels and nerves: 22- Distal palmar anastomosis between the palmar metacarpal and digital veins; 23- Medial proper digital artery; 24- Medial proper digital vein, 24a- roots; 25- Medial proper digital nerve; 26- Lateral proper digital artery; 27- Lateral proper digital vein, 27a- roots; 28- Lateral proper digital nerve; 29- Medial (venous) ungular superficial and deep plexi; 30- Lateral (venous) ungular superficial and deep plexi;

Ungular cartilages and superficial structures: 31- Medial ungular cartilage; 32- Lateral ungular cartilage; 33- Digital cushion, 33a- medial lobe, 33b- lateral lobe, 33c- body (cuneal part); 34- Coronal cushion and corium; 35- Parietal corium; 36- Solar corium; 37- Corium of the frog; 38- Hoof wall, 38a- medial quarter, 38b- lateral quarter; 38c- medial bar, 38d- lateral bar; 39- Sole, 39a- medial sole angle, 39b- lateral sole angle; 40- Frog (junction between body and branches), 40a- medial sulcus, 40b- lateral sulcus; 41- Skin.

G.1 PHYSICAL ASPECT

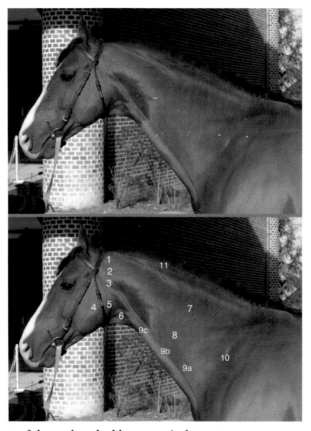

Fig. G.1 **Physical aspect of the neck: palpable anatomical structures.**

1- Nuchal region; 2- Atlas wing; 3- Parotid region; 4- Masseteric region; 5- Margin (angle) of the mandible; 6- Throat (larynx region); 7- Dorsal cervical region (dorsal cervical muscles: extensor muscles); 8- Vertebral axis; 9- Ventral cervical region (ventral cervical muscles: flexor muscles), 9a- brachiocephalicus muscle, 9b- jugular sulcus, 9c- sternocephalicus muscle; 10- Cranial margin of the shoulder; 11- Mane.

G.2 NUCHAL AREA

G.2.1 Radiographic anatomy

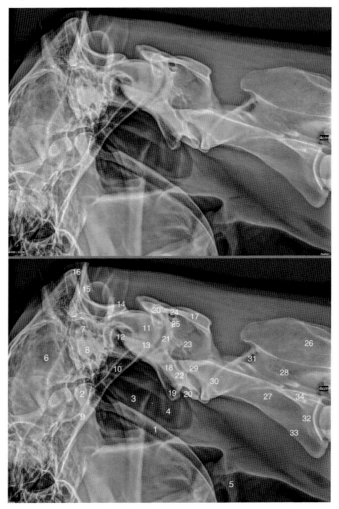

Fig. G.2 **Lateral radiographic view of the nuchal area.**

Head: 1- Branch (ramus) of the mandible; 2- Condyle process of the mandible; 3- Hyoid (stylo-hyoideum); 4- Guttural pouch; 5- Larynx; 6- Cerebral cavity; 7- Cerebellar cavity; 8- Petrosa part of the temporal bone; 9- Sphenoid bone; 10- Occipital bone (basilar part); 11- Occipital condyles; 12- Ventral condylar fossae; 13- Paracondylar process; 14- Foramen magnum opened at the nuchal face of the occipital bone; 15- External occipital crest; 16- External occipital protuberance;

Atlas: 17- Dorsal arch; 18- Ventral arch; 19- Ventral tubercle; 20- Transverse process (atlas wing); 21- Cranial articular fossa; 22- Fovea dentis; 23- Vertebral canal; 24- Lateral vertebral foramen (foramen intervertebral for the first cervical nerve); 25- Alar foramen;

Axis: 26- Spinous process; 27- Vertebral body; 28- Vertebral canal; 29- Dens; 30- Lateral expansion; 31- Lateral vertebral (intervertebral) foramen; 32- Vertebral fossa; 33- Ventral crest of the body; 34- Transverse processes.

G.3 DISSECTED SPECIMEN

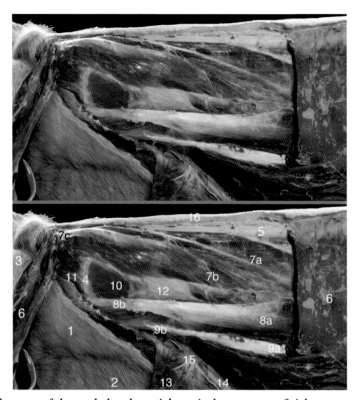

FIG. G.3 **Lateral aspect of the nuchal and cranial cervical areas: superficial structures.**

1- Parotid region; 2- Masseteric region; 3- Left ear; 4- Margin of the atlas wing; 5- Nuchal ligament (funiculus); 6- Splenius muscle (cranial part, cut and reclined cranially); 7- Semispinalis capitis muscle, 7a- dorsal part (biventer cervicis muscle), 7b- ventral part (complexus muscle), 7c- nuchal tendon; 8- Longissimus capitis muscle, 8a- muscle body, 8b- tendon; 9- Longissimus atlantis muscle, 9a- muscle body, 9b- tendon; 10- Obliquus capitis caudalis muscle; 11- Obliquus capitis cranialis muscle; 12- Deep cervical fascia; 13- Omotransversarius muscle; 14- Brachiocephalicus muscle; 15- Ventral rami of the first and second cervical nerves; 16- Skin of the mane.

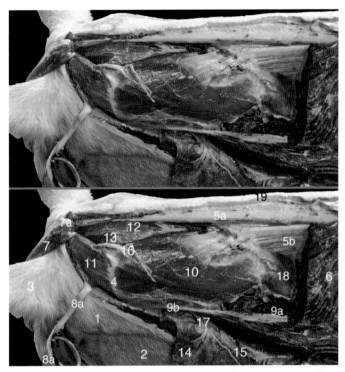

Fig. G.4 **Dorsolateral aspect of the nuchal and cranial cervical areas: intermediate structures.**

1- Parotid region; 2- Masseteric region; 3- Left ear; 4- Margin of the atlas wing; 5- Nuchal ligament, 5a- funiculus, 5b- lamina; 6- Splenius muscle (cranial part, cut and removed); 7- Semispinalis capitis muscle (cranial part, cut and reclined cranially); 8- Longissimus capitis muscle (cranial part, cut and reclined cranially), 8a- muscle body, 8b- tendon; 9- Longissimus atlantis muscle, 9a- muscle body, 9b- tendon; 10- Obliquus capitis caudalis muscle; 11- Obliquus capitis cranialis muscle; 12- Rectus capitis dorsalis major muscle; 13- Rectus capitis dorsalis minor muscle; 14- Omotransversarius muscle; 15- Brachiocephalicus muscle; 16- Dorsal rami of the first cervical nerves; 17 - Ventral rami of the first and second cervical nerves; 18- Multifidus colli muscle; 19- Skin of the mane.

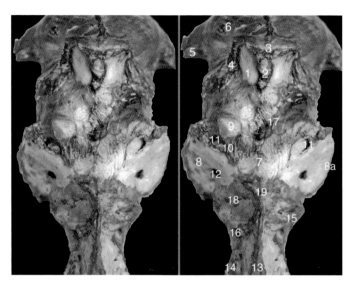

Fig. G.5 **Dorsal aspect of the nuchal area: deep structures.**

Head: 1- Nuchal face of the occipital bone; 2- External occipital crest; 3- External occipital protuberance; 4- Nuchal crest; 5- Zygomatic arch; 6- Temporal muscle;

Atlas: 7- Dorsal arch; 8- Atlas wing, 8a- margin; 9- Cranial margin; 10- Lateral vertebral foramen (foramen intervertebral for the first cervical nerve); 11- Alar foramen; 12- Transverse foramen;

Axis: 13- Spinous process; 14- Transverse process; 15- Lateral expansion of the cranial articular surface; 16- Lateral vertebral (intervertebral) foramen;

Joint structures: 17- Dorsal atlantooccipital membrane; 18- Dorsal atlantoaxial membrane; 19- Dorsal atlantoaxial ligament.

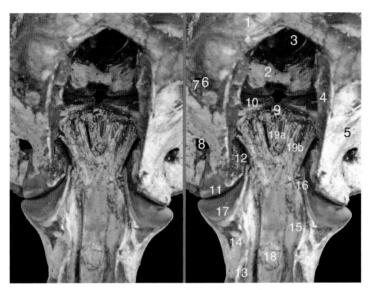

Fig. G.6 **Dorsal aspect of the nuchal area: vertebral canal opened.**

Occipital bone: 1- Nuchal face of the occipital bone; 2- Basilar part of the occipital bone; 3- Foramen magnum;

Atlas: 4- Dorsal arch (cut); 5- Atlas wing; 6- Lateral vertebral foramen (foramen intervertebral for the first cervical nerve); 7- Alar foramen; 8- Transverse foramen; 9- Ventral arch; 10- Cranial articular surface for the occipital condyle (ventral part); 11- Caudal articular surface for the axis; 12- Fovea dentis;

Axis: 13- Vertebral pedicle (cut to remove the arch); 14- Vertebral body; 15- Vertebral canal; 16- Dens; 17- Lateral expansion of the cranial articular surface;

Joint structures: 18- Dorsal longitudinal ligament; 19- Dentis longitudinal ligament; 19a- median part, 19b- lateral part.

G.4 CROSS-SECTION

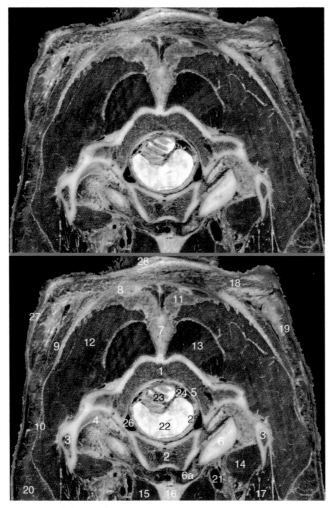

Fig. G.7 **Transverse section of the nuchal area.**

Bone and joints: 1- Occipital bone (squamous part); 2- Basilar part of the occipital bone; 3- Paracondylar process; 4- Ventral condylar fossa; 5- Foramen magnum; 6- Cranial margin of the atlas, 6a- Atlantooccipital joint cavity; 7- Nuchal ligament (funiculus);

Muscles: 8- Splenius muscle (cranial aponeurosis); 9- Brachiocephalicus muscle; 10- Tendon of the longissimus capitis muscle; 11- Tendon of the semispinalis capitis muscle; 12- Obliquus capitis cranialis muscle; 13- Rectus capitis dorsalis major and rectus capitis dorsalis minor muscles; 14- Rectus capitis lateralis muscle; 15- Rectus capitis ventralis muscle; 16- Fat; 17- Digastric muscle; 18- Cervicoauricular muscles; 19- Parotidoauricular muscle; 20- Parotid gland; 21- Occipital vein; 22- Brain stem (medulla oblongata); 23- Vermis of the cerebrum; 24- Cerebellomedullaris cistern; 25- Dura mater; 26- Basilar sinus (veins).

G.5 MIDDLE AND CAUDAL CERVICAL AREAS

G.5.1 Radiographic anatomy

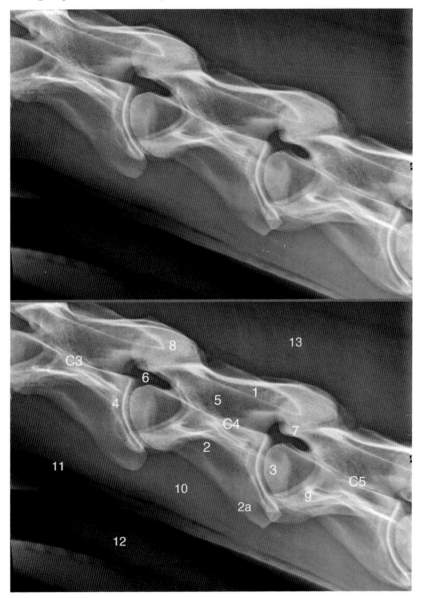

Fig. G.8 **Lateral radiographic view of the middle cervical area (from the third cervical vertebra (C3) to the fifth one (C5)).**

C3- Third cervical vertebra; C4- Fourth cervical vertebra; C5- Fifth cervical vertebra;

1- Vertebral arch; 2- Vertebral body; 3- Vertebral head; 4- Vertebral fossa; 5- Vertebral canal; 6- Intervertebral foramen; 7- Cranial articular process; 8- Caudal articular process; 9- Transverse process; 10- Shadow of the longus colli muscle; 11- Oesophagus; 12- Trachea; 13- Dorsal cervical muscles.

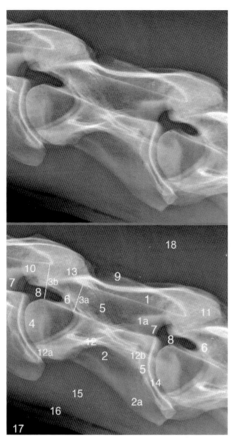

Fig. G.9 **Lateral radiographic view of the fourth cervical vertebra (C4).**

1- Vertebral arch, 1a- vertebral pedicule; 2- Vertebral body, 2a- ventral crest; 3- Vertebral foramen (canal), 3a- intravertebral median diameter, 3b- intervertebral median diameter; 4- Vertebral head (cranial extremity); 5- Vertebral fossa (caudal extremity); 6- Cranial vertebral incisura; 7- Caudal vertebral incisura; 8- Intervertebral foramen; 9- Spinal process; 10- Cranial articular process; 11- Caudal articular process; 12- Transverse process, 12a- ventral tubercle, 12b- dorsal tubercle, 12c- Transverse foramen; 13- Articular process joint; 14- Vertebral symphysis with the intervertebral disc; 15- Shadow of the longus colli muscle; 16- Oesophagus; 17- Trachea; 18- Dorsal cervical muscles.

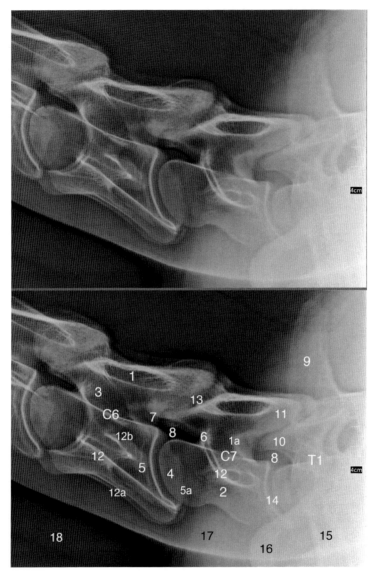

Fig. G.10 Lateral radiographic view of the caudal cervical area (from the fifth cervical vertebra to the first thoracic vertebra).

C6- Sixth cervical vertebra; C7- Seventh cervical vertebra; T1-First thoracic vertebra;

1- Vertebral arch, 1a- vertebral pedicule; 2- Vertebral body; 3- Vertebral foramen (vertebral canal); 4- Vertebral head (cranial extremity); 5- Vertebral fossa (caudal extremity), 5a- margin; 6- Cranial vertebral incisura; 7- Caudal vertebral incisura; 8- Intervertebral foramen; 9- Spinal process of T1 (C7 does not have a spinal process on this horse); 10- Cranial articular process (of T1); 11- Caudal articular process (of C7); 12- Transverse process, 12a- ventral lamina (C6), 12b- transverse foramen; 13- Articular process joint; 14- Vertebral symphysis with the intervertebral disc; 15- First rib; 16- Tuberculum supraglenoidale of the right scapula; 17- Shadow of the longus colli muscle; 18-Trachea.

G.5.2 Dissected specimen

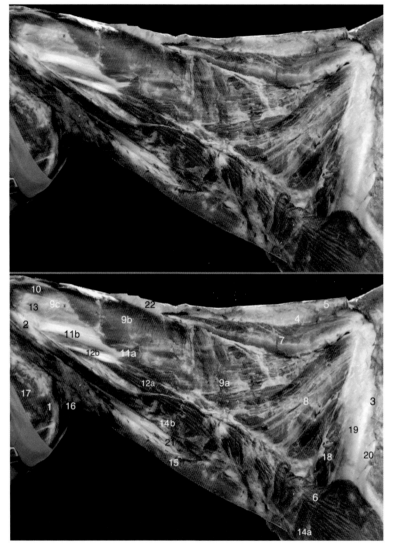

Fig. G.11 **Lateral aspect of the cervical area: superficial structures.**

1- Branch (ramus) of the mandible; 2- Margin of the atlas wing; 3- Spine of the scapula; 4- Nuchal ligament (funiculus); 5- Trapezius muscle (cervical part, cut and reclined); 6- Omotransversarius muscle; 7- Rhomboideus cervicis muscle; 8- Serratus (ventralis) cervicis muscle; 9- Splenius muscle, 9a- splenius cervicis muscle, 9b- splenius capitis muscle, 9c- cranial aponeurosis; 10- Semispinalis capitis muscle; 11- Longissimus capitis muscle, 11a- muscle body, 11b- tendon; 12- Longissimus atlantis muscle, 12a- muscle body, 12b- tendon; 13- Caudal obliquus capitis muscle; 14- Brachiocephalicus muscle, 14a- cleidobrachialis muscle, 14b- cleidocervicalis muscle; 15- Sternocephalicus muscle; 16- Omohyoideus muscle; 17- Masseter muscle; 18- Suclavius muscle; 19- Supraspinatus muscle; 20- Infraspinatus muscle; 21- Jugular vein; 22- Fat of the mane.

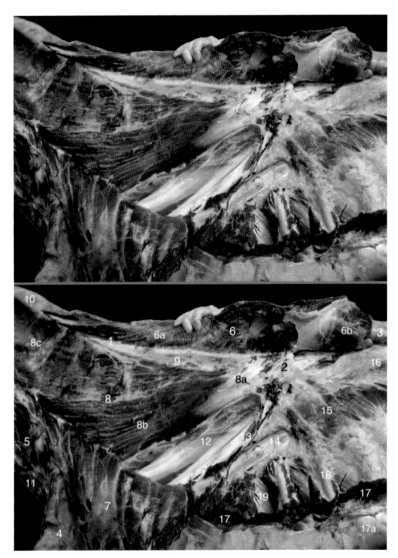

Fig. G.12 **Lateral aspect of the cervical area: intermediate structures.**

1- Nuchal ligament (funiculus); 2- Dorsoscapular ligament; 3- Trapezius muscle (thoracic part); 4- Omotransversarius muscle (reclined); 5- Brachiocephalicus muscle; 6- Rhomboideus muscle, 6a- cervical part, 6b- thoracic part; 7- Serratus (ventralis) cervicis muscle (reclined); 8- Splenius muscle, 8a- caudal aponeurosis, 8b- splenius cervicis, 8c- splenius capitis; 9- Semispinalis capitis muscle; 10- Fat of the mane; 11- Sternocephalicus muscle; 12- Longissimus cervicis muscle; 13- Longissimus thoracis muscle; 14- Iliocostalis thoracis muscle; 15- Serratus dorsalis cranialis muscle; 16- Thoracolumbar fascia; 17- Serratus ventralis thoracis muscle (cut), 17a- fibroelastic aponeurosis; 18- Rib; 19- Intercostalis externus muscle.

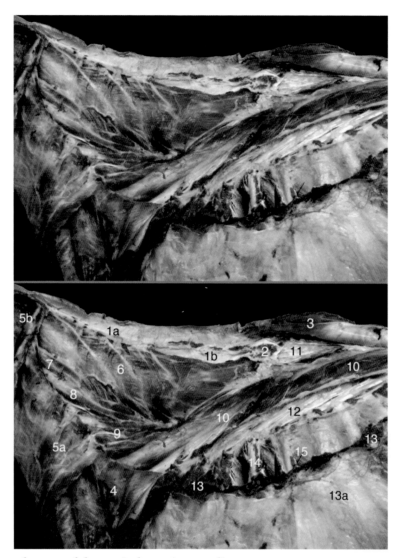

Fig. G.13 **Lateral aspect of the cervical area: intermediate structures.**

1- Nuchal ligament, 1a- funiculus, 1b- lamina; 2- Dorsoscapular ligament; 3- Rhomboideus cervicis muscle; 4- Serratus cervicis (ventralis) muscle (reclined); 5- Splenius muscle, 5a- splenius cervicis (reclined), 5b- splenius capitis; 6- Semispinalis capitis muscle (complexus muscle); 7- Longissimus capitis muscle; 8- Longissimus atlantis muscle; 9- Longissimus cervicis muscle; 10- Longissimus thoracis muscle; 11- Spinalis thoracis muscle; 12- Iliocostalis thoracis muscle; 13- Serratus ventralis thoracis muscle (cut), 13a- fibroelastic aponeurosis; 14- Rib; 15- Intercostalis externus muscle.

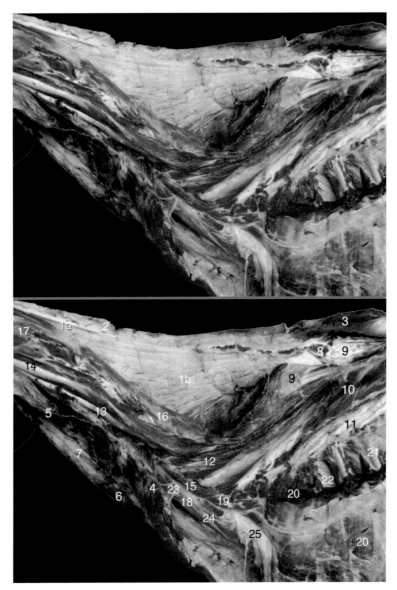

Fig. G.14 **Lateral aspect of the cervical area: deep structures.**

1- Nuchal ligament, 1a- funiculus, 1b- lamina; 2- Fat of the mane; 3- Rhomboideus cervicis muscle; 4- Omotransversarius muscle (cut); 5- Brachiocephalicus muscle; 6- Sternocephalicus muscle; 7- Jugular vein; 8- Dorsoscapular ligament; 9- Spinalis thoracis muscle; 10- Longissimus thoracis muscle; 11- Iliocostalis thoracis muscle; 12- Longissimus cervicis muscle; 13- Longissimus atlantis muscle; 14- Longissimus capitis muscle; 15- Iliocostalis cervicis muscle; 16- Multifidus cervicis muscle; 17- Obliquus capitis caudalis muscle; 18- Scalenus ventralis muscle; 19- Scalenus medius muscle; 20- Serratus ventralis thoracis muscle; 21- Rib; 22- Intercostalis externus muscle; 23- Ventral ramus of the sixth cervical nerve; 24- Root of the phrenic nerve; 25- Brachial plexus.

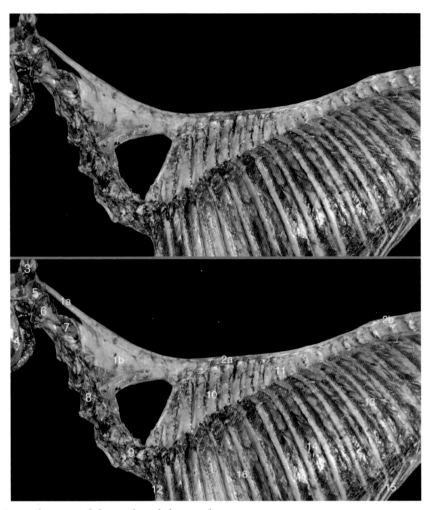

Fig. G.15 **Lateral aspect of the neck and thorax: deep structures.**

1- Nuchal ligament, 1a- funiculus, 1b- lamina; 2- Supraspinal ligament, 2a- cranial thoracic (elastic) part, 2b- lumbar (ligamentous) part; 3- Left ear; 4- Mandible; 5- Atlantooccipital joint; 6- Atlas (C1); 7- Axis (C2); 8- Fourth cervical vertebra (C4); 9- Seventh cervical vertebra (C7); 10- Fifth thoracic spinal process; 11- Interspinal ligament; 12- First rib (R1); 13- Thirteenth rib (R13); 14- Intercostal muscle; 15- Costal arch; 16- Intercostal nerve.

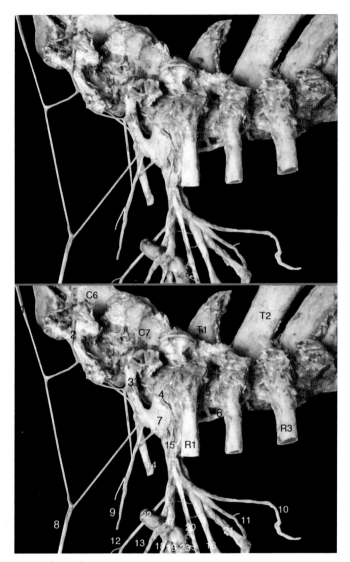

Fig. G.16 **Brachial plexus: lateral aspect.**

C6- Sixth cervical vertebra; C7- Seventh cervical vertebra; T1-First thoracic vertebra (spinal process); T2- Second thoracic vertebra (spinal process); R1- First rib; R3- Third rib.

1- Ventral ramus of the fifth cervical nerve (contributing to the phrenic nerve); 2- Ventral ramus of the sixth cervical nerve (contributing to the phrenic nerve and brachial plexus); 3- Ventral ramus of the seventh cervical nerve; 4- Ventral ramus of the eighth cervical nerve; 5- Ventral ramus of the first thoracic nerve; 6- Ventral ramus of the second thoracic nerve; 7- Brachial plexus; 8- Phrenic nerve; 9- Subclavius nerve; 10- Thoracodorsal nerve; 11- Lateral thoracic nerve; 12- Cranial pectoral nerves; 13- Caudal pectoral nerve (for the pectoralis profundus (ascendens) muscle); 14- Suprascapular nerve; 15- Subscapular nerves; 16- Axillary nerve; 17- Axillary ansa (loop) (around the subclavia artery); 18- Musculocutaneus nerve; 19- Median nerve; 20- Ulnar nerve; 21- Radial nerve; 22- Subclavia artery; 23- Axillary artery.

G.5.3 Cross-sections

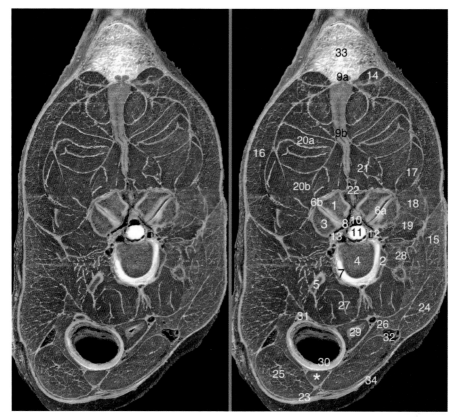

Fig. G.17 **Transverse section of the cervical area at the level of the C3–C4 intervertebral joint.**

C3- Third cervical vertebra, C4- Fourth cervical vertebra.

Bones and joints: 1- Caudal articular process of C3; 2- Vertebral fossa (margin) of C3; 3- Cranial articular process of C4; 4- Vertebral head (cranial extremity) of C4; 5- Transverse process (ventral tubercle) of C4; 6- Articular process joint, 6a- joint space, 6b- articular capsule; 7- Intervertebral disc; 8- Vertebral foramen (canal); 9- Nuchal ligament, 9a- funiculus, 9b- lamina;

Nervous structures: 10- Dura mater; 11- Spinal cord; 12- Internal vertebral plexus (veins); 13- Fourth cervical nerve in the intervertebral foramen;

Muscles: 14- Rhomboideus cervicis muscle; 15- Omotransversarius muscle; 16- Splenius muscle; 17- Longissimus capitis muscle; 18- Longissimus atlantis muscle; 19- Longissimus cervicis muscle; 20- Semispinalis capitis muscle, 20a- biventer capitis muscle (dorsal part), 20b- complexus muscle (ventral part); 21- Multifidus cervicis muscle; 22- Spinalis cervicis muscle; 23- Cutaneus colli muscle; 24- Brachiocephalicus muscle; 25- Sternocephalicus muscle; *- Sternohyoideus and sternothyroideus muscles; 26- Omohyoideus muscle; 27- Longus colli muscle; 28- Intertranversarii muscles;

Other structures: 29- Oesophagus; 30- Trachea; 31- Common carotid artery; 32- External jugular vein; 33- Fat of the mane; 34- Skin.

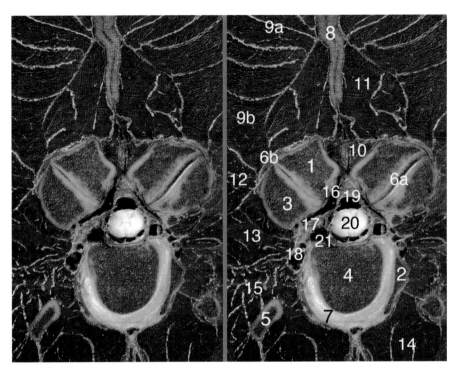

Fig. G.18 **Transverse section of the cervical area at the level of the C3–C4 intervertebral joint.**

C3- Third cervical vertebra, C4- Fourth cervical vertebra.

Bones and joints: 1- Caudal articular process of C3; 2- Vertebral fossa (margin) of C3; 3- Cranial articular process of C4; 4- Vertebral head (cranial extremity) of C4; 5- Transverse process of C4 (ventral tubercle); 6- Articular process joint, 6a- joint space, 6b- articular capsule; 7- Intervertebral disc; 8- Nuchal ligament (lamina);

Muscles: 9- Semispinalis capitis muscle, 9a- biventer capitis muscle (dorsal part), 9b- complexus muscle (ventral part); 10- Spinalis cervicis muscle; 11- Multifidus cervicis muscle; 12- Longissimus atlantis muscle; 13-Longissimus cervicis muscle; 14- Longus colli muscle; 15- Intertranversarii muscles;

Nervous structures and associated structures: 16- Vertebral foramen (canal); 17- Fourth cervical nerve in the intervertebral foramen; 18- Vertebral artery and vein; 19- Dura mater separating the epidural space filled with fat and the subdural (subarachnoidean) space; 20- Spinal cord; 21- Internal vertebral plexus (veins).

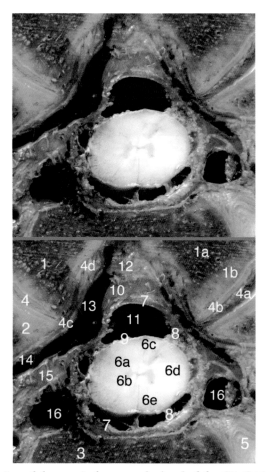

Fig. G.19 **Transverse section of the cervical area at the level of the C3–C4 intervertebral joint focused on the vertebral canal.**

C3- Third cervical vertebra, C4- Fourth cervical vertebra.

Bones and joints: 1- Caudal articular process of C3, 1a- spongious bone, 1b- subchondral bone; 2- Cranial articular process of C4; 3- Vertebral head (cranial extremity) of C4; 4- Articular process joint, 4a- joint space, 4b- articular cartilage, 4c- articular capsule, 4d- insertion (enthesis) of the articular capsule; 5- Intervertebral disc;

Nervous structures and associated structures: 6- Spinal cord, 6a- dorsal horn of the grey mater, 6b- ventral horn of the grey mater, 6c- dorsal funiculus of the white mater, 6d- lateral funiculus of the white mater, 6c- ventral funiculus of the white mater; 7- Dura mater; 8- Arachnoid; 9- Pia mater; 10- Epidural space; 11- Subdural (subarachnoidean) space; 12- Flavum (intervertebral) ligament; 13- Vertebral foramen (canal); 14- Intervertebral foramen; 15- Fourth cervical nerve; 16- Internal vertebral plexus (veins).

THE BACK (THORACOLUMBAR REGIONS)

H.1 PHYSICAL ASPECT

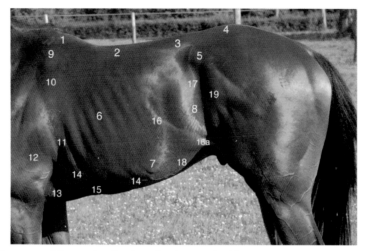

Fig. H.1 **Lateral aspect of the equine back and pelvis: palpable anatomical structures.**

1- Withers; 2- Thoracic area; 3- Lumbar area; 4- Point of the croup (tuber sacrale); 5- Angle of the croup (tuber coxae); 6- Thorax (the ribs can be seen on this fit horse); 7- Costal arch; 8- Abdomen; 9- Trapezius muscle (thoracic part); 10- Latissimus dorsi muscle; 11- Serratus ventralis thoracis muscle; 12- Triceps brachii muscle; 13- Pectoralis profundus (ascendens) muscle; 14- External thoracic vein; 15- Xyphoid area; 16- Cutaneous trunci muscle, 16a- caudal attachment on the thigh (stifle plica); 17- Flank (obliquus abdominis muscles); 18- Rectus abdominis muscle; 19- Cranial margin of the thigh (tensor fascia latae).

H.2 RADIOGRAPHIC ANATOMY

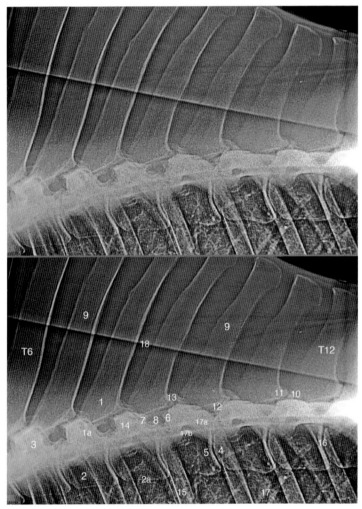

Fig. H.2 **Lateral radiographic view of the mid-thoracic area from the sixth thoracic vertebra (T6) to the twelfth thoracic vertebra (T12) from the left side. Cranial is to the left.**

1- Vertebral arch, 1a- vertebral pedicle; 2- Vertebral body, 2a- ventral crest; 3- Vertebral foramen (canal); 4- Vertebral head (cranial extremity); 5- Vertebral fossa (caudal extremity); 6- Cranial vertebral notch; 7- Caudal vertebral notch; 8- Intervertebral foramen; 9- Spinal process; 10- Cranial articular process; 11- Caudal articular process; 12- Articular process joint; 13- Mamillary process; 14- Transverse process (articulating with the corresponding rib); 15- Ninth rib; 16- Vertebral symphysis with a thin intervertebral disc; 17- Lungs, 17a and 17b- dorsal margin of the left and right lungs; 18- Border of the shadow of an aluminium filter used to compensate the thickness difference between the narrow dorsal midline and the epaxial muscles ventrally.

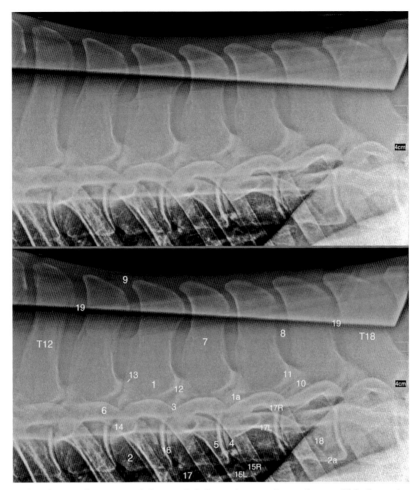

Fig. H.3 **Lateral radiographic view of the caudal thoracic area from the twelfth thoracic vertebra (T12) to the eighteenth thoracic vertebra (T18) from the left side. Cranial is to the left.**

1- Vertebral arch, 1a- vertebral pedicle; 2- Vertebral body, 2a- ventral crest; 3- Vertebral foramen (canal); 4- Vertebral head (cranial extremity); 5- Vertebral fossa (caudal extremity); 6- Intervertebral foramen; 7- Spinal process; 8- Interspinal space (syndesmosis); 9- Shadow of the supraspinal ligament; 10- Cranial articular process; 11- Caudal articular process; 12- Articular process joint; 13- Mamillary process; 14- Costal fovea (articulating with the corresponding rib); 15- Fifteenth ribs, 15L- left rib, 15R- right rib; 16- Vertebral symphysis with the intervertebral disc; 17- Lungs, 17L- dorsal margin of the left lung, 17R- dorsal margin of the right lung; 18- Shadow of the diaphragm and liver; 19- Border of the shadow of an aluminium filter used to compensate the thickness difference between the dorsal and ventral parts of the epaxial muscles.

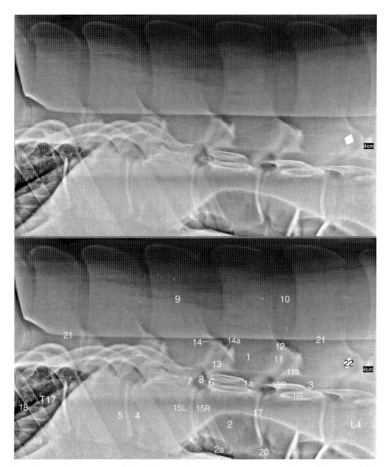

Fig. H.4 Lateral radiographic view of the thoracolumbar junction and lumbar area from the seventeenth thoracic vertebra (T17) to the fourth lumbar vertebra (L4) from the left side. Cranial is to the left.

1- Vertebral arch, 1a- vertebral pedicle; 2- Vertebral body, 2a- ventral crest; 3- Vertebral foramen (canal); 4- Vertebral head (cranial extremity); 5- Vertebral fossa (caudal extremity); 6- Cranial vertebral notch; 7- Caudal vertebral notch; 8- Intervertebral foramen; 9- Spinal process of the first lumbar vertebra; 10- Interspinal space (syndesmosis); 11- Cranial articular process, 11b- subchondral bone; 12- Caudal articular process; 13- Articular process joint; 14- Mamillary process, 14a-crest; 15- Eighteenth ribs, 15L- left rib, 15R- right rib; 16- Transverse processes of the second lumbar vertebra, 16L- left, 16R- right; 17- Vertebral symphysis with the intervertebral disc; 18- Lungs; 19- Shadow of the diaphragm and liver; 20- Base of the caecum; 21- Border of the shadow of an aluminium filter used to compensate the thickness difference between the dorsal and ventral parts of the epaxial muscles; 22- Radiopaque marker placed on the right tuber coxae.

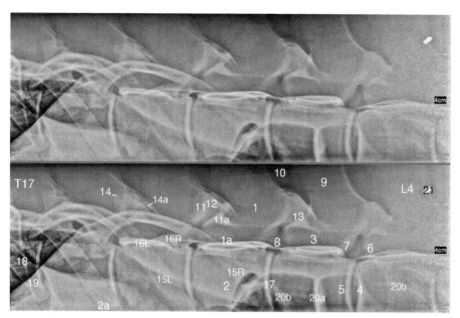

Fig. H.5 Lateral radiographic view of the thoracolumbar junction and lumbar area from the seventeenth thoracic vertebra (T17) to the fourth lumbar vertebra (L4) from the left side. The head of the fifth lumbar vertebra is imaged on the right. Cranial is to the left.

1- Vertebral arch, 1a- vertebral pedicle; 2- Vertebral body, 2a- ventral crest; 3- Vertebral foramen (canal); 4- Vertebral head (cranial extremity); 5- Vertebral fossa (caudal extremity); 6- Cranial vertebral notch; 7- Caudal vertebral notch; 8- Intervertebral foramen; 9- Spinal process of the third lumbar vertebra; 10- Interspinal space (syndesmosis); 11- Cranial articular process of the second lumbar vertebra, 11b- subchondral bone; 12- Caudal articular process of the first lumbar vertebra; 13- Articular process joint; 14- Mamillary process of the first lumbar vertebra, 14a-crest; 15- Eighteenth ribs, 15L- left rib, 15R- right rib; 16- Transverse processes of the first lumbar vertebra, 16L- left, 16R- right; 17- Vertebral symphysis with the intervertebral disc; 18- Lungs; 19- Shadow of the diaphragm and liver; 20- Base of the caecum, 20a- semilunar plica, 20b- haustra; 21- Radiopaque marker placed on the right tuber coxae.

H.3 DISSECTED SPECIMEN

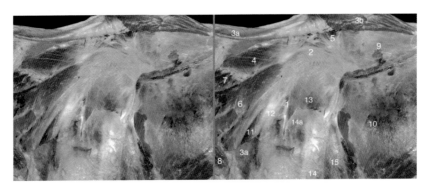

Fig. H.6 **Lateral aspect of the dissected withers: superficial and intermediate structures. Cranial is to the left.**

1- Spine of the scapula; 2- Cartilage of the scapula; 3- Trapezius muscle, 3a- cervical part, 3b- thoracic part; 4- Rhomboideus cervicalis muscle; 5- Rhomboideus thoracis muscle; 6- Serratus ventralis cervicis muscle; 7- Splenius muscle; 8- Omotransversarius muscle; 9- Thoracolumbar fascia covering the thoracic spinalis and longissimus muscles; 10- Latissimus dorsi muscle attaching to the thoracolumbar fascia; 11- Subclavius muscle; 12- Supraspinatus muscle; 13- Infraspinatus muscle; 14- Deltoideus muscle, 14a- aponeurosis covering the infraspinatus muscle; 15- Triceps brachii muscle (long head).

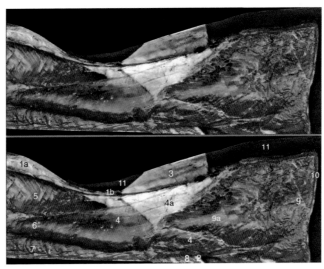

Fig. H.7 **Dorsolateral aspect of the dissected back (thoracolumbar region): superficial structures. Cranial is to the left.**

1- Supraspinal ligament, 1a- wide, thin and elastic in the withers, 1b- mid-thoracic part; 2- Left eighteenth rib; 3- Thoracolumbar fascia (reclined on the right side); 4- Erector spinae muscle, 4a- superficial aponeurosis; 5- Spinalis thoracis muscle; 6- Longissimus thoracis muscle; 7- Iliocostalis thoracis muscle; 8- Intercostal muscle; 9- Gluteus medius muscle, 9a- lumbar part; 10- Gluteal fascia; 11- Skin (on the right side).

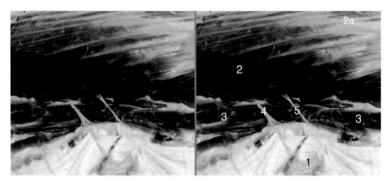

Fig. H.8 **Lateral aspect of the thoracolumbar junction: superficial structures. Cranial is to the left.**

1- Thoracolumbar fascia (reclined laterally and ventrally); 2- Erector spinae muscle, 2a- superficial aponeurosis; 3- Iliocostalis thoracis muscle; 4 and 5- Cutaneous branches of the lateral rami of the dorsal rami of the last thoracic nerves going through the thoracolumbar fascia to reach the skin.

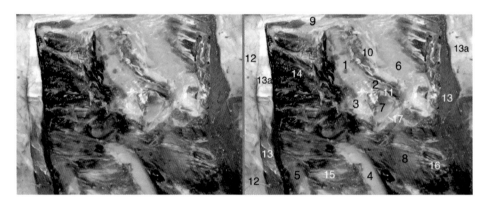

Fig. H.9 **Dorsolateral aspect of the thoracolumbar junction: deep structures. Cranial is to the left.**

1- Spinal process of the last (eighteenth) thoracic vertebra (T18); 2- Caudal articular process of T18; 3- Vertebral pedicle of T18; 4- Last (eighteenth) rib; 5- Seventeenth rib; 6- Spinal process of the first lumbar vertebra (L1); 7- Cranial articular process of L1; 8- Transverse process of L1; 9- Supraspinal ligament; 10- Thoracolumbar interspinal ligament; 11- Thoracolumbar articular process joint; 12- Thoracolumbar fascia; 13- Erector spinae muscle, 13a- superficial aponeurosis; 14- Multifidus muscle; 15- Intercostal muscles; 16- Intertransverse muscle and ligament; 17- Nerve ramus for the articular process joint.

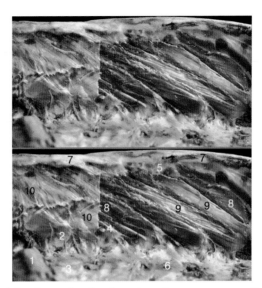

Fig. H.10 **Lateral aspect of the thoracolumbar junction: deep structures. Cranial is to the left.**

1- Left last (eighteenth) rib; 2- Articular process of the first lumbar vertebra (L1); 3- Transverse process of L1; 4- Mamillary process of the second lumbar vertebra; 5- Spinal process of the third lumbar vertebra (L3); 6- Transverse process of L3; 7- Supraspinal ligament; 8- Multifidus muscle fasciculi; 9- Multifidus aponeuroses; 10- Multifidus fascia.

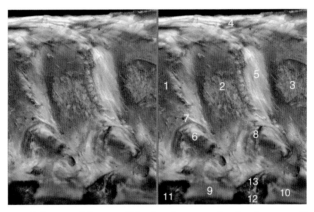

Fig. H.11 **Lateral aspect of the cranial part of the lumbar vertebral column: articular structures. Cranial is to the left.**

1- Spinal process of the first lumbar vertebra (L1); 2- Spinal process of the second lumbar vertebra (L2); 3- Spinal process of the third lumbar vertebra (L3); 4- Supraspinal ligament; 5- Interspinal ligament; 6- Cranial articular process of L2; 7- Caudal articular process of L1; 8- Articular process joint; 9- Transverse process of L2; 10- Transverse process of L3; 11- Vertebral body of L1; 12- Second lumbar intervertebral disc; 13- Intervertebral foramen.

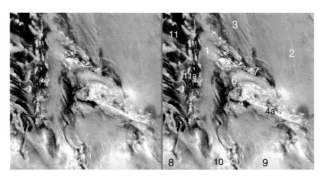

Fig. H.12 **Lateral aspect of the cranial part of the lumbar vertebral column: articular structures. Cranial is to the left.**

1- Spinal process of the first lumbar vertebra (L1); 2- Spinal process of the second lumbar vertebra (L2); 3- Interspinal ligament; 4- Cranial articular process of L2, 4a- crest; 5- Caudal articular process of L1; 6- Joint capsule of the articular process joint; 7- Flavum (interarcual) ligament; 8- Transverse process of L1; 9- Transverse process of L2; 10- Intertransverse ligament; 11- Multifidus muscle, 11a- section plane.

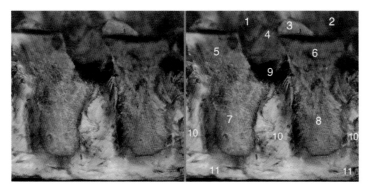

Fig. H.13 **Ventrolateral aspect of the cranial part of the lumbar vertebral column: articular structures. Cranial is to the left.**

1- Spinal process of the first lumbar vertebra (L1); 2- Spinal process of the second lumbar vertebra (L2); 3- Cranial articular process of L2; 4- Caudal articular process of L1; 5- Transverse process of L1; 6- Transverse process of L2; 7- Vertebral body of L1; 8- Vertebral body of L2; 9- Intervertebral foramen for the first lumbar artery, vein and nerve; 10- Intervertebral discs; 11- Ventral longitudinal ligament.

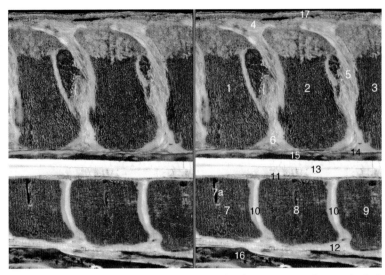

Fig. H.14 **Median section of the thoracolumbar vertebral column. Cranial is to the left.**

1- Spinal process of the seventeenth thoracic vertebra (T17); 2- Spinal process of the eighteenth thoracic vertebra (T18); 3- Spinal process of the first lumbar vertebra (L1); 4- Supraspinal ligament; 5- Interspinal ligament; 6- Flavum (interarcual) ligament; 7- Vertebral body of T17; 8- Vertebral body of T18; 9- Vertebral body of L1; 10- Intervertebral discs; 11- Dorsal longitudinal ligament; 12- Ventral longitudinal ligament; 13- Spinal cord; 14- Dura mater in the vertebral canal; 15- Subdural (subarachnoidean) space; 16- Aorta; 17- Skin.

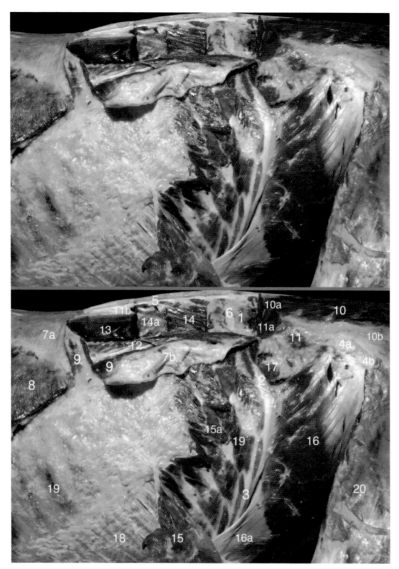

Fig. H.15 Dorsolateral aspect of the dissected back (thoracolumbar region) and abdominal wall: superficial structures. Cranial is to the left.

1- Spinal process of the first lumbar vertebra; 2- Last (eighteenth) rib; 3- Costal arch; 4- Tuber coxae, 4a- cranial part; 4b- caudal part; 5- Supraspinal ligament; 6- Interspinal ligament; 7-Thoracolumbar fascia, 7a- connected to the latissimus dorsi muscle, 7b- connected to the serratus dorsalis caudalis muscle; 8- Latissimus dorsi muscle; 9- Serratus dorsalis caudalis muscle; 10- Gluteus medius muscle, 10a- lumbar part, 10b- gluteal fascia; 11- Erector spinae muscle, 11a- section plane, 11b- superficial aponeurosis; 12- Iliocostalis thoracis muscle; 13- Longissimus thoracis muscle; 14- Multifidus muscle, 14a- multifidus fascia; 15- Obliquus externus abdominis muscle, 15a- section plane; 16- Obliquus internus abdominis muscle, 16a- aponeurosis; 17- Retractor costae muscle; 18- Tunica flava abdominis; 19- Intercostal muscles; 20- Tensor fascia latae muscle.

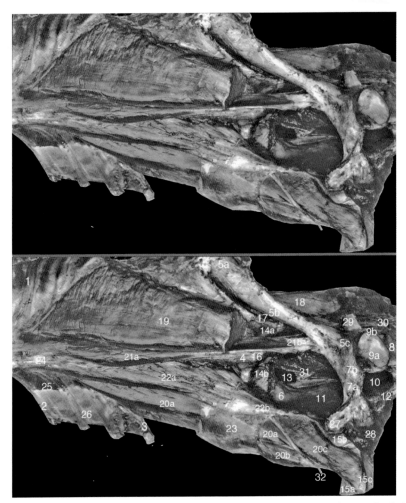

Fig. H.16 **Ventrolateral aspect of the roof of the abdomen and pelvis. Cranial is to the left.**

1- Left fifteenth rib; 2- Right fifteenth rib; 3- Right eighteenth rib; 4- Sixth lumbar vertebra (body); 5- Left ilium, 5a- tuber coxae, 5b- neck, 5c- body; 6- Right ilium neck; 7- Left pubis, 7a- cranial branch, 7b- body; 8- Left ischium; 9- Left acetabulum, 9a- lunar surface, 9b- margin; 10- Left obturator foramen; 11- Right acetabular area (medial aspect); 12- Pelvic symphysis; 13- Right major ischiatic foramen; 14- Transverse processes of the first sacral vertebra (sacral wing), 14a- left one, 14b- right one; 15- Right femur, 15a- body, 15b- head (in the right acetabulum), 15c- lesser trochanter; 16- Lumbosacral disc (L6 disc); 17- Left sacroiliac joint; 18- Membranous part of the left dorsal sacroiliac ligament; 19- Left major psoas muscle (cut); 20- Right iliopsoas muscle, 20a- major psoas muscle, 20b- iliac muscle (lateral part), 20c- iliac muscle (medial part); 21- Left minor psoas muscle, 21a- muscle body, 20b- tendon inserted on the tuberculum of the minor psoas of the ilium neck; 22- Right minor psoas muscle, 22a- muscle body, 22b- tendon; 23- Iliac fascia; 24- Ventral longitudinal ligament covering the lumbar vertebral bodies; 25- Intercostal muscle; 26- Intercostal nerve; 27- Prepubic tendon (insertion of the rectus abdominis on the pubis); 28- Obturator externus muscle; 29- Proximal tendon of the rectus femoris muscle; 30- Left sciatic nerve; 31- Right sciatic nerve; 32- Right femoral nerve.

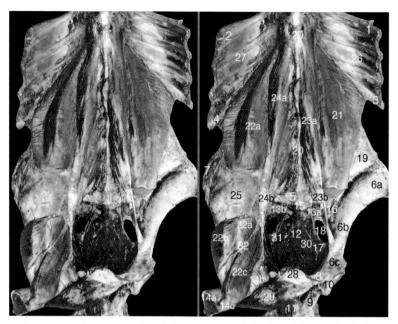

Fig. H.17 **Ventral aspect of the roof of the abdomen and pelvis. Cranial is to the left.**

1- Left fifteenth rib; 2- Right fifteenth rib; 3- Left eighteenth rib; 4- Right eighteenth rib; 5- Sixth lumbar vertebra (body); 6- Left ilium, 6a- tuber coxae, 6b- neck, 6c- body; 7- Right tuber coxae; 8- Left pubis (body); 9- Left ischium; 10- Left acetabulum; 11- Pelvic symphysis; 12- Sacrum; 13- First sacral vertebra (sacral wings), 13a- left transverse process, 13b- right transverse process; 14- Right femur, 14a- body, 14b- head (in the right acetabulum*), 14c- lesser trochanter; 15- Lumbosacral disc (L6 disc); 16- Left sacroiliac joint; 17- Left sacrosciatic ligament; 18- Major ischiatic foramen; 19- Iliocostal ligament; 20- Ventral longitudinal ligament covering the lumbar vertebral bodies; 21- Left major psoas muscle (cut); 22- Right iliopsoas muscle, 22a- major psoas muscle, 22b- iliac muscle (lateral part), 22c- iliac muscle (medial part); 23- Left minor psoas muscle, 23a- muscle body, 23b- tendon inserted on the tuberculum of the minor psoas of the ilium neck; 24- Right minor psoas muscle, 24a- muscle body, 24b- tendon; 25- Iliac fascia; 26-Intercostal muscle; 27- Intercostal nerve; 28- Prepubic tendon (insertion of the rectus abdominis on the pubis); 29- Obturator externus muscle; 30- Left sciatic nerve; 31- Right sciatic nerve; 32- Right femoral nerve.

H.4 CROSS-SECTIONS

H.4.1 Median and paramedian sections

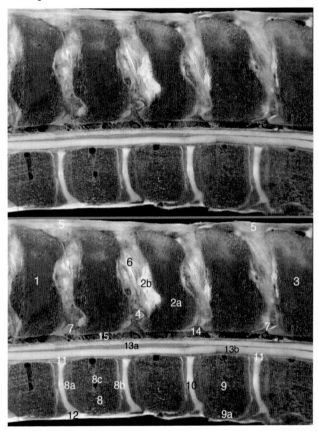

Fig. H.18 Median section of the thoracolumbar vertebral column from the fifteenth thoracic vertebra to the first lumbar vertebra. Cranial is to the left.

1- Spinal process of the fifteenth thoracic vertebra; 2- Spinal process of the seventeenth thoracic vertebra, 2a- spongy bone, 2b- compact bone; 3- Spinal process of the first lumbar vertebra; 4- Caudal articular process of the sixteenth thoracic vertebra (T16); 5- Supraspinal ligament; 6- Interspinal ligament; 7- Flavum (interarcual) ligament; 8- Vertebral body of T16, 8a- vertebral head, 8b- vertebral fossa, 8c- basivertebral vein; 9- Vertebral body of the eighteenth thoracic vertebra, 9a- ventral crest; 10- Intervertebral disc; 11- Dorsal longitudinal ligament; 12- Ventral longitudinal ligament; 13- Spinal cord, 13a- grey matter, 13b- white matter; 14- Dura mater in the vertebral canal; 15- Subdural (subarachnoidean) space.

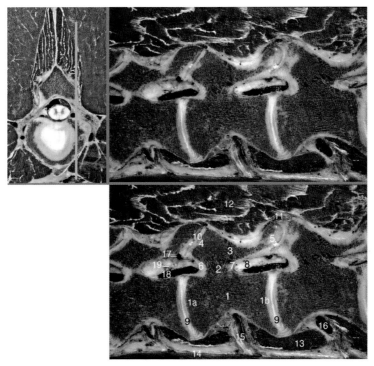

Fig. H.19 Paramedian section of the thoracolumbar area. Cranial is to the left.

1- Vertebral body of the seventeenth thoracic vertebra (T17), 1a- head, 1b- compact bone of the vertebral fossa; 2- Pedicle of T17; 3- Arch of T17; 4- Cranial articular process; 5- Caudal articular process; 6- Cranial vertebral notch; 7- Caudal vertebral notch; 8- Intervertebral foramen; 9- Intervertebral discs; 10- Articular process joint; 11- Joint capsule of the articular process joint; 12- Multifidus muscle; 13- Psoas minor muscle; 14- Aorta; 15- Dorsal intercostal artery; 16- Dorsal intercostal vein; 17- Spinal ramus (of the dorsal ramus of the dorsal intercostal artery); 18- Intervertebral vein; 19- Radices of the intervertebral thoracic nerve (in fat).

H.4.2 Transverse sections

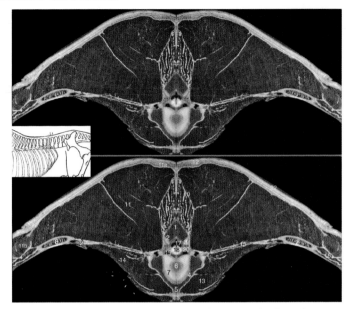

Fig. H.20 Transverse section of the thoracolumbar area between the last thoracic vertebra and the first lumbar vertebra.

1- Vertebral arch of the eighteenth thoracic vertebra (T18); 2- Caudal articular process of T18; 3- Articular process joint between T18 and the first lumbar vertebra (L1); 4- Vertebral fossa of T18; 5- Ventral crest of T18; 6- Vertebral head of L1; 7- Intervertebral disc between T18 and L1; 8- Eighteenth (last) rib; 9- Multifidus muscle; 10- Multifidus fascia; 11- Erector spinae muscle, 11a- aponeurosis, 11b- iliocostalis lumborum muscle; 12- Thoracolumbar fascia; 13- Psoas minor muscle; 14- Psoas major muscle; 15- Costotransverse muscle; 16- Intercostal muscles; 17- Vertebral canal; 18- Spinal cord; 19- Internal vertebral plexus; 20- Intervertebral foramen; 21- Dorsal costoabdominal artery, vein and nerve; 22- Skin.

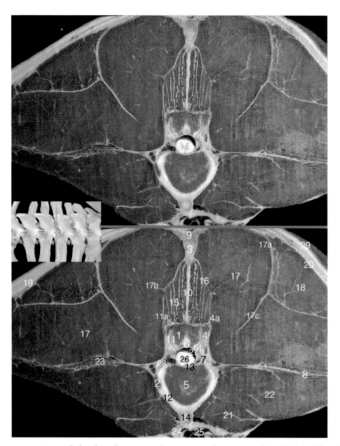

Fig. H.21 **Transverse section of the lumbar area between the second and third lumbar vertebrae.**

1- Caudal articular process of the second lumbar vertebra (L2); 2- Vertebral fossa of L2; 3- Spinal process of the third lumbar vertebra (L3); 4- Cranial articular process of L3, 4a- mamillary process; 5- Vertebral head of L3; 6- Vertebral canal; 7- Intervertebral foramen; 8- Transverse process of L3; 9- Supraspinal ligament; 10- Interspinal ligament; 11- Articular process joint between L2 and L3, 11a- articular capsule; 12- Intervertebral disc; 13- Dorsal longitudinal ligament; 14- Ventral longitudinal ligament; 15- Multifidus muscle; 16- Multifidus fascia; 17- Erector spinae muscle, 17a- superficial aponeurosis, 17b and 17c- intramuscular aponeuroses; 18- Gluteus medius muscle; 19- Thoracolumbar fascia; 20- Gluteal fascia; 21- Psoas minor muscle; 22- Psoas major muscle; 23- Intertransverse ligament and muscle; 24- Tendon (crus) of the diaphragm; 25- Aorta; 26- Spinal cord; 27- Dura mater and subdural (subarachnoidean) space; 28- Lumbar vein (ramus spinals) and nerve (in the intervertebral foramen); 29- Skin.

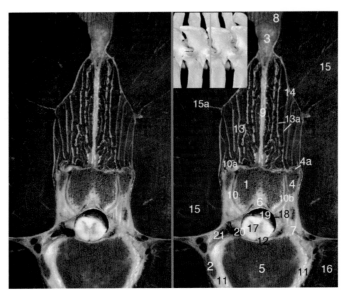

Fig. H.22 **Transverse section of the lumbar area between the second and third lumbar vertebrae.**

1- Caudal articular process of the second lumbar vertebra (L2); 2- Vertebral fossa of L2; 3- Spinal process of the third lumbar vertebra (L3); 4- Cranial articular process of L3, 4a- mamillary process; 5- Vertebral head of L3; 6- Vertebral canal and epidural fat; 7- Intervertebral foramen; 8- Supraspinal ligament; 9- Interspinal ligament; 10- Articular process joint between L2 and L3, 10a- articular capsule; 11- Intervertebral disc; 12- Dorsal longitudinal ligament; 13- Multifidus muscle, 13a- fascicular aponeuroses; 14- Multifidus fascia; 15- Erector spinae muscle, 15a- intramuscular aponeurosis; 16- Psoas major muscle; 17- Spinal cord; 18- Dura mater; 19- Subdural (subarachnoidean) space; 20- Internal vertebral (venous) plexus; 21- Lumbar vein (ramus spinals) and nerve (in the intervertebral foramen).

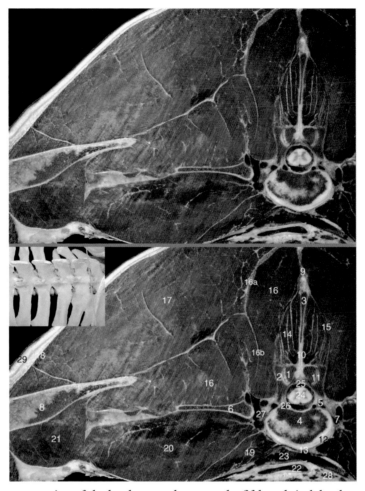

Fig. H.23 Transverse section of the lumbar area between the fifth and sixth lumbar vertebrae.

1- Caudal articular process of the fifth lumbar vertebra (L5); 2- Cranial articular process of the sixth lumbar vertebra (L6); 3- Spinal process of L6; 4- Vertebral head of L6; 5- Intervertebral foramen; 6- Transverse process of L6; 7- Intertransverse foramen; 8- Ilium; 9- Supraspinal ligament; 10- Interspinal ligament; 11- Articular process joint between L5 and L6; 12- Intervertebral disc; 13- Ventral longitudinal ligament; 14- Multifidus muscle; 15- Multifidus fascia; 16- Erector spinae muscle, 16a- superficial aponeurosis, 16b- intramuscular aponeurosis; 17- Gluteus medius muscle; 18- Gluteal fascia; 19- Psoas minor muscle; 20- Psoas major muscle; 21- Iliac muscle (lateral part); 22- Aorta (collapsed); 23- Caudal vena cava (collapsed); 24- Spinal cord; 25- Dura mater separating the epidural space and the subdural (subarachnoidean) space; 26- Internal vertebral (venous) plexus; 27- Lumbar artery, vein and nerve (in the intertransverse foramen); 28- Medial iliac lymph nodes; 29- Skin.

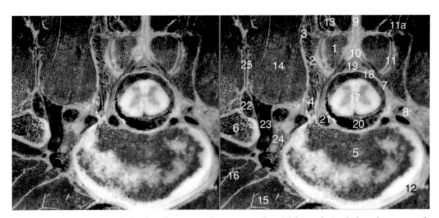

Fig. H.24 **Transverse section of the lumbar area between the fifth and sixth lumbar vertebrae.**

1- Caudal articular process of the fifth lumbar vertebra (L5); 2- Cranial articular process of the sixth lumbar vertebra (L6); 3- Mamillary process; 4- Vertebral pedicle of L6; 5- Vertebral head of L6; 6- Transverse process of L6; 7- Vertebral canal; 8- Intervertebral foramen; 9- Interspinal ligament; 10- Flavum ligament in the interarcual space; 11- Articular process joint between L5 and L6, 11a- articular capsule; 12- Fifth lumbar intervertebral disc; 13- Multifidus muscle; 14- Erector spinae muscle, 15- Psoas minor muscle; 16- Psoas major muscle; 17- Spinal cord; 18- Dura mater; 19- Epidural space and fat; 20- Subdural (subarachnoidean) space; 21- Internal vertebral (venous) plexus; 22- Lumbar artery; 23- Lumbar vein (in the intertransverse foramen); 24- Ventral ramus of the fifth lumbar nerve (contributing to the femoral, obturator and sciatic nerves); 25- Dorsal ramus of the fifth lumbar nerve.

CHAPTER I

THE PELVIS

I.1 PHYSICAL ASPECT

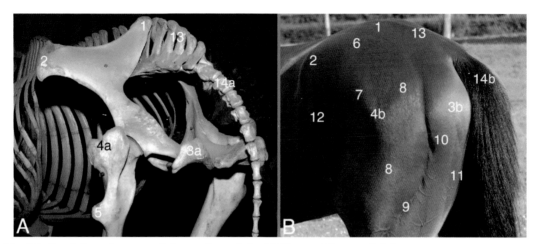

Fig. I.1 **Caudolateral aspect of the equine pelvis. (A) Bones; (B) superficial aspect.**

1- Sacral tuber; 2- Tuber coxae; 3a- Tuber ischiadicum, 3b- point of the croup; 4a- Greater trochanter, 4b- Hip; 5- Third trochanter; 6- Gluteus medius muscle; 7- Gluteus superficialis muscle; 8- Gluteofemoralis muscle; 9- Biceps femoris muscle; 10- Semitendinosus muscle; 11- Semimembranosus muscle; 12- Tensor fascia latae muscle; 13- Sacrum (median sacral crest); 14a- Caudal vertebrae, 14b- Tail.

I.2 BONES

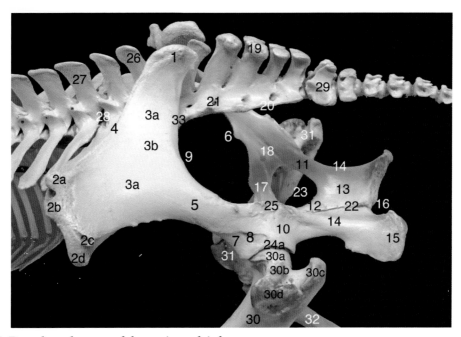

Fig. I.2 **Dorsolateral aspect of the equine pelvic bones.**

Ilium: 1- Sacral tuber; 2- Tuber coxae, 2a- dorsocranial cuspid, 2b- ventrocranial cuspid, 2c- dorsocaudal cuspid, 2d-ventrocaudal cuspid; 3- Ilium wing, 3a- gluteal face, 3b- accessory gluteal line; 4- Ilium crest, 5- Ilium neck; 6- Psoas minor muscle tubercle; 7- Ilium body; 8- Lateral rectus femoris muscle area; 9- Major sciatic incisura;

Ischium: 10- Ischium body; 11- Lateral (acetabular) ramus; 12- Medial ramus; 13- Ischium table; 14- Minor sciatic incisura; 15- Tuber ischiadicum (ischiatic tuberosity); 16- Ischiatic arch;

Pubis: 17- Cranial ramus; 18- Obturator sulcus;

Sacrum: 19- Median sacral crest (five spinal processes); 20- Lateral sacral crest (fused transverse processes); 21- Dorsal sacral foramen;

Pelvis and connected bones: 22- Pelvic symphysis; 23- Obturator foramen; 24- Acetabulum, 24a- Acetabular margin; 25- Ischiatic spine (sciatic crest); 26- Spinal process of the sixth lumbar vertebra; 27- Fourth lumbar vertebra; 28- Intervertebral foramen; 29- First caudal vertebra; 30- Left femur, 30a- head, 30b- neck, 30c- major trochanter (caudal part); 30d- major trochanter (cranial part); 31- Right femur; 32- Right tibia; 33- Sacroiliac joint.

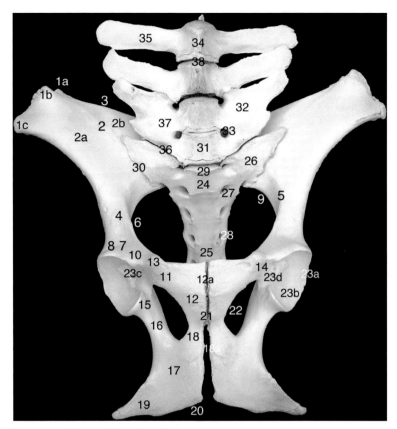

Fig. I.3 **Ventral aspect of the equine pelvic bones.**

Ilium: 1- Tuber coxae, 1a- dorsocranial cuspid, 1b- ventrocranial cuspid, 1c- ventrocaudal cuspid; 2- Ilium wing, 2a- iliac face, 2b- sacropelvic face (insertion of the interosseous sacroiliac ligament); 3- Ilium crest; 4- Ilium neck; 5- Arch line; 6- Psoas minor muscle tubercle; 7- Ilium body; 8- Medial rectus femoris muscle area; 9- Major sciatic incisura;

Pubis: 10- Pubis body; 11- Cranial ramus; 12- Caudal ramus, 12a- symphysial face; 13- Pubis pecten; 14- Accessory ligament sulcus;

Ischium: 15- Ischium body; 16- Lateral (acetabular) ramus; 17- Ischium table; 18- Medial ramus, 18a- symphysial face; 19- Tuber ischiadicum (ischiatic tuberosity); 20- Ischiatic arch;

Pelvis: 21- Pelvic symphysis; 22- Obturator foramen; 23- Acetabulum, 23a- acetabular margin, 23b- lunar surface, 23c- acetabular fossa, 23d- acetabular notch;

Sacrum: 24- First sacral vertebra; 25- Fourth sacral vertebra; 26- Sacral wing; 27- First ventral (intervertebral) sacral foramen; 28- Third ventral (intervertebral) sacral foramen; 29- Promontory; 30- Sacroiliac joint;

Lumbar spine: 31- Sixth lumbar vertebra (L6); 32- Transverse process of the fifth lumbar vertebra (L5, fused with L6); 33- Lumbar ventral intervertebral foramen; 34- Third lumbar vertebra (L3, ventral crest); 35- Transverse process of L3; 36- Intertransverse lumbosacral joint; 37- Intertransverse synostosis between L5 and L6; 38- Intervertebral symphysis between L3 and L4.

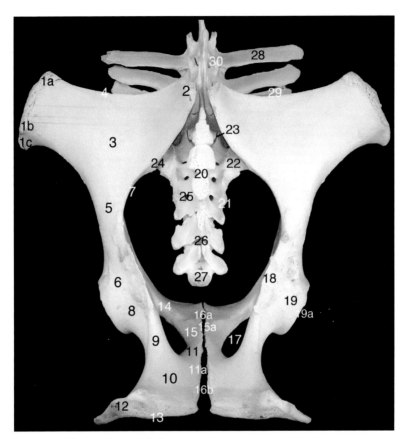

Fig. I.4 **Dorsal aspect of the equine pelvic bones.**

Ilium: 1- Tuber coxae, 1a- dorsocranial cuspid, 1b- dorsocaudal cuspid, 1c- ventrocaudal cuspid; 2- Sacral tuber; 3- Ilium wing; 4- Ilium crest; 5- Ilium neck; 6- Ilium body; 7- Major sciatic incisura;

Ischium: 8- Ischium body; 9- Lateral (acetabular) ramus; 10- Ischium table; 11- Medial ramus, 11a- symphysial face; 12- Tuber ischiadicum (ischiatic tuberosity); 13- Ischiatic arch;

Pubis: 14- Cranial ramus; 15- Caudal ramus, 15a- symphysial face;

Pelvis: 16- Pelvic symphysis, 16a- cranial (pubic part), 16b- caudal (ischiatic) part; 17- Obturator foramen; 18- Ischiatic spine (sciatic crest); 19- Acetabulum, 19a- acetabular margin;

Sacrum: 20- Median sacral crest; 21- Lateral sacral crest; 22- Transverse process of the first sacral vertebra (sacral wing); 23- Right lumbosacral articular process joint; 24- Sacroiliac joint; 25- Third dorsal (intervertebral) sacral foramen; 26- Sacral canal (caudal opening); 27- First caudal vertebra (vertebral body);

Lumbar spine: 28- Transverse process of the third lumbar vertebra (L3); 29- Transverse process of the fifth lumbar vertebra (L5); 30- Right articular process joint between L3 and L4.

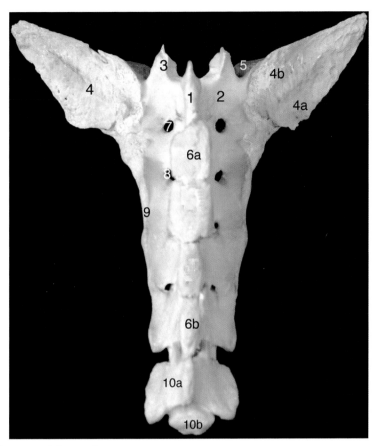

Fig. I.5 **Dorsal aspect of the equine sacrum.**

1- Spinal process of the first sacral vertebra (S1); 2- Vertebral arch of S1; 3- Left cranial articular process of S1; 4- Transverse process of the first sacral vertebra (sacral wing), 4a- auricular surface (contributing to the sacroiliac joint), 4b- insertion surface of the interosseous sacroiliac ligament; 5- Articular surface of the intertransverse lumbosacral joint seen through the cranial intervertebral incisura; 6- Median sacral crest, 6a- spinal process of the second sacral vertebra, 6b- spinal process of the fifth sacral vertebra; 7- First dorsal (intervertebral) sacral foramen; 8- Second dorsal (intervertebral) sacral foramen; 9- Lateral sacral crest; 10- First caudal vertebra, 10a- vertebral arch, 10b- vertebral body.

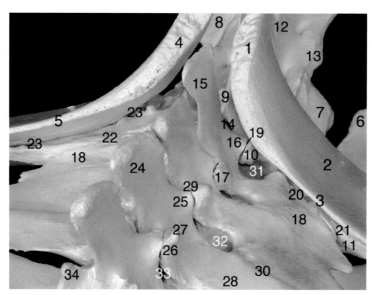

Fig. I.6 **Craniolaterodorsal aspect of the lumbosacroiliac area.**

Coxal bones: 1- Sacral tuber of the left ilium; 2- Ilium wing of the left ilium; 3- Ilium crest of the left ilium; 4- Sacral tuber of the right ilium; 5- Ilium crest of the right ilium; 6- Left ischium (angle between ilium arch and pelvic symphysis); 7- Right ischium (angle between ilium arch and pelvic symphysis); 8- Right tuber ischiadicum;

Sacrum: 9- Spinal process of the first sacral vertebra (S1); 10- (Cranial) articular process of S1; 11- Left transverse process of S1 (sacral wing); 12- Median sacral crest; 13- Lateral sacral crest; 14- Interarcual space between the last lumbar vertebra (L6) and S1;

Lumbar vertebrae and sacroiliac joints: 15- Spinal process of L6; 16- Caudal articular process of L6; 17- Cranial articular process of L6; 18- Transverse process of L6 (fused with the transverse process of the fifth lumbar vertebra (L5)); 19- Left lumbosacral articular process joint; 20- Left lumbosacral intertransverse joint; 21- Left sacroiliac joint; 22- Right lumbosacral intertransverse joint; 23- Right sacroiliac joint; 24- Spinal process of the fourth lumbar vertebra (L4); 25- Caudal articular process of L4; 26- Cranial articular process of L4; 27- Mammillary process; 28- Transverse process of L4; 29- Left articular process joint between L3 and L4; 30- Left intertransverse joint between L4 and L5; 31- Dorsal lumbosacral intertransverse foramen; 32- Dorsal intertransverse foramen between L4 and L5; 33- Left intervertebral foramen between L3 and L4; 34- Right cranial articular process of the third lumbar vertebra.

I.3 DISSECTED SPECIMEN

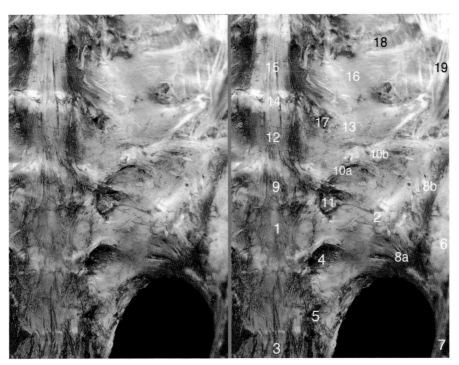

Fig. I.7 **Ventral aspect of the roof of the pelvis: bones and ligaments.**

1- Body of the first sacral vertebra (S1); 2- Transverse process of S1 (sacral wing); 3- Body of the third sacral vertebra (S3); 4- First ventral (intervertebral) sacral foramen; 5- Second ventral (intervertebral) sacral foramen; 6- Ilium wing; 7- Ilium neck; 8- Sacroiliac joint covered by the ventral sacroiliac ligament, 8a- caudomedial part, 8b- craniolateral part (covered by the iliopsoas muscle); 9- Lumbosacral intervertebral disc (sixth lumbar (L6) disc); 10- Lumbosacral intertransverse joint, 10a- joint space, 10b- lumbosacral intertransverse ligament; 11- Ventral ramus of the sixth lumbar nerve; 12- Body of the sixth lumbar vertebra (L6); 13- Transverse process of L6 (fused with L5 transverse process); 14- Fifth lumbar intervertebral disc; 15- Body of the fifth lumbar vertebra (L5); 16- Transverse process of L5 (fused with L6 transverse process); 17- Ventral intertransverse foramen between L5 and L6; 18- Intertransverse ligament; 19- Iliolumbar ligament.

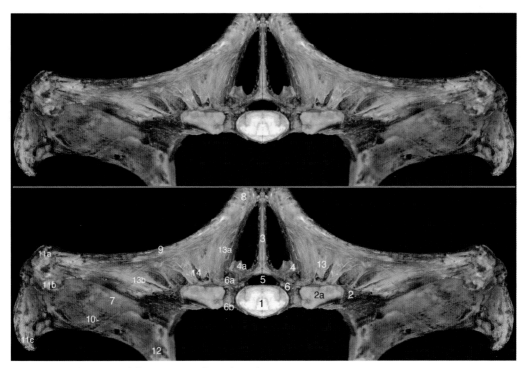

Fig. I.8 **Cranial aspect of the equine pelvis: dorsal part.**

1- Vertebral body of the first sacral vertebra (S1); 2- Transverse process of S1 (sacral wing), 2a- articular surface of the intertransverse lumbosacral joint; 3- Spinal process of S1; 4- Left (cranial) articular process of S1, 4a- articular surface of the right articular process of S1; 5- Sacral (vertebral) canal; 6- Lumbosacral intervertebral foramen, 6a- dorsal opening (dorsal intertransverse foramen), 6b- ventral opening (ventral intertransverse foramen); 7- Iliac wing; 8- Right sacral tuber; 9- Right iliac crest; 10- Iliac face; 11- Right tuber coxae, 11a- dorsocranial cuspid, 11b- ventrocranial cuspid, 11c- ventrocaudal cuspid; 12- Right ilium neck; 13- Interosseous sacro-iliac ligament, 13a- caudomedial part, 13b- craniolateral part; 14- Sacroiliac fat.

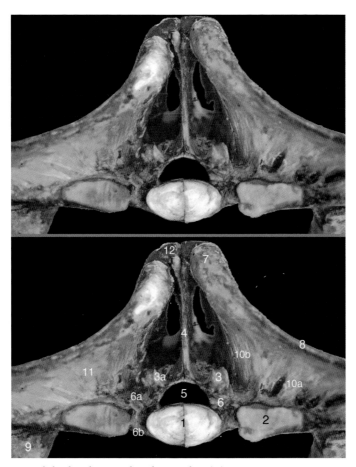

Fig. I.9 **Cranial aspect of the lumbosacral and sacroiliac joints.**

1- Vertebral body of the first sacral vertebra (S1); 2- Articular surface of the intertransverse lumbosacral joint; 3- Left cranial articular process of S1, 3a- articular surface of the right articular process of S1; 4- Spinal process of S1; 5- Sacral (vertebral) canal; 6- Lumbosacral intervertebral foramen, 6a- dorsal opening (dorsal intertransverse foramen), 6b- ventral opening (ventral intertransverse foramen); 7- Left sacral tuber; 8- Left iliac crest; 9- Right ilium neck; 10- Interosseous sacroiliac ligament, 10a- craniolateral part, 10b- caudomedial part; 11- Sacroiliac fat; 12- Gluteus muscle fibers.

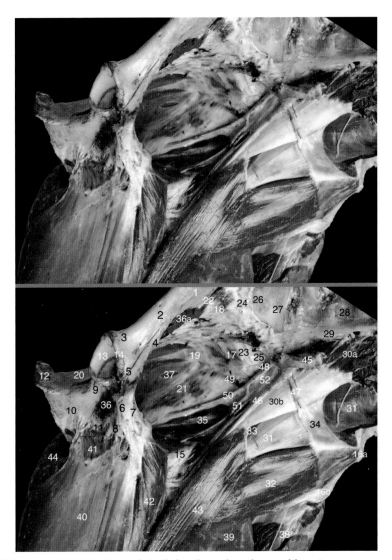

Fig. I.10 **Medial aspect of the equine pelvis (left side with right coxal bone).**

Right coxal bone: 1- Ilium wing; 2- Ilium neck; 3- Ilium body; 4- Psoas minor muscle tubercle; 5- Pubis body; 6- Cranial ramus of the pubis; 7- Pubis pecten; 8- Caudal ramus of the right pubis; 9- Ischium body; 10- Ischium table; 11- Medial ramus of the right ischium; 12- Tuber ischiadicum (ischiatic tuberosity); 13- Right acetabulum (lunar surface); 14- Acetabular labrum;

Left coxal bone: 15- Cranial ramus of the left pubis; 16- Left tuber coxae, 16a- ventrocranial cuspid, 16b- ventrocaudal cuspid;

Sacrum, lumbar spine and joints: 17- First sacral vertebra; 18- Right sacral wing; 19- Third sacral vertebra; 20- Right sacrosciatic ligament; 21- Left sacrosciatic ligament; 22- Right sacroiliac joint; 23- Lumbosacral (L6) intervertebral disc and promontorium; 24- Right intertransverse lumbosacral joint; 25- Sixth lumbar vertebra (L6); 26- Transverse process of L6 fused with the transverse process of the fifth lumbar vertebra (L5); 27- Transverse process of L5; 28- Third lumbar vertebra (L3); 29- Ventral longitudinal ligament;

Muscles: 30- Psoas minor muscle, 30a- muscle body, 30b- tendon; 31- Psoas major muscle; 32- Iliac muscle, lateral part; 33- Iliac muscle, medial part; 34- Iliac fascia; 35- Left obturator internus muscle (iliac part); 36- Right obturator internus muscle, 36a- iliac part; 37- Gluteus medius muscle (seen through the sacrosciatic ligament); 38- Tensor fascia latae muscle; 39- Quadriceps femoris muscle; 40- Gracilis muscle; 41- Median aponeurosis between the left and right gracilis muscles; 42- Pectineus muscle; 43- Sartorius muscle; 44- Semimembranosus muscle;

Vessels: 45- Aorta; 46- External iliac artery; 47- Deep circumflex iliac artery; 48- Internal iliac artery; 49- Caudal gluteal artery and vein; 50- Cranial gluteal artery and vein (medial rami); 51- Obturator artery and vein; 52- Common iliac vein.

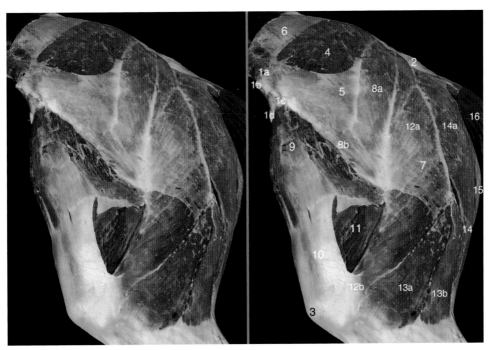

Fig. I.11 **Lateral aspect of the pelvis: superficial structures. Cranial is to the left.**

1- Tuber coxae, 1a- dorsocranial cuspid, 1b- ventrocranial cuspid, 1c- dorsocaudal cuspid, 1d- ventrocaudal cuspid; 2- Median sacral crest (spinal processes of the sacrum); 3- Patella; 4- Gluteus medius muscle; 5- Gluteal fascia; 6- Thoracolumbar fascia; 7- Femoral fascia; 8- Gluteus superficialis muscle, 8a- proximal (sacral) part, 8b- distal (iliac) part; 9- Tensor fascia latae muscle; 10- Fascia latae; 11- Quadriceps femoris muscle (vastus lateralis); 12- Gluteofemoralis muscle, 12a- sacral part, 12b- distal tendon inserting on the patella; 13- Biceps femoris muscle, 13a- cranial head, 13b- caudal head; 14- Semitendinosus muscle, 14a- supraischiatic part; 15- Semimembranosus muscle; 16- Tail.

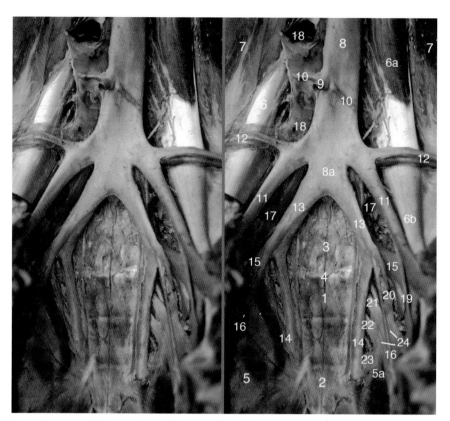

Fig. I.12 **Ventral aspect of the equine pelvis: vessels and nerves.**

1- First sacral vertebra (S1); 2- Third sacral vertebra; 3- Sixth lumbar vertebra (L6); 4- Lumbosacral (L6) intervertebral disc and promontorium; 5- Right sacrosciatic ligament; 6- Psoas minor muscle, 6a- muscle body, 6b- tendon; 7- Psoas major muscle; 8- Aorta, 8b- quadrifurcation; 9- Caudal mesenteric artery; 10- Renal arteries; 11- External iliac artery; 12- Deep circumflex iliac artery and vein; 13- Internal iliac artery; 14- Caudal gluteal artery and vein; 15- Cranial gluteal artery; 16- Obturator artery; 17- Common iliac vein; 18- Caudal vena cava; 19- Obturator nerve; 20- Ventral ramus of the sixth lumbar nerve; 21- Ventral ramus of the first sacral nerve; 22- Ventral ramus of the second sacral nerve; 23- Ventral ramus of the third sacral nerve; 24- Lumbosacral truncus, origin of the sciatic nerve.

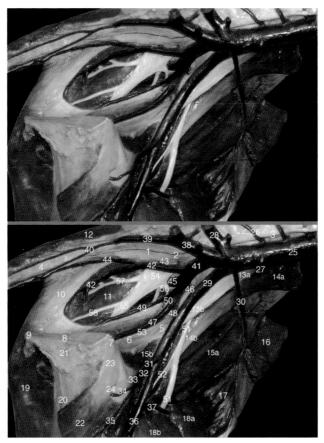

Fig. I.13 **Medial aspect of the equine pelvis: vessels and nerves – Courtesy of the Fragonard Museum, Ecole Nationale Vétérinaire d'Alfort; Anatomical plaster specimen made by E. Petitcolin (c. 1900).**

1- Sacrum; 2- Lumbosacral intervertebral disc and promontorium; 3- Ventral longitudinal ligament and lumbar spine; 4- Caudal vertebrae; 5- Left ilium neck; 6- Acetabular area; 7- Pubis pecten; 8- Pelvic symphysis; 9- Ischiatic arch; 10- Left sacrosciatic ligament (cut); 11- Gluteus medius muscle; 12- Caudal muscles; 13- Psoas minor muscle, 13a- muscle body, 13b- tendon; 14- Psoas major muscle, 14a- muscle body, 14b- tendon; 15- Iliac muscle, 15a- lateral part, 15b- medial part; 16- Obliquus internus abdominis muscle; 17- Tensor fascia latae muscle; 18- Quadriceps femoris muscle, 18a- rectus femoris muscle, 18b- vastus medialis muscle; 19- Semimembranosus muscle; 20- Gracilis muscle; 21- Median aponeurosis; 22- Rectus abdominis muscle; 23- Prepubic tendon; 24- Internal inguinal ring; 25- Aorta; 26- Lumbar artery; 27- Caudal mesenteric artery; 28- Right external iliac artery; 29- Left external iliac artery; 30- Deep circumflex iliac artery; 31- Deep femoral artery; 32- Medial femoral circumflex artery; 33- Pudendoepigastric trunk; 34- Internal pudendal artery; 35- Caudal epigastric artery; 36- Femoral artery; 37- Lateral femoral circumflex artery; 38- Right internal iliac artery; 39- Right caudal gluteal artery; 40- Caudal arteries; 41- Left internal iliac artery; 42- Left caudal gluteal artery; 43- Sacral artery; 44- Caudal arteries; 45- Cranial gluteal artery; 46- Iliolumbar artery; 47- Obturator artery; 48- Iliacofemoral artery; 49- Internal pudendal artery; 50- Umbilical artery; 51- Femoral nerve; 52- Saphenous nerve (origin); 53- Obturator nerve; 54- Lumbosacral trunk; 55- Sciatic nerve; 56- Cranial gluteal nerve; 57- Caudal gluteal nerve; 58- Caudal femoral cutaneous nerve.

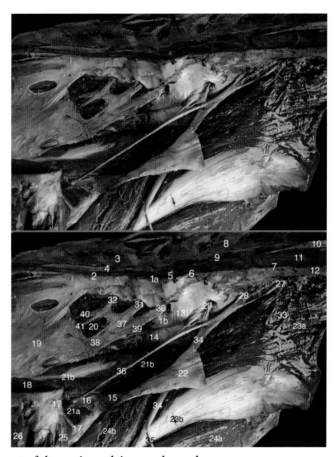

Fig. I.14 **Medial aspect of the equine pelvis: muscles and nerves.**

1- First sacral vertebra, 1a- body, 1b- transverse process (sacral wing); 2- Body of the third sacral vertebra; 3- Spinal process of the second sacral vertebra; 4- Sacral canal and cauda equina; 5- Lumbosacral intervertebral disc and promontorium; 6- Body of the sixth lumbar vertebra; 7- Body of the fourth lumbar vertebra; 8- Spinal process of the fifth lumbar vertebra; 9- Vertebral canal; 10- Spinal cord in the vertebral canal; 11- Intervertebral disc between the third and fourth lumbar vertebrae; 12- Ventral longitudinal ligament; 13- Left lumbosacral intertransverse joint; 14- Left sacroiliac joint; 15- Ilium neck (tubercle of the psoas minor muscle); 16- Acetabular area; 17- Pubis; 18- Pelvic symphysis (cut); 19- Left sacrosciatic ligament; 20- Gluteus medius muscle; 21- Obturator internus muscle, 21a- muscle body, 21b- iliac part; 22- Psoas minor muscle (tendon); 23- Psoas major muscle, 23a- muscle body, 23b- tendon; 24- Iliac muscle, 24a- lateral part, 24b- medial part; 25- Pectineus muscle; 26- Gracilis muscle; 27- Ventral ramus of the third lumbar nerve; 28- Ventral ramus of the fourth lumbar nerve; 29- Ventral ramus of the fifth lumbar nerve; 30- Ventral ramus of the sixth lumbar nerve; 31- Ventral ramus of the first sacral nerve; 32- Ventral ramus of the second sacral nerve; 33- Muscle ramus of the ventral ramus of the third lumbar nerve; 34- Femoral nerve; 35- Saphenous nerve (displaced cranially); 36- Obturator nerve; 37- Lumbosacral trunk; 38- Sciatic nerve; 39- Cranial gluteal nerve; 40- Caudal gluteal nerve; 41- Caudal femoral cutaneous nerve.

I.4 CROSS-SECTIONS

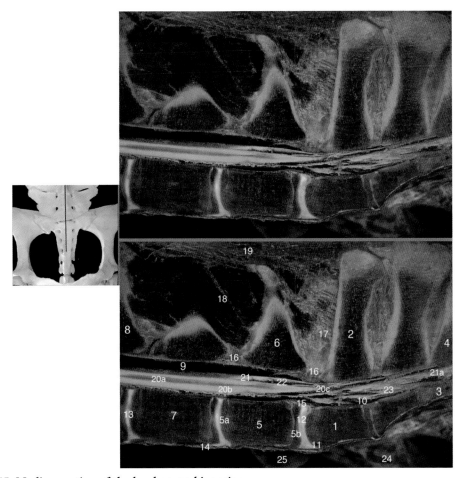

Fig. I.15 **Median section of the lumbosacral junction.**

1- Body of the first sacral vertebra; 2- Spinal process of the first sacral vertebra; 3- Body of the third sacral vertebra; 4- Spinal process of the third sacral vertebra; 5- Body of the sixth lumbar vertebra (L6), 5a- vertebral head (with growing cartilage), 5b- vertebral fossa (with growing cartilage); 6- Spinal process of L6; 7- Body of the fifth lumbar vertebra; 8- Spinal process of the fourth lumbar vertebra; 9- Vertebral canal (lumbar part); 10- Sacral canal; 11- Promontorium; 12- Sixth (lumbosacral) intervertebral disc; 13- Fourth lumbar intervertebral disc; 14- Ventral longitudinal ligament; 15- Dorsal longitudinal ligament; 16- Flavum (interarcual) ligament; 17- Interspinal ligament; 18- Multifidus muscle; 19- Erector spinae muscle; 20- Spinal cord, 20a- grey matter; 20b- white matter, 20c- filum terminale; 21- Dura matter, 21a- filum of the spinal dura matter; 22- Subdural (subarachnoidean) space; 23- Cauda equina; 24- Right ilium neck; 25- Right tuber coxae (ventral cuspids).

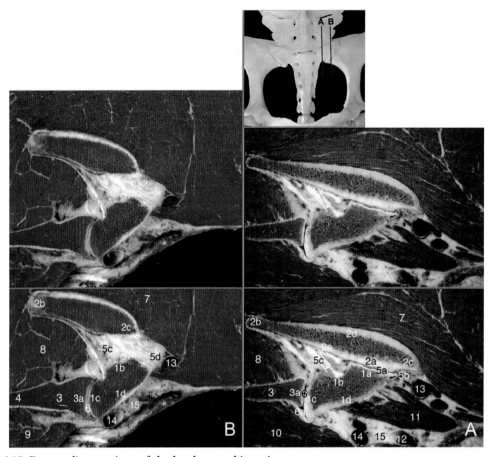

Fig. I.16 **Paramedian sections of the lumbosacral junction.**

1- Transverse process of the first sacral vertebra (sacral wing), 1a- auricular surface, 1b- dorsal surface (insertion of the interosseous sacroiliac ligament), 1c- articular surface of the lumbosacral intertransverse joint, 1d- ventral surface; 2- Iliac wing, 2a- auricular surface; 2b- iliac crest, 2c- caudal border, 2d- gluteal face and compact bone, 2e- sacropelvic face and compact bone; 3- Transverse process of the sixth lumbar vertebra (L6), 3a- articular surface of the lumbosacral intertransverse joint; 4- Transverse process of the fifth lumbar vertebra (fused with L6); 5- Sacroiliac joint, 5a- joint space, 5b- ventral sacroiliac ligament, 5c- interosseous sacroiliac ligament, 5d- junction between the ventral and interosseous sacroiliac ligaments; 6- Lumbosacral intertransverse joint, 6a- ventral lumbosacral intertransverse ligament; 7- Gluteus medius muscle; 8- Erector spinae muscle; 9- Psoas major muscle (lateral part); 10- Psoas major muscle (medial part); 11- Obturator internus muscle (sacroiliac part); 12- Obturator artery; 13- Cranial gluteal artery and veins; 14- Iliolumbar artery and vein; 15- Fat.

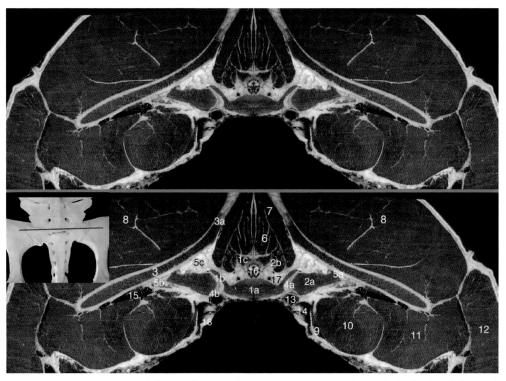

Fig. I.17 **Transverse section of the lumbosacroiliac junction passing through the body of the sixth lumbar vertebra (L6).**

1- Sixth lumbar vertebra (L6), 1a- body, 1b- transverse process, 1c- caudal articular process; 2- First sacral vertebra (S1), 2a- transverse process, 2b- cranial articular process; 3- Iliac wing, 3a- base of the sacral tuber; 4- Lumbosacral intertransverse joint, 4a- joint space, 4b- ventral lumbosacral intertransverse ligament; 5- Sacroiliac joint, 5a- joint space, 5b- ventral sacroiliac ligament, 5c- interosseous sacroiliac ligament; 6- Multifidus muscle; 7- Dorsolateral sacrocaudal muscle; 8- Gluteus medius muscle; 9- Psoas minor muscle and tendon; 10- Psoas major muscle; 11- Lateral part of the iliac muscle; 12- Tensor fascia latae muscle; 13- Internal iliac artery; 14- Common iliac vein; 15- Iliolumbar artery and vein; 16- Sacral canal with end of the spinal cord, dural cone and origin of the cauda equina; 17- Dorsal ramus of the sixth lumbar nerve; 18- Ventral ramus of the fifth lumbar nerve.

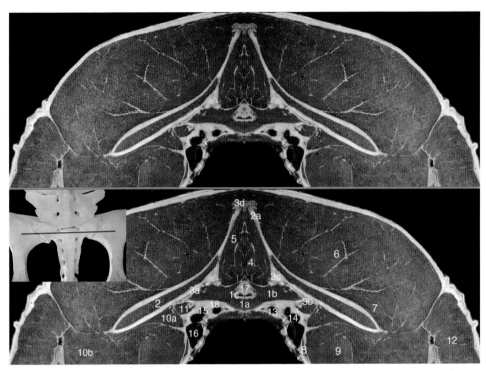

Fig. I.18 Transverse section of the lumbosacroiliac junction passing through the body of the first sacral vertebra (S1).

1- First sacral vertebra (S1), 1a- vertebral body, 1b-transverse process (sacral wing), 1c- sacral canal; 2- Iliac wing, 2a- sacral tuber; 3- Sacroiliac joint, 3a- joint space, 3b- ventral sacroiliac ligament, 3c- interosseous sacroiliac ligament, 3d- dorsal sacroiliac ligament; 4- Multifidus muscle; 5- Dorsolateral sacrocaudal muscle; 6- Gluteus medius muscle; 7- Gluteus accessorius muscle; 8- Psoas minor muscle and tendon; 9- Psoas major muscle; 10- Iliac muscle, 10a- medial part, 10b- lateral part; 11- Obturator internus muscle (sacroiliac part); 12- Tensor fascia latae muscle; 13- Caudal gluteal artery; 14- Cranial gluteal artery; 15- Branch coming from the ventral ramus of the fifth lumbar nerve; 16- Common iliac vein; 17- Origin of the cauda equina; 18- Ventral ramus of the sixth lumbar nerve.

THE HIP AND THIGH

J.1 PHYSICAL ASPECT

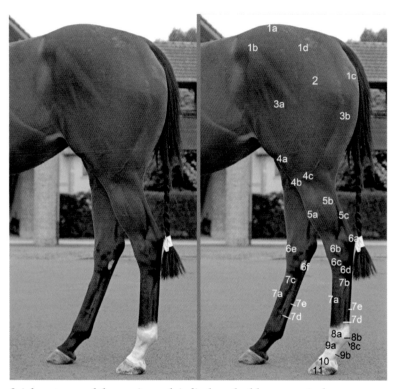

Fig. J.1 Superficial anatomy of the equine pelvic limb: palpable anatomical structures.

1- Croup (pelvis), 1a- croup angle (sacral tuber), 1b- hip angle (tuber coxae), 1c- point of the croup (tuber ischiadicum), 1d- gluteal muscles; 2- Hip (coxofemoral joint); 3- Thigh (femoral region), 3a- cranial femoral muscles, 3b- caudal femoral muscles; 4- Stifle (femorotibiopatellar joint), 4a- patella, 4b- tibial tuberosity, 4c- head of the fibula; 5- Crus (tibial area), 5a- cranial tibial muscles, 5b- caudal tibial muscles, 5c- common calcanean tendon; 6- Hock (tarsus), 6a- point of the hock, 6b- lateral malleolus (distal end of the fibula), 6c- lateral trochlear ridge of the talus, 6d- head of the fourth metatarsal bone, 6e- medial malleolus (tibia), 6f- chestnut; 7- Metatarsus, 7a- cannon bone (third metatarsal bone), 7b- fourth metatarsal bone, 7c- second metatarsal bone, 7d- suspensory ligament (third interosseous muscle), 7e- digital flexor tendons; 8- Fetlock, 8a- lateral collateral ligament, 8b- base of the proximal sesamoid bone, 8c- ergot; 9- Pastern, 9a- extensor branch of the suspensory ligament, 9b- digital flexor tendons; 10- Coronet, 11- Foot.

J.2 SUPERFICIAL STRUCTURES

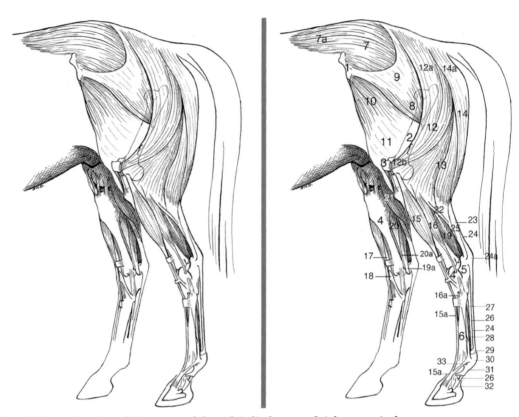

Fig. J.2 **Lateral and medial aspects of the pelvic limb: superficial anatomical structures.**

1- Tuber coxae; 2- Femur; 3- Patella; 4- Talus; 5- Calcaneus; 6- Third metatarsal bone; 7- Gluteus medius, 7a- lumbar part; 8- Gluteus superficialis; 9- Gluteal fascia; 10- Tensor fascia latae muscle; 11- Lata fascia; 12- Gluteofemoralis muscle, 12a- Supraischiatic part, 12b- Tendon inserting on the patella; 13- Biceps femoris (with two heads); 14- Semitendinosus muscle, 14a- Supraischiatic part; 15- Long digital extensor muscle, 15a- distal tendon; 16- Lateral digital extensor muscle, 16a- tendon; 17- Peroneus tertius muscle; 18- Tibialis cranialis muscle (tendon); 19- Lateral digital flexor muscle, 19a- tendon; 20- Medial digital flexor muscle, 20a- tendon; 21- Gastrocnemius muscle (medial head); 22- Soleus muscle; 23- Gastrocnemius tendon; 24- Superficial digital flexor tendon, 24a- calcanean cap; 25- Common calcanean tendon; 26- Deep digital flexor tendon; 27- Accessory ligament of the deep digital flexor tendon; 28- Third interosseous muscle (suspensory ligament); 29- Manica flexoria; 30- Plantar annular ligament; 31- Proximal digital annular ligament; 32- Distal digital annular ligament; 33- Extensor branch of the third interosseous muscle.

J.3 THE HIP (COXOFEMORAL REGION) AND THIGH

J.3.1 Physical aspect

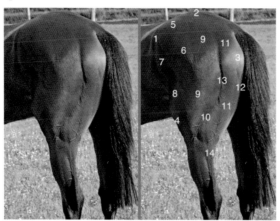

Fig. J.3 **Caudolateral aspect of the proximal pelvic limb: superficial anatomical structures.**

1- Tuber coxae; 2- Sacral tuber; 3- Point of the croup (tuber ischiadicum); 4- Patella; 5- Gluteus medius; 6- Gluteus superficialis; 7- Tensor fascia latae muscle; 8- Quadriceps femoris; 9- Gluteofemoralis muscle; 10- Biceps femoris (with two heads); 11- Semitendinosus muscle; 12- Semimembranosus muscle; 13- Intermuscular sulcus; 14- Origin of the common calcanean tendon.

J.3.2 Radiographic anatomy

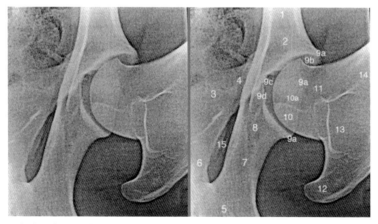

Fig. J.4 **Distomedial radiographic view of the coxofemoral joint (horse lying under general anesthesia).**

1- Ilium neck; 2- Ilium body; 3- Pubis; 4- Cranial ramus of the pubis; 5- Ischium table; 6- (Medial) ramus of the ischium; 7- Lateral (acetabular) ramus of the ischium; 8- Body of the ischium; 9- Acetabulum, 9a- acetabular margin, 9b- lunar surface, 9c- acetabular fossa, 9d- incisura (ventral); 10- Femoral head, 10a- fovea capitis; 11- Femoral neck; 12- Major trochanter (top); 13- Trochanteric fossa; 14- Body of the femur; 15- Obturator foramen.

J.3.3 Dissected specimen

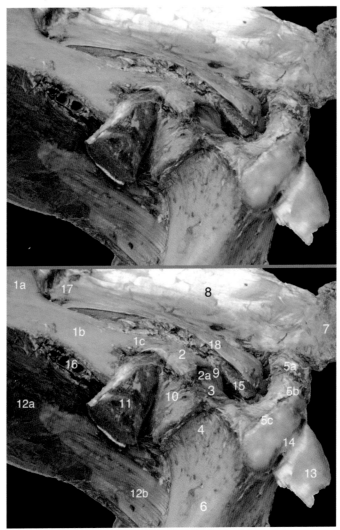

Fig. J.5 **Lateral aspect of the coxofemoral joint: deep structures.**

1- Ilium, 1a- wing, 1b- neck, 1c-body; 2- Acetabulum, 2a- lunar surface; 3- Femoral head; 4- Femoral neck; 5- Major trochanter, 5a- caudal part (top), 5b- trochanteric notch, 5c- cranial part (convexity); 6- Body of the femur; 7- Ischium; 8- Sacrosciatic ligament; 9- Acetabular labrum; 10- Articular capsule of the coxofemoral joint; 11- Rectus femoris muscle (sagittal head of the quadriceps femoris muscle); 12- Iliacus muscle (lateral part), 12a- tendon; 13- Tendon of the gluteus accessorius muscle; 14- Trochanteric bursa (opened); 15- Obturator internus muscle; 16- Iliacofemoral artery and vein; 17- Lumbosacral truncus; 18- Sciatic nerve.

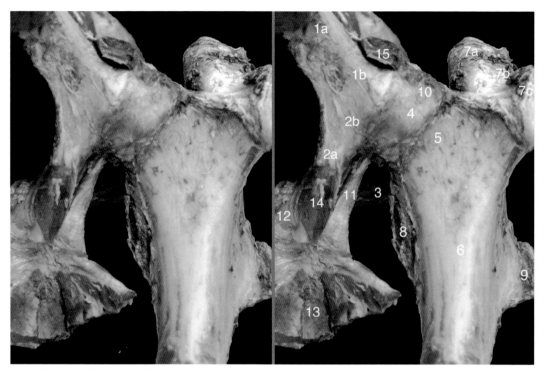

Fig. J.6 **Cranial aspect of the coxofemoral joint: deep structures.**

1- Ilium, 1a- neck, 1b-body; 2- Pubis, 2a- cranial ramus, 2b- body; 3- Ischium (partly covered by the obturator externus muscle; 4- Femoral head (covered by the articular capsule of the coxofemoral joint); 5- Femoral neck; 6- Body of the femur; 7- Greater trochanter, 7a- caudal part (top), 7b- trochanteric notch, 7c- cranial part (convexity); 8- Lesser trochanter; 9- Third trochanter; 10- Articular capsule of the coxofemoral joint; 11- Accessory ligament; 12- Prepubic tendon; 13- Rectus abdominis muscle; 14- Pectineus muscle; 15- Rectus femoris (sagittal head of the quadriceps femoris): proximal insertion (cut).

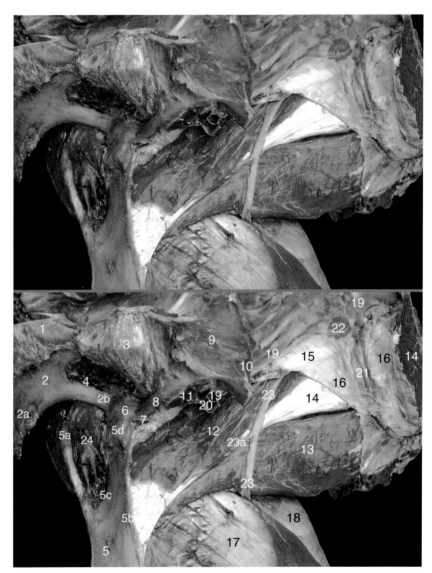

Fig. J.7 **Distomedial aspect of the coxofemoral joint.**

1- Right ischium; 2- Left ischium, 2a- tuber ischiadicum, 2b- lateral (acetabular) ramus; 3- Pelvic symphysis; 4- Obturator foramen; 5- Femur, 5a- greater trochanter, 5b- lesser trochanter, 5c- trochanteric fossa, 5d- femoral head covered by the articular capsule of the coxofemoral joint; 6- Articular capsule of the coxofemoral joint; 7- Transverse ligament of the acetabulum; 8- Accessory ligament of the femur; 9- Prepubic tendon; 10- Rectus abdominis muscle (cut); 11- Pectineus muscle (cut); 12- Iliac muscle (medial part); 13- Iliac muscle (lateral part); 14- Psoas major muscle; 15- Psoas minor muscle; 16- Iliac fascia; 17- Medial head of the quadriceps femoris muscle; 18- Rectus femoris muscle (sagittal head of the quadriceps femoris muscle); 19- External iliac artery; 20- External iliac vein; 21- Deep circumflex iliac artery; 22- Medial iliac lymph nodes; 23- Femoral nerve, 23a- ramus for the iliopsoas muscle; 24- Obturator internus and gemelli muscles.

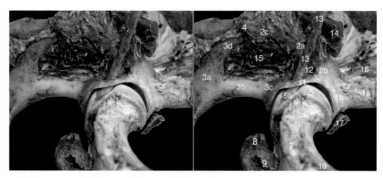

Fig. J.8 **Distomedial aspect of the coxofemoral joint: deep structures.**

1- Left ilium, 1a- neck, 1b- body; 2- Left pubis, 2a- cranial ramus, 2b- body, 2c- caudal ramus; 3- Left ischium, 3a- tuber ischiadicum, 3b- lateral (acetabular) ramus, 3c- body, 3d- (medial) ramus; 4- Pelvic symphysis; 5- Femoral head, 5a- fovea capitis; 6- Femoral neck; 7- Lesser trochanter; 8- Greater trochanter; 9- Trochanteric fossa; 10- Body of the femur; 11- Transverse ligament of the acetabulum; 12- Capitis ligament (of the femur); 13- Accessory ligament (of the femur); 14- Pectineus muscle; 15- Obturator muscles in the obturator foramen; 16- Sacroiliac part of the obturator internus muscle; 17- Rectus femoris muscle (sagittal head of the quadriceps femoris muscle), proximal insertion (cut).

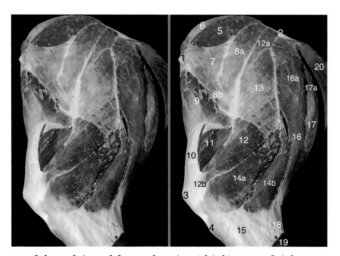

Fig. J.9 **Lateral aspect of the pelvis and femoral region (thigh): superficial structures. Cranial is to the left.**

1- Tuber coxae; 2- Median sacral crest (spinous processes of the sacrum); 3- Patella; 4- Tibial tuberosity; 5- Gluteus medius muscle; 6- Thoracolumbar fascia; 7- Gluteal fascia; 8- Gluteus superficialis muscle, 8a- proximal (sacral) part, 8b- distal part; 9- Tensor fascia latae muscle; 10- Lata fascia; 11- Vastus lateralis of the quadriceps femoris muscle; 12- Gluteofemoralis muscle, 12a- sacral part, 12b- distal tendon inserting on the patella; 13- Femoral fascia; 14- Biceps femoris muscle, 14a- cranial head, 14b- caudal head; 15- Crural fascia; 16- Semitendinosus muscle, 16a- supraischiatic part; 17- Semimembranosus muscle, 17a- supraischiatic part; 18- Common calcanean tendon; 19- Skin; 20- Tail.

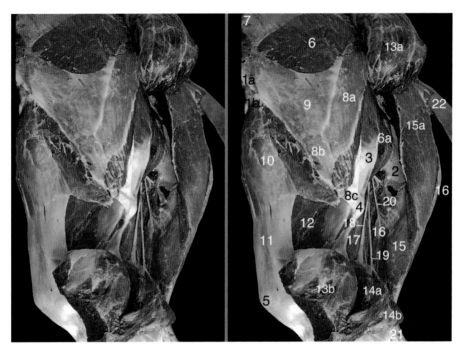

Fig. J.10 **Lateral aspect of the pelvis and femoral region (thigh): intermediate structures. Cranial is to the left.**

1- Tuber coxae, 1a- cranial cuspids, 1b- caudal cuspids; 2- Ischium; 3- Greater trochanter of the femur; 4- Third trochanter of the femur; 5- Patella; 6- Gluteus medius muscle, 6a- post-trochanteric part; 7- Thoracolumbar fascia; 8- Gluteus superficialis muscle, 8a- proximal (sacral) part, 8b- distal part, 8c- tendon; 9- Gluteal fascia; 10- Tensor fascia latae muscle; 11- Fascia lata; 12- Vastus lateralis of the quadriceps femoris muscle; 13- Gluteofemoralis muscle (cut), 13a- proximal part (reclined), 13b- distal part (reclined); 14- Biceps femoris muscle (cut and reclined), 14a- cranial head, 14b- caudal head; 15- Semitendinosus muscle, 15a- supraischiatic part; 16- Semimembranosus muscle; 17- Adductor magnus muscle; 18- Tibial nerve; 19- Common fibular nerve; 20- Muscle rami (for the caudal femoral and deep pelvic muscles) of the sciatic nerve; 21- Common calcanean tendon; 22- Tail.

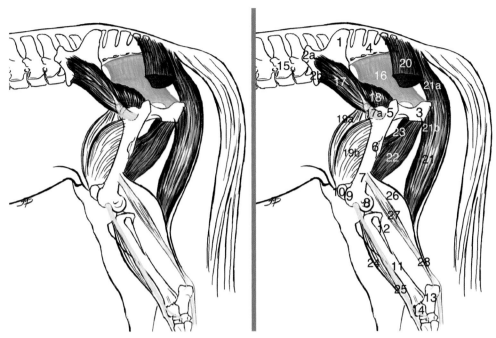

Fig. J.11 Lateral aspect of the pelvis and femoral region (thigh): deep structures. Cranial is to the left.

1- Sacral tuber; 2- Tuber coxae, 2a- cranial cuspids, 2b- caudal cuspids; 3- Ischium; 4- Sacrum; 5- Greater trochanter of the femur; 6- Third trochanter of the femur; 7- Supracondylar fossa of the femur; 8- Femoral condyles; 9- Femoral trochlea; 10- Patella; 11- Tibia; 12- Fibula; 13- Calcaneus; 14- Talus; 15- Fourth lumbar vertebra; 16- Sacrosciatic ligament; 17- Gluteus accessorius muscle, 17a- tendon; 18- Gluteus profundus muscle; 19- Quadriceps femoris muscle, 19a- rectus femoris muscle, 19b- vastus lateralis muscle; 20- Gluteofemoralis muscle (proximal part, cut); 21- Semitendinosus muscle, 21a- supraischiatic part, 21b- ischiatic origin; 22- Adductor magnus muscle; 23- Quadratus femoris muscle; 24- Tibialis cranialis muscle; 25- Peroneus tertius muscle; 26- Gastrocnemius muscle (profile); 27- Superficial digital flexor muscle; 28- Common calcanean tendon.

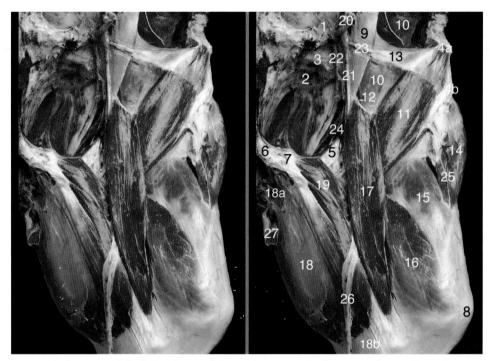

Fig. J.12 **Medial aspect of the left pelvis and femoral region (thigh). Cranial is to the right.**

1- Fifth lumbar vertebra; 2- Second sacral vertebra; 3- Lumbosacral intervertebral disc; 4- Tuber coxae, 4a- cranial cupids, 4b- caudal cupids; 5- Ilium (body); 6- Right pubis; 7- Pelvic symphysis; 8- Patella; 9- Psoas minor muscle; 10- Psoas major muscle; 11- Iliac muscle (lateral part); 12- Iliac muscle (medial part); 13- Iliac fascia; 14- Tensor fascia latae muscle; 15- Quadriceps femoris muscle (rectus femoris muscle); 16- Quadriceps femoris muscle (vastus medialis muscle); 17- Sartorius muscle; 18- Gracilis muscle; 19- Pectineus muscle; 20- Aorta; 21- External iliac artery; 22- Internal iliac artery; 23- Deep circumflex iliac artery; 24- Obturator nerve; 25- Lateral cutaneous femoral nerve; 26- Saphenous artery, vein and nerve; 27- Penis (cut).

J.3.4 Cross-sections

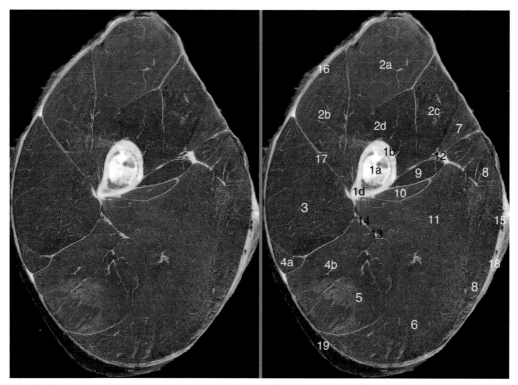

Fig. J.13 **Transverse section of the femoral area (thigh). Cranial is to the top, lateral is to the left.**

1- Femur, 1a- medullary cavity, 1b- cortex, 1c- base of the third trochanter; 2- Quadriceps femoris muscle, 2a- rectus femoris muscle, 2b- vastus lateralis muscle, 2c- vastus medialis muscle, 2d- vastus intermedius muscle; 3- Gluteofemoralis muscle; 4- Biceps femoris muscle, 4a- cranial head, 4b- caudal head; 5- Semitendinosus muscle; 6- Semimembranosus muscle; 7- Sartorius muscle; 8- Gracilis muscle; 9- Pectineus muscle; 10- Adductor brevis muscle; 11- Adductor magnus muscle; 12- Femoral artery and vein; 13- Tibial nerve; 14- Common fibular nerve; 15- Saphenous vein and nerve; 16- Lata fascia; 17- Lateral femoral septum; 18- Femoral fascia; 19- Skin.

THE STIFLE

K.1 PHYSICAL ASPECT

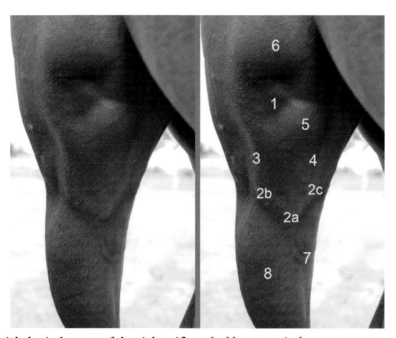

Fig. K.1 **Cranial physical aspect of the right stifle: palpable anatomical structures.**

1- Patella; 2- Tibial tuberosity, 2a- distal part, 2b- lateral branch, 2c- medial branch; 3- Lateral patellar ligament over the lateral ridge of the femoral trochlea; 4- Medial patellar ligament; 5- Tuberculum of the femoral trochlea; 6- Quadriceps femoris muscle; 7- Tibia; 8- Cranial crural muscles.

K.2 BONE AND RADIOGRAPHIC ANATOMY

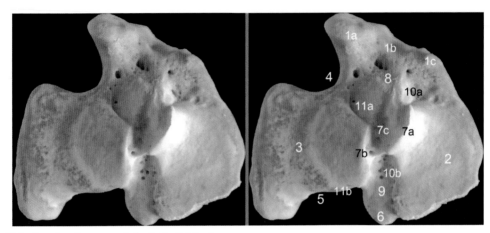

Fig. K.2 **Proximal aspect of the left tibial plateau.**

1- Tibial tuberosity, 1a- lateral branch, 1b- sulcus, 1c- medial branch; 2- Medial tibial condyle; 3- Lateral tibial condyle; 4- Extensor sulcus; 5- Popliteal notch; 6- Tubercle of the caudal cruciate ligament; 7- Intercondylar eminence (tibial spine), 7a- medial intercondylar tubercle, 7b- lateral intercondylar tubercle, 7c- central intercondylar area (insertion of the cranial cruciate ligament); 8- Cranial intercondylar area; 9- Caudal intercondylar area; 10- Insertion surfaces for the medial meniscus, 10a- craniomedial meniscotibial ligament, 10b- caudomedial meniscotibial ligament; 11- Insertion surfaces for the lateral meniscus, 11a- craniolateral meniscotibial ligament, 11b- caudolateral meniscotibial ligament.

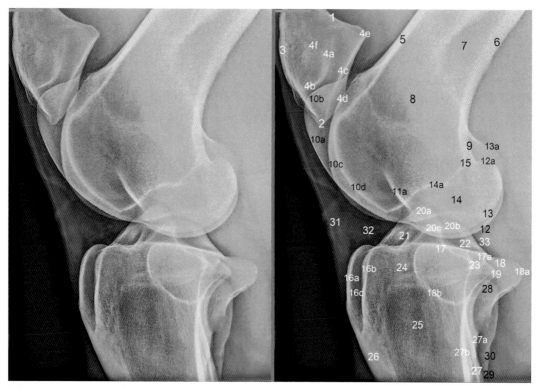

FIG. K.3 **Lateromedial radiographic view of the left stifle.**

Patella: 1- Base, 2- Apex; 3- Cranial face; 4- Articular surface, 4a- proximomedial part; 4b- disto-medial part; 4c- lateral part; 4d- sagittal ridge, 4e- proximal margin, 4f- spongy bone.

Femur: 5- Cranial cortex; 6- Caudal cortex; 7- Supracondylar fossa; 8- Distal metaphysis; 9- Popliteal face; 10- Femoral trochlea, 10a- medial trochlear ridge, 10b- tubercle; 10c- lateral trochlear ridge, 10d- trochlea groove; 11- Extensor fossa, 11a- bottom; 12- Medial femoral con-dyle, 12a- caudal margin; 13- Lateral femoral condyle, 13a- caudal margin; 14- Intercondylar fossa, 14a- bottom; 15- Intercondylar line;

Tibia: 16- Tibial tuberosity, 16a- lateral branch, 16b- medial branch, 16c- sulcus; 17- Medial tibial condyle, 17a- caudal margin; 18- Lateral tibial condyle, 18a- caudal margin; 18b- cranio-distal profile; 19- Insertion tubercle of the caudal cruciate ligament; 20- Intercondylar eminence, 20a- medial intercondylar tubercle, 20b- lateral intercondylar tubercle, 20c- central intercon-dylar area; 21- Cranial intercondylar area; 22- Caudal intercondylar area; 23- Popliteal notch; 24- Extensor sulcus; 25- Extensor fossa; 26- Tibial crest; 27- Caudal cortex, 27a- caudolateral cortex (irregular on this horse), 27b- caudomedial cortex;

Fibula: 28- Head, 29- Body; 30- Fibrous non-union gap;

Soft tissues: 31- Shadow of the medial and lateral patellar ligaments; 32- Infrapatellar fat pad; 33- Shadow of the menisci.

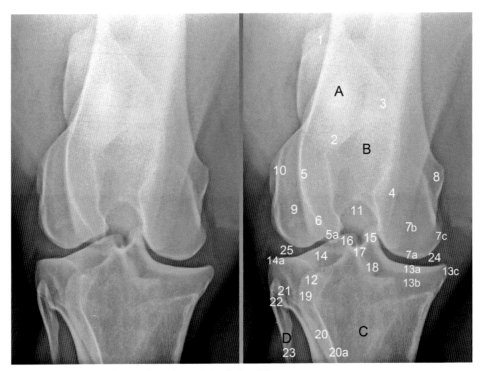

Fig. K.4 **Caudocranial radiographic view of the left stifle.**

A- Patella: 1- Base, 2- Apex; 3- Medial angle;

B- Femur: 4- Medial trochlear ridge; 5- Lateral trochlear ridge, 5a- distal profile; 6- Extensor fossa (bottom); 7- Medial femoral condyle, 7a- subchondral bone, 7b- spongy bone, 7c- medial margin; 8- Medial femoral epicondyle; 9- Lateral femoral condyle; 10- Lateral femoral epicondyle; 11- Intercondylar fossa;

C- Tibia: 12- Tibial tuberosity; 13- Medial tibial condyle, 13a- medial margin, 13b- subchondral bone, 13c- spongy bone; 14- Lateral tibial condyle, 14a- lateral margin; 15- Medial intercondylar tubercle; 16- Lateral intercondylar tubercle; 17- Central intercondylar area; 18- Caudal and cranial intercondylar areas (superimposed); 19- Extensor sulcus; 20- Extensor fossa, 20a- bottom;

D- Fibula: 21- Tibiofibular joint; 22- Head of the fibula; 23- Body of the fibula;
Soft tissues: 24- Shadow of the medial meniscus; 25- Shadow of the lateral meniscus.

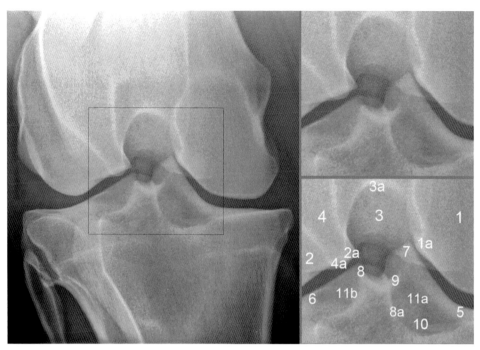

Fig. K.5 **Caudocranial radiographic view of the left stifle: zoom on the intercondylar structures.**

Femur: 1- Medial femoral condyle, 1a- axial margin; 2- Lateral femoral condyle, 2a- axial margin; 3- Intercondylar fossa, 3a- bottom with dense bone; 4- Lateral trochlea ridge, 4a- distal profile;

Tibia: 5- Medial tibial condyle (subchondral bone); 6- Lateral tibial condyle; 7- Medial intercondylar tubercle; 8- Lateral intercondylar tubercle, 8a caudal margin; 9- Central intercondylar area (insertion of the cranial cruciate ligament); 10- Caudal intercondylar area (insertion of the caudomedial meniscotibial ligament); 11- Cranial intercondylar area, 11a- insertion of the craniomedial meniscotibial ligament, 11b- insertion of the craniolateral meniscotibial ligament.

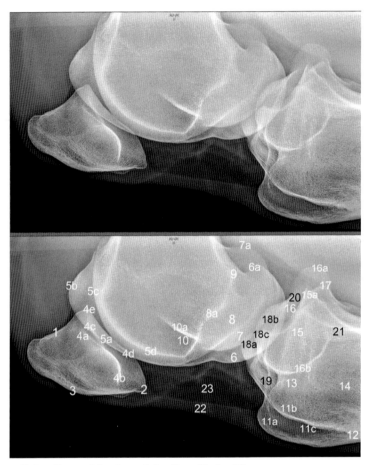

Fig. K.6 **Lateromedial radiographic view of the flexed left stifle.**

Patella: 1- Base; 2- Apex; 3- Cranial face; 4- Articular surface, 4a- proximomedial part, 4b- disto-medial part, 4c- lateral part, 4d- sagittal ridge, 4e- proximal margin;

Femur: 5- Femoral trochlea, 5a- medial trochlear ridge, 5b- tubercle, 5c- lateral trochlear ridge, 5d- groove; 6- Medial femoral condyle, 6a- caudal margin; 7- Lateral femoral condyle, 7a- caudal margin; 8- Intercondylar fossa, 8a- bottom with dense bone; 9- Intercondylar line; 10- Extensor fossa, 10a- bottom with dense bone;

Tibia: 11- Tibial tuberosity, 11a- lateral branch, 11b- medial branch, 11c- sulcus; 12- Tibial crest; 13- Extensor sulcus; 14- Extensor fossa; 15- Medial tibial condyle, 15a- caudal margin; 16- Lateral tibial condyle, 16a- caudal margin, 16b- craniodistal profile; 17- Insertion tubercle of the caudal cruciate ligament; 18- Intercondylar eminence, 18a- medial intercondylar tubercle, 18b- lateral intercondylar tubercle, 18c- central intercondylar area; 19- Cranial intercondylar area; 20- Caudal intercondylar area;

Fibula: 21- Head;

Soft tissues: 22- Shadow of the lateral and medial patellar ligament; 23- Infrapatellar fat pad.

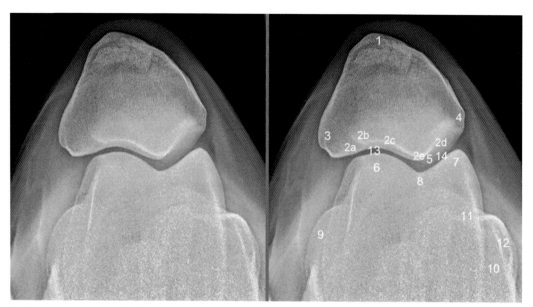

Fig. K.7 **Proximodistal radiographic view of the flexed right stifle.**

Patella: 1- Cranial surface; 2- Articular surface, 2a- proximomedial part, 2b- distomedial part, 2c- subchondral bone, 2d- lateral part, 2e- sagittal ridge; 3- Medial angle; 4- Lateral aspect; 5- Apex;

Femur: 6- Medial trochlear ridge; 7- Lateral trochlear ridge; 8- Femoral trochlear groove; 9- Medial femoral condyle; 10- Lateral femoral condyle; 11- Extensor fossa; 12- Collateral fossa;

Femoropatellar joint: 13- Medial part; 14- Lateral part.

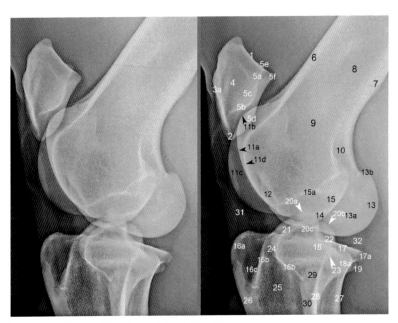

Fig. K.8 **Caudolateral radiographic view of the left stifle.**

Patella: 1- Base; 2- Apex; 3- Cranial face, 3a- compact bone; 4- Spongy bone; 5- Articular surface, 5a- proximomedial part, 5b- distomedial part, 5c- lateral part, 5d- sagittal ridge, 5e- proximomedial margin, 5f- proximolateral margin;

Femur: 6- Craniolateral cortex; 7- Caudomedial cortex; 8- Supracondylar fossa; 9- Distal metaphysis; 10- Popliteal face; 11- Femoral trochlea, 11a- medial trochlear ridge, 11b- tubercle, 11c- lateral trochlear ridge, 11d- trochlea groove; 12- Extensor fossa; 13- Medial femoral condyle, 13a- axial margin, 13b- caudal margin; 14- Lateral femoral condyle; 15- Intercondylar fossa, 15a- bottom;

Tibia: 16- Tibial tuberosity, 16a- lateral branch, 16b- medial branch, 16c- sulcus; 17- Medial tibial condyle, 17a- caudomedial margin; 18- Lateral tibial condyle, 18a- caudal margin; 18b- craniodistal margin; 19- Insertion tubercle of the caudal cruciate ligament; 20- Intercondylar eminence, 20a- medial intercondylar tubercle, 20b- lateral intercondylar tubercle, 20c- central intercondylar area; 21- Cranial intercondylar area; 22- Caudal intercondylar area; 23- Popliteal notch; 24- Extensor sulcus; 25- Extensor fossa; 26- Tibial crest; 27- Caudomedial cortex; 28- Caudolateral cortex;

Fibula: 29- Head; 30- Body;

Soft tissues: 31- Shadow of the lateral patellar ligament; 32- Shadow of the medial meniscus.

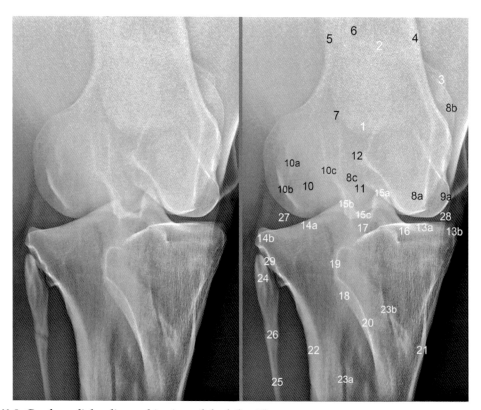

Fig. K.9 **Caudomedial radiographic view of the left stifle.**

Patella: 1- Base; 2- Apex; 3- Medial angle;

Femur: 4- Craniomedial cortex; 5- Caudolateral cortex; 6- Supracondylar fossa; 7- Popliteal face; 8- Femoral trochlea, 8a- medial trochlear ridge, 8b- tubercle, 8c- lateral trochlear ridge; 9- Medial femoral condyle, 9a- medial margin; 10- Lateral femoral condyle, 10a- collateral fossa, 10b- popliteal fossa, 10c- axial margin; 11- Intercondylar fossa; 12- Intercondylar line;

Tibia: 13- Medial tibial condyle, 13a- subchondral bone, 13b- craniomedial margin; 14- Lateral tibial condyle, 14a- subchondral bone, 14b- caudolateral margin; 15- Intercondylar eminence, 15a- medial intercondylar tubercle, 15b- lateral intercondylar tubercle, 15c- central intercondylar area; 16- Cranial intercondylar area; 17- Caudal intercondylar area; 18- Tibial tuberosity and crest; 19- Extensor sulcus (bottom); 20- Extensor fossa (bottom); 21- Craniomedial cortex; 22- Caudolateral cortex; 23- Vascular channels, 23a- common location, 23b- unusual location;

Fibula: 24- Head; 25- Body; 26- Fibrous non-union gap;

Soft tissues and joints: 27- Shadow of the lateral meniscus; 28- Shadow of the medial meniscus; 29- Tibiofibular joint.

K.3 DISSECTED SPECIMEN

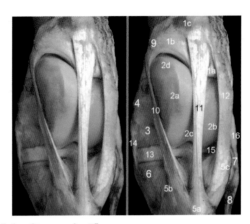

Fig. K.10 **Cranial aspect of the dissected stifle.**

1- Patella, 1a- apex, 1b- medial angle, 1c- dorsal face; 2- Femoral trochlea, 2a- medial trochlear ridge, 2b- lateral trochlear ridge, 2c- groove, 2d- tubercle; 3- Medial femoral condyle; 4- Medial femoral epicondyle; 5- Tibial tuberosity, 5a- distal part, 5b- medial branch, 5c- lateral branch; 6- Medial tibial condyle; 7- Lateral tibial condyle; 8- Fibula; 9- Medial parapatellar fibrocartilage; 10- Medial patellar ligament; 11- Intermediate patellar ligament; 12- Lateral patellar ligament; 13- Medial meniscus; 14- Medial collateral ligament; 15- Lateral meniscus; 16- Lateral collateral ligament.

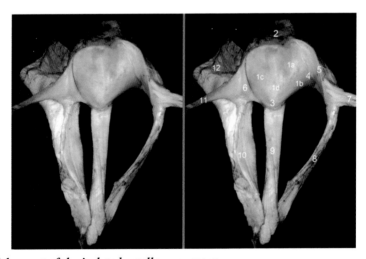

Fig. K.11 **Caudal aspect of the isolated patellar apparatus.**

1- Articular surface of the patella, 1a- proximomedial part, 1b- distomedial part, 1c- lateral part; 2- Base of the patella; 3- Apex of the patella; 4- Medial angle of the patella; 5- Medial parapatellar fibrocartilage; 6- Lateral parapatellar fibrocartilage; 7- Medial femoropatellar ligament; 8- Medial patellar ligament; 9- Intermediate patellar ligament; 10- Lateral patellar ligament; 11- Lateral femoropatellar ligament; 12- Distal tendon of the gluteofemoral muscle.

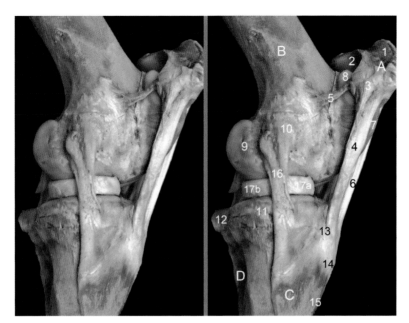

Fig. K.12 **Medial aspect of the dissected stifle.**

A- Patellar apparatus: 1- Base; 2- Articular surface; 3- Medial parapatellar fibrocartilage; 4- Medial patellar ligament; 5- Medial femoropatellar ligament; 6- Intermediate patellar ligament;

B- Femur: 7- Medial trochlear ridge; 8- Tubercle of the femoral trochlea; 9- Medial femoral condyle; 10- Medial femoral epicondyle;

C- Tibia: 11- Medial tibial condyle; 12- Lateral tibial condyle; 13- Tibial tuberosity (medial branch); 14- Tibial tuberosity (distal part); 15- Tibial crest;

D- Fibula;

E- Medial femorotibial joint: 16- Medial collateral ligament; 17- Medial meniscus, 17a- cranial horn, 17b- caudal horn.

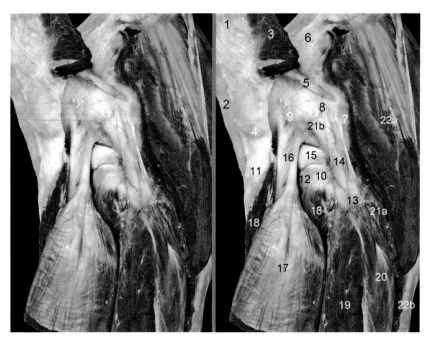

Fig. K.13 **Lateral aspect of the dissected stifle: superficial structures.**

1- Patella; 2- Infrapatellar fat pad; 3- Gluteofemoralis tendon; 4- Lateral patellar ligament; 5- Lateral femoropatellar ligament; 6- Femur; 7- Lateral femoral condyle; 8- Lateral femoral epicondyle; 9- Extensor fossa of the femur; 10- Lateral tibial condyle; 11- Tibial tuberosity (lateral branch); 12- Extensor sulcus of the tibia; 13- Fibula; 14- Lateral collateral ligament; 15- Lateral meniscus (cranial horn); 16- Common proximal tendon of the long digital extensor and peroneus tertius muscles; 17- Long digital extensor muscle; 18- Tibialis cranialis muscle; 19- Lateral digital extensor muscle; 20- Lateral digital flexor muscle; 21- Popliteus muscle, 21a- muscle body; 21b- tendon; 22- Gastrocnemius muscle (lateral head), 22a- muscle body, 22b- Common calcanean tendon.

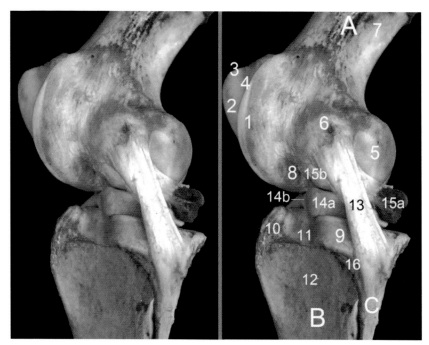

Fig. K.14 **Lateral aspect of the dissected stifle: deep structures.**

A- Femur: 1- Lateral trochlea ridge; 2- Medial trochlea ridge; 3- Tubercle of the femoral trochlea; 4- Groove of the femoral trochlea; 5- Lateral femoral condyle; 6- Lateral femoral epicondyle; 7- Supracondylar fossa of the femur; 8- Extensor fossa of the femur;

B- Tibia: 9- Lateral tibial condyle; 10- Tibial tuberosity (lateral branch); 11- Extensor sulcus of the tibia; 12- Extensor fossa of the tibia;

C- Fibula;

D- Lateral femorotibial joint: 13- Lateral collateral ligament; 14- Lateral meniscus, 14a-cranial horn, 14b- craniolateral meniscotibial ligament; 15- Popliteus muscle, 15a- body (proximal part), 15b- tendon (inserted in the popliteal fossa of the femur); 16- Tibiofibular joint.

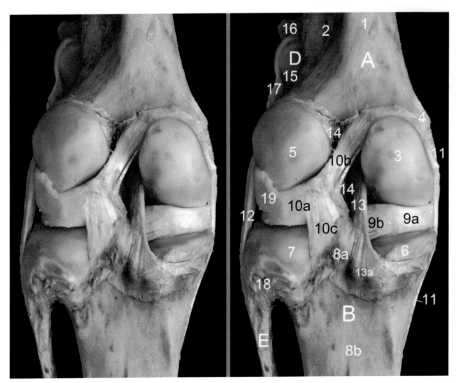

Fig. K.15 **Caudal aspect of the dissected stifle placed in extension.**

A- Femur: 1- Body (diaphysis); 2- Supracondylar fossa of the femur; 3- Medial femoral condyle; 4- Medial femoral epicondyle; 5- Lateral femoral condyle;

B- Tibia: 6- Medial tibial condyle; 7- Lateral tibial condyle; 8a- Popliteal notch, 8b- Insertion surface of the popliteus muscle;

C- Menisci and ligaments: 9- Medial meniscus, 9a- caudal horn, 9b- caudomedial meniscotibial ligament; 10- Lateral meniscus, 10a- caudal horn, 10b- meniscofemoral ligament, 10c- caudolateral meniscotibial ligament; 11- Medial collateral ligament; 12- Lateral collateral ligament; 13- Caudal cruciate ligament, 13a- tibial tubercle; 14- Cranial cruciate ligament;

D- Patella: 15- Articular surface (lateral part); 16- Base; 17- Lateral patellar ligament;

E- Fibula: 18- Tibiofibular joint;

F- Muscle: 19- Popliteus tendon (cut).

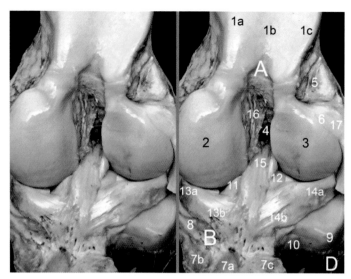

Fig. K.16 **Cranial aspect of the flexed stifle.**

A- Femur: 1- Femoral trochlea, 1a- medial trochlear ridge, 1b- groove, 1c- lateral trochlear ridge; 2- Medial femoral condyle; 3- Lateral femoral condyle; 4- Intercondylar fossa; 5- Extensor fossa of the femur; 6- Popliteal fossa;

B- Tibia: 7- Tibial tuberosity, 7a- medial branch, 7b- sulcus, 7c- lateral branch; 8- Medial tibial condyle; 9- Lateral tibial condyle; 10- Extensor sulcus of the tibia; 11- Medial intercondylar tubercle; 12- Lateral intercondylar tubercle;

C- Menisci and ligaments: 13- Medial meniscus, 13a- cranial horn, 13b- craniomedial meniscotibial ligament; 14- Lateral meniscus, 14a- cranial horn, 14b- craniolateral meniscotibial ligament; 15- Cranial cruciate ligament; 16- Caudal cruciate ligament;

D- Fibula;

E- Muscle: 17- Popliteus tendon (cut).

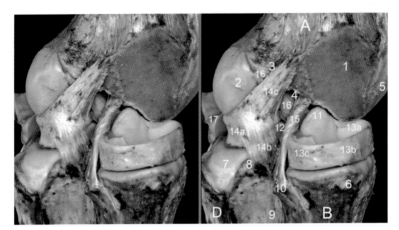

Fig. K.17 **Caudomedial aspect of the dissected stifle after resection of the medial femoral condyle.**

A- Femur: 1- Medial femoral condyle (cut); 2- Lateral femoral condyle; 3- Intercondylar line; 4- Intercondylar fossa; 5- Medial trochlear ridge (cut distally);

B- Tibia: 6- Medial tibial condyle; 7- Lateral tibial condyle; 8- Popliteal notch; 9- Insertion surface of the popliteus muscle; 10- Tubercle of the caudal cruciate ligament; 11- Medial intercondylar tubercle; 12- Lateral intercondylar tubercle;

C- Menisci and ligaments: 13- Medial meniscus, 13a- cranial horn, 13b- body, 13c- caudal horn; 14- Lateral meniscus, 14a- caudal horn, 14b- caudolateral meniscotibial ligament, 14c- meniscofemoral ligament; 15- Caudal cruciate ligament; 16- Cranial cruciate ligament;

D- Fibula;

E- Muscle: 17- Popliteus tendon (cut).

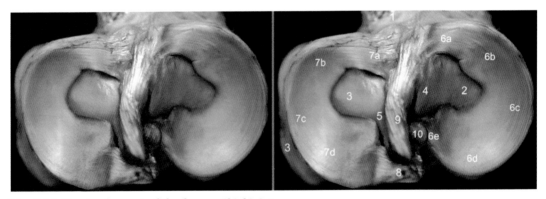

Fig. K.18 **Proximal aspect of the femorotibial joint.**

1- Tibial tuberosity; 2- Medial tibial condyle; 3- Lateral tibial condyle; 4- Medial intercondylar tubercle; 5- Lateral intercondylar tubercle; 6- Medial meniscus, 6a- craniomedial meniscotibial ligament, 6b- cranial horn, 6c- body, 6d- caudal horn, 6e- caudomedial meniscotibial ligament; 7- Lateral meniscus, 7a- craniolateral meniscotibial ligament, 7b- cranial horn, 7c- body, 7d- caudal horn; 8- Meniscofemoral ligament; 9- Cranial cruciate ligament; 10- Caudal cruciate ligament.

K.4 CROSS-SECTIONS

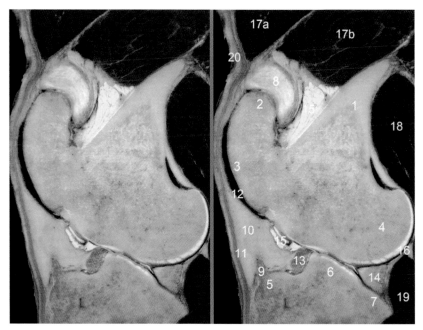

Fig. K.19 **Medial parasagittal section of the stifle.**

1- Femur; 2- Tubercle of the femoral trochlea; 3- Medial trochlear ridge; 4- Medial femoral condyle; 5- Tibial tuberosity (medial branch); 6- Base of the medial intercondylar tubercle; 7- Caudal intercondylar area; 8- Medial parapatellar fibrocartilage; 9- Medial patellar ligament; 10- Infrapatellar fat pad; 11 Patellar fascia; 12- Synovial cavity of the femoropatellar joint; 13- Craniomedial meniscotibial ligament; 14- Caudal horn of the medial meniscus; 15- Medial recess of the medial femorotibial joint (distended); 16- Caudal recess of the medial femorotibial joint; 17- Quadriceps femoris muscle, 17a- rectus femoris muscle, 17b- vastus medialis muscle; 18- Medial head of the gastrocnemius muscle; 19- Popliteus muscle; 20- Skin.

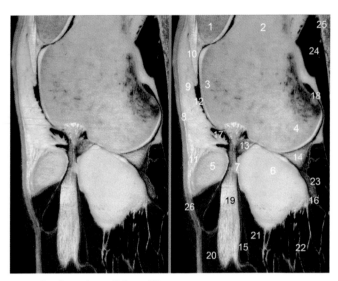

Fig. K.20 **Lateral parasagittal section of the stifle.**

1- Patella; 2- Femur; 3- Lateral ridge of the femoral trochlea; 4- Lateral femoral condyle; 5- Tibial tuberosity (lateral branch); 6- Lateral tibial condyle; 7- Extensor sulcus of the tibia; 8- Patellar fascia; 9- Infrapatellar fat pad; 10- Lateral patellar ligament (origin); 11- Lateral patellar ligament (end); 12- Synovial cavity of the femoropatellar joint; 13- Junction between the cranial horn of the lateral meniscus and craniolateral meniscotibial ligament; 14- Caudal horn of the lateral meniscus; 15- Subextensor recess; 16- Subpopliteal recess; 17- Cranial recess of the lateral femorotibial joint; 18- Caudal recess of the lateral femorotibial joint; 19- Common proximal tendon of the long digital extensor and peroneus tertius muscles; 20- Long digital extensor muscle body; 21- Tibialis cranialis muscle; 22- Lateral digital flexor muscle; 23- Popliteus tendon and muscle; 24- Gastrocnemius muscle (lateral head); 25- Superficial digital flexor muscle (fibrous); 26- Skin.

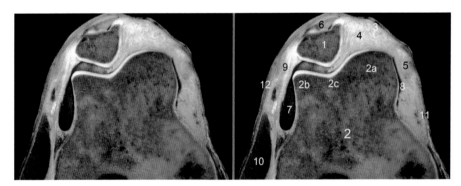

Fig. K.21 **Transverse section of the stifle proximal to the apex of the patella.**

1- Patella; 2- Femur, 2a- medial trochlear ridge, 2b- lateral trochlear ridge, 2c- groove of the femoral trochlea; 3- Patellar fascia; 4- Infrapatellar fat pad; 5- Medial patellar ligament; 6- Intermediate patellar ligament; 7- Lateral recess of the femoropatellar joint; 8- Medial recess of the femoropatellar joint; 9- Tendon of the gluteofemoral muscle; 10- Biceps femoris muscle; 11- Femoral fascia; 12- Skin.

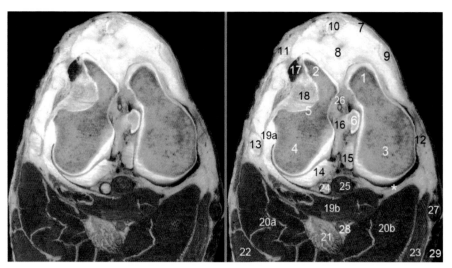

Fig. K.22 **Transverse section of the stifle passing through the intercondylar fossa of the femur.**

1- Medial ridge of the femoral trochlea; 2- Lateral ridge of the femoral trochlea; 3- Medial femoral condyle; 4- Lateral femoral condyle; 5- Extensor fossa; 6- Medial intercondylar tubercle; 7- Patellar fascia; 8- Infrapatellar fat pad; 9- Medial patellar ligament; 10- Intermediate patellar ligament; 11- Lateral patellar ligament; 12- Medial collateral ligament; *- Caudal femorotibial membrane and caudal recess of the medial femorotibial joint; 13- Lateral collateral ligament; 14- Meniscofemoral ligament; 15- Caudal cruciate ligament; 16- Cranial cruciate ligament; 17- Subextensor recess; 18- Common proximal tendon of the long digital extensor and peroneus tertius muscles; 19- Popliteus muscle, 19a- tendon, 19b- muscle body, 19c- subpopliteal recess; 20- Gastrocnemius muscle, 20a- lateral head, 20b- medial head; 21- Superficial digital flexor muscle (fibrous); 22- Biceps femoris muscle; 23- Gracilis muscle; 24- Popliteal artery; 25- Popliteal vein; 26- Middle genu artery; 27- Saphenous vein; 28- Tibial nerve with the caudal femoral artery and vein; 29- Skin.

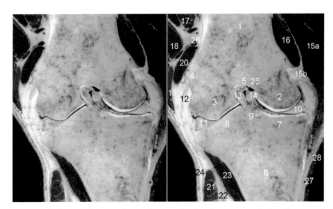

Fig. K.23 **Frontal section of the stifle passing through the intercondylar fossa of the femur.**

1- Femur; 2- Medial femoral condyle; 3- Lateral femoral condyle; 4- Lateral femoral epicondyle; 5- Intercondylar fossa; 6- Tibia; 7- Medial tibial condyle; 8- Lateral tibial condyle; 9- Caudal intercondylar area; 10- Medial meniscus; 11- Lateral meniscus; 12- Lateral collateral ligament; 13- Cranial cruciate ligament; 14- Caudal cruciate ligament; 15- Semimembranosus muscle, 15a- muscle body, 15b- femoral insertion; 16- Adductor magnus muscle; 17- Vastus lateralis muscle; 18- Gluteofemoralis muscle; 19- Biceps femoris muscle; 20- Gastrocnemius muscle (lateral head); 21- Long digital extensor muscle; 22- Peroneus tertius muscle; 23- Tibialis cranialis muscle; 24- Crural fascia; 25- Genu middle artery; 26- Genu lateral proximal artery; 27- Saphenous artery (ramus); 28- Skin.

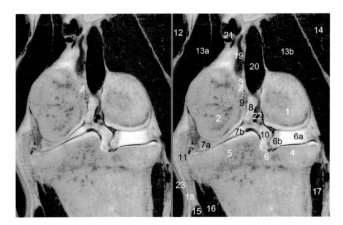

Fig. K.24 **Frontal section of the stifle passing through the femoral condyles.**

1- Medial femoral condyle; 2- Lateral femoral condyle; 3- Intercondylar line; 4- Medial tibial condyle; 5- Lateral tibial condyle; 6- Caudal intercondylar area; 6- Medial meniscus, 6a- caudal horn, 6b- caudomedial meniscotibial ligament; 7- Lateral meniscus, 7a- body, 7b- caudal horn; 8- Meniscofemoral ligament; 9- Cranial cruciate ligament; 10- Caudal cruciate ligament; 11- Lateral collateral ligament; 12- Biceps femoris; 13- Gastrocnemius muscle, 13a- lateral head, 13b- medial head; 14- Semimembranosus muscle; 15- Long digital extensor muscle; 16- Lateral digital flexor muscle; 17- Popliteus muscle; 18- Crural fascia; 19- Popliteal artery; 20- Popliteal vein; 21- Genu lateral proximal artery and vein; 22- Middle genu artery; 23- Skin.

CHAPTER L

THE CRUS

L.1 PHYSICAL ASPECT

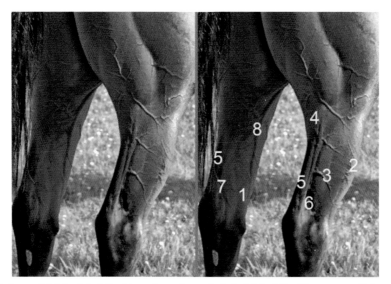

Fig. L.1 **Caudolateral (right hind limb) and caudomedial (left hind limb) aspects of the crus.**

1- Tibia; 2- Cranial tibial area; 3- Caudal tibial area; 4- Gastrocnemius muscle body (distal part); 5- Common calcanean tendon; 6- Lateral sulcus of the hock; 7- Medial sulcus of the hock; 8- Saphenous vein.

L.2 BONE ANATOMY

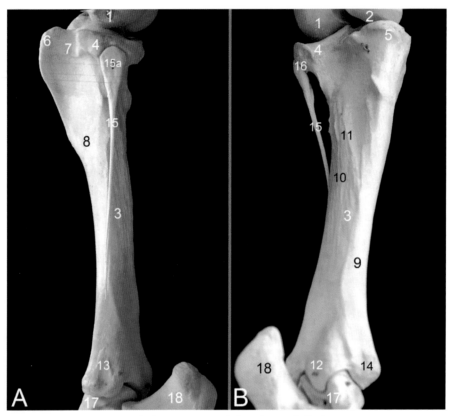

Fig. L.2 **Lateral (A) and caudomedial (B) aspects of the tibia and fibula.**

1- Lateral femoral condyle; 2- Medial femoral condyle; 3- Body of the tibia; 4- Lateral tibial condyle; 5- Medial tibial condyle; 6- Tibial tuberosity (lateral branch); 7- Extensor sulcus; 8- Lateral face; 9- Medial face; 10- Caudal face; 11- Popliteal line; 12- Tibial cochlea; 13- Lateral malleolus; 14- Medial malleolus; 15- Fibula (body), 15a- head of the fibula; 16- Tibiofibular joint; 17- Talus; 18- Calcaneus.

L.3 DISSECTED SPECIMEN

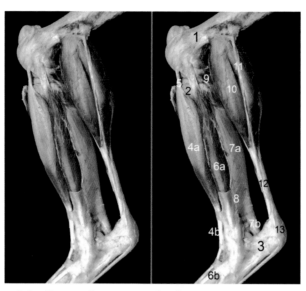

Fig. L.3 **Lateral aspect of the dissected crus: superficial structures.**

1- Distal femur; 2- Lateral tibial condyle; 3- Calcaneus; 4- Long digital extensor muscle, 4a- muscle body, 4b- distal tendon; 5- Common proximal tendon of the long digital extensor and peroneus tertius muscles; 6- Lateral digital extensor muscle, 6a- muscle body, 6b- tendon; 7- Lateral digital flexor muscle, 7a- muscle body, 7b- tendon; 8- Crural fascia (deep layer); 9- Popliteus muscle; 10- Gastrocnemius muscle (lateral head); 11- Crural fascia (superficial layer, most of it having been removed); 12- Common calcanean tendon; 13- Calcanean cap of the superficial digital flexor tendon.

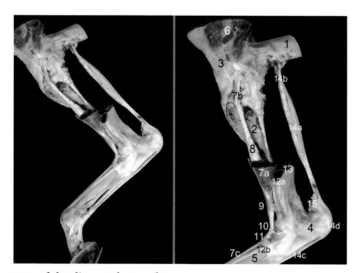

Fig. L.4 **Lateral aspect of the dissected crus: deep structures.**

1- Distal femur; 2- Tibia; 3- Patella; 4- Calcaneus; 5- Third metatarsal bone; 6- Quadriceps femoris muscle; 7- Long digital extensor muscle, 7a- muscle body, 7b- common proximal tendon of the long digital extensor and peroneus tertius muscles, 7c- distal tendon; 8- Peroneus tertius muscle; 9- Proximal (tibial) extensor retinaculum; 10- Intermediate (tarsal) extensor retinaculum; 11- Distal (metatarsal) extensor retinaculum; 12- Lateral digital extensor muscle, 12a- muscle body, 12b- tendon; 13- Lateral digital flexor muscle; 14- Superficial digital flexor muscle, 14a- muscle body (atrophied), 14b- proximal tendon, 14c- distal tendon, 14d- calcanean cap; 15- Gastrocnemius tendon and femoral tendon of the biceps femoris muscle (cut).

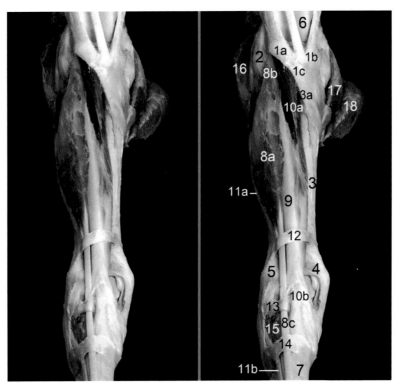

Fig. L.5 **Cranial aspect of the right dissected crus. Lateral is to the left.**

1- Tibial tuberosity, 1a- lateral branch, 1b- medial branch, 1c distal part; 2- Lateral tibial condyle; 3- Body of the tibia, 3a- tibial crest; 4- Medial malleolus; 5- Lateral malleolus; 6- Femoral trochlea; 7- Third metatarsal bone; 8- Long digital extensor muscle, 8a- muscle body, 8b- common proximal tendon of the long digital extensor and peroneus tertius muscles, 8c- distal tendon; 9- Peroneus tertius muscle; 10- Cranial tibial muscle, 10a- body, 10b- distal tendons; 11- Lateral digital extensor muscle, 11a- muscle body, 11b- distal tendon; 12- Proximal (tibial) extensor retinaculum; 13- Intermediate (tarsal) extensor retinaculum; 14- Distal (metatarsal) extensor retinaculum; 15- Short digital extensor muscle; 16- Lateral head of the gastrocnemius muscle; 17- Medial head of the gastrocnemius muscle; 18- Distal part of the semitendinosus muscle body.

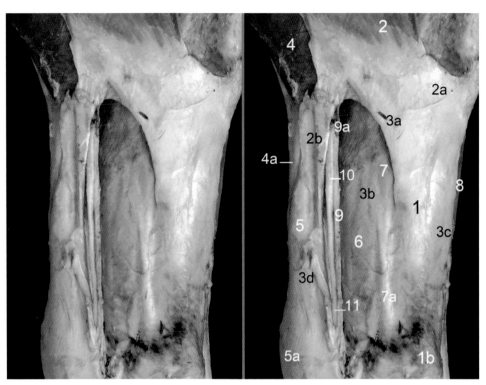

Fig. L.6 **Medial aspect of the dissected crus: superficial structures.**

1- Tibia; 2- Semitendinosus muscle, 2a- tibial tendon, 2b, calcanean tendon; 3- Crural fascia, 3a- superficial layer, 3b- deep layer, 3c- dorsal part, 3d- proper layer (around the common calcanean tendon); 4- Gastrocnemius muscle (medial head), 4a- tendon; 5- Superficial digital flexor tendon, 5a- calcanean cap; 6- Lateral digital flexor muscle; 7- Medial digital flexor muscle, 7a- tendon covered by the crural fascia; 8- Long digital extensor muscle; 9- Caudal root of the saphenous vein, 9a- anastomosis with the caudal femoral vein; 10- Tibial nerve; 11- Origin of the plantar nerves.

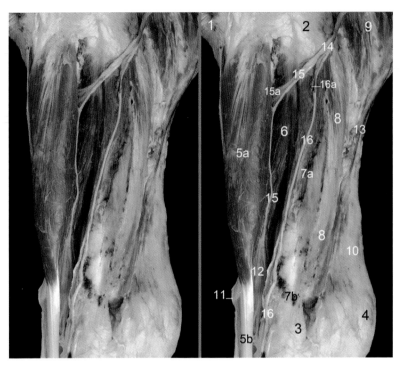

Fig. L.7 **Lateral aspect of the dissected crus: fibular nerves.**

1- Tibial tuberosity; 2- Lateral collateral ligament of the femorotibial joint; 3- Lateral malleo-lus (distal end of the fibula); 4- Point of the hock; 5- Long digital extensor muscle, 5a- muscle body, 5b- distal tendon; 6- Tibialis cranialis muscle; 7- Lateral digital extensor muscle, 7a- muscle body, 7b- tendon (covered by the crural fascia); 8- Lateral digital flexor muscle; 9- Gastrocnemius muscle (lateral head); 10- Common calcanean tendon; 11- Tibial (proximal) extensor retinaculum (cut and reclined); 12- Cranial tibial vein; 13- Lateral saphenous vein; 14- Common fibular (pero-neal) nerve; 15- Deep fibular (peroneal) nerve, 15a- muscle rami; 16- Superficial fibular (peroneal) nerve, 16a- muscle ramus.

L.4 CROSS-SECTIONS

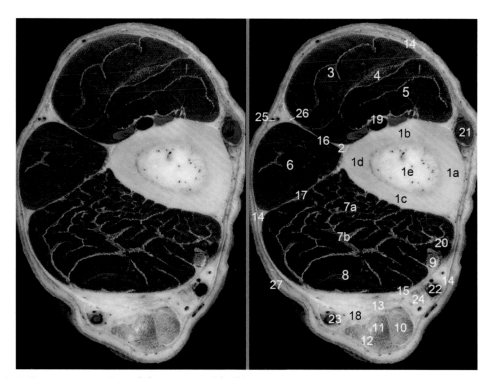

Fig. L.8 **Transverse section of the crus at mid-tibia.**

Bones: 1- Tibia, 1a- medial cortex and face, 1b- cranial cortex and face, 1c- caudal cortex and face, 1d- lateral cortex and border, 1e- medullary cavity; 2- Fibula;

Muscles and associated structures: 3- Long digital extensor muscle; 4- Peroneus tertius muscle (fibrous); 5- Tibialis cranialis muscle; 6- Lateral digital extensor muscle; 7- Lateral digital flexor muscle, 7a- striated muscle fibres, 7b- intramuscular aponeuroses; 8- Tibialis caudalis muscle; 9- Medial digital flexor tendon; 10- Superficial digital flexor tendon; 11- Gastrocnemius tendon, medial head; 12- Gastrocnemius tendon, lateral head; 13- Common calcanean tendon of the biceps femoris and semitendinosus muscles; 14- Crural fascia, superficial layer; 15- Crural fascia, deep layer; 16- Cranial crural septum; 17- Caudal crural septum; 18- Crural fascia, proper layer (around the common calcanean tendon);

Vessels and nerves: 19- Cranial tibial artery and veins; 20- Caudal tibial artery and vein; 21- Medial saphenous vein (cranial root); 22- Caudal root of the medial saphenous vein communicating to the caudal femoral vein; 23- Lateral saphenous vein; 24- Tibial nerve; 25- Superficial fibular (peroneal) nerve; 26- Deep fibular (peroneal) nerve; 27- Skin.

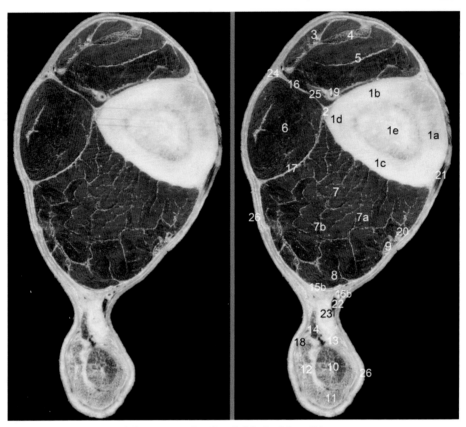

Fig. L.9 **Transverse section of the crus at the distal third of the tibia.**

Bones: 1- Tibia, 1a- medial cortex and face, 1b- cranial cortex and face, 1c- caudal cortex and face, 1d- lateral cortex and border, 1e- medullary cavity; 2- Fibula (fibrous);

Muscles and associated structures: 3- Long digital extensor muscle; 4- Peroneus tertius muscle (fibrous); 5- Tibialis cranialis muscle; 6- Lateral digital extensor muscle; 7- Lateral digital flexor muscle, 7a- striated muscle fibres, 7b- intramuscular aponeuroses; 8- Tibialis caudalis muscle; 9- Medial digital flexor tendon; 10- Superficial digital flexor tendon; 11- Gastrocnemius tendon, medial head; 12- Gastrocnemius tendon, lateral head; 13- Common calcanean tendon of the biceps femoris and semitendinosus muscles; 14- Soleus muscle; 15- Crural fascia, 15a- superficial layer, 15b- deep layer; 16- Cranial crural septum;

Vessels and nerves: 17- Caudal crural septum; 18- Crural fascia, proper layer (around the common calcanean tendon); 19- Cranial tibial artery (satellite veins are empty); 20- Caudal tibial artery (satellite vein is empty); 21- Medial saphenous vein (cranial root); 22- Caudal root of the medial saphenous vein communicating to the caudal femoral vein; 23- Tibial nerve; 24- Superficial fibular (peroneal) nerve; 25- Deep fibular (peroneal) nerve; 26- Skin.

THE TARSUS

M.1 PHYSICAL ASPECT

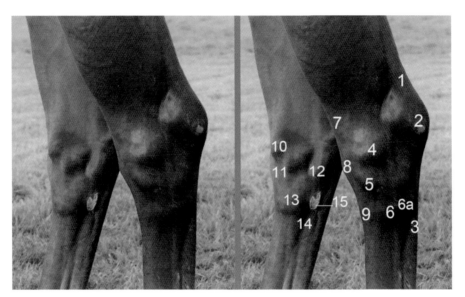

Fig. M.1 **Lateral and medial aspects of the equine hock: palpable anatomical structures.**

1- Common calcanean tendon; 2- Point of the hock; 3- Digital flexor tendons; 4- Lateral malleolus (distal part of the fibula); 5- Lateral ridge of the trochlea of the talus; 6- Tarsometatarsal junction, 6a- head of the lateral splint bone (fourth metatarsal bone); 7- Proximal plica of the hock (tibial retinaculum); 8- Tendons of the tarsal flexor muscles (peroneus tertius and tibialis cranialis muscles) over the medial ridge of the trochlea of the talus; 9- Distal plica of the hock (metatarsal retinaculum); 10- Medial malleolus of the tibia; 11- Dorsal recess of the tarsocrural joint; 12- Sustentaculum tali and lateral digital flexor tendon; 13- Distal tarsus; 14- Distomedial sulcus of the hock (over the proximal insertion of the suspensory ligament); 15- Chestnut.

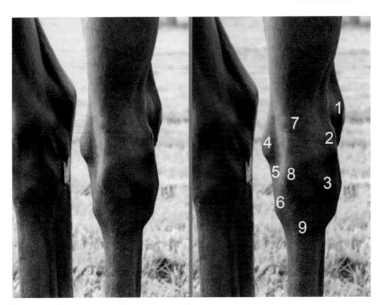

Fig. M.2 **Dorsal aspect of the equine hock: palpable anatomical structures.**

1- Point of the hock; 2- Lateral malleolus (distal part of the fibula); 3- Lateral ridge of the trochlea of the talus; 4- Medial malleolus of the tibia; 5- Dorsal recess of the tarsocrural joint (the dorsal root of the saphenous vein is empty); 6- Distal tarsus; 7- Proximal plica of the hock (tibial retinaculum); 8- Tendons of the tarsal flexor muscles (peroneus tertius and tibialis cranialis muscles) over the medial ridge of the trochlea of the talus; 9- Distal plica of the hock (metatarsal retinaculum).

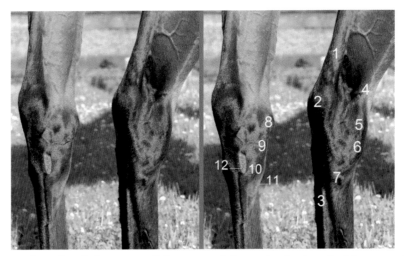

Fig. M.3 **Plantarolateral and plantaromedial aspects of the equine hock: palpable anatomical structures.**

1- Common calcanean tendon; 2- Point of the hock; 3- Digital flexor tendons; 4- Lateral digital extensor tendon; 5- Lateral malleolus (distal part of the fibula); 6- Lateral ridge of the trochlea of the talus; 7- Head of the lateral splint bone (fourth metatarsal bone); 8- Medial malleolus of the tibia; 9- Medial collateral ligament; 10- Distal tarsus; 11- Dorsal root of the saphenous vein; 12- Chestnut.

M.2 RADIOGRAPHIC ANATOMY

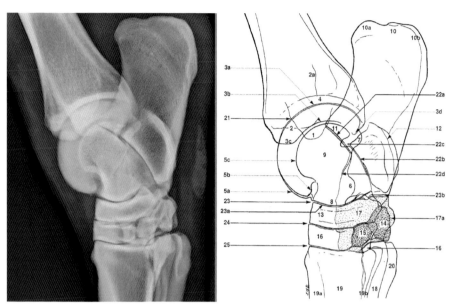

Fig. M.4 **Lateromedial radiographic view of the left tarsus.**

Tibia: 1- Medial malleolus; 2- Lateral malleolus (distal part of the fibula), 2a- caudal lobe; 3- Tibial cochlea, 3a- grooves, 3b- intermediate ridge, 3c- dorsal extremity of the intermediate ridge, 3d- plantar extremity of the intermediate ridge; 4- subchondral bone;

Talus: 5- Trochlea of the talus, 5a- medial trochlear ridge, 5b- lateral trochlear ridge, 5c- intermediate groove; 6- Distal tubercle; 7- Proximal tubercle; 8- Head of the talus; 9- Body of the talus;

Calcaneus: 10- Tuber calcanei, 10a- dorsal lobe, 10b- plantar lobe; 11- Coracoid process; 12- Sustentaculum tali;

Distal tarsus: 13- Central tarsal bone; 14- First tarsal bone; 15- Second tarsal bone; 16- Third tarsal bone; 17- Fourth tarsal bone, 17a- plantar tubercle;

Metatarsus: 18- Second metatarsal bone; 19- Third metatarsal bone, 19a- dorsal cortex, 19b- plantar cortex; 20- Fourth metatarsal bone;

Joints: 21- Tarsocrural joint; 22- Talocalcaneal joint, 22a- lateral part, 22b- medial part, 22c- tarsal sinus; 22d- lateral talocalcaneal joint space; 23- Proximal intertarsal (mediotarsal) joint; 24- Distal intertarsal (centrodistal) joint; 25- Tarsometatarsal joint.

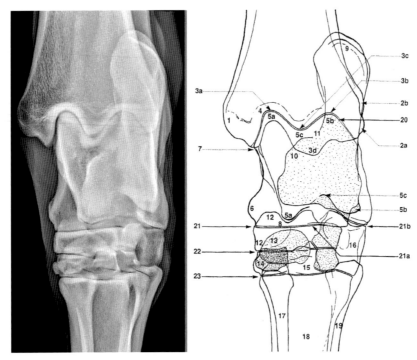

Fig. M.5 **Dorsoplantar radiographic view of the left tarsus.**

Tibia: 1- Medial malleolus; 2- Lateral malleolus (distal part of the fibula), 2a- cranial lobe, 2b- caudal lobe; 3- Tibial cochlea, 3a- medial groove, 3b- lateral groove, 3c- intermediate ridge, 3d- dorsal extremity of the intermediate ridge; 4- subchondral bone;

Talus: 5- Trochlea of the talus, 5a- medial trochlear ridge, 5b- lateral trochlear ridge, 5c- intermediate groove; 6- Distal tubercle; 7- Proximal tubercle; 8- Head of the talus;

Calcaneus: 9- Tuber calcanei; 10- Sustentaculum tali; 11- Gliding surface for the lateral digital flexor tendon;

Distal tarsus: 12- Central tarsal bone; 13- First tarsal bone; 14- Second tarsal bone; 15- Third tarsal bone; 16- Fourth tarsal bone;

Metatarsus: 17- Second metatarsal bone; 18- Third metatarsal bone; 19- Fourth metatarsal bone;

Joints: 20- Tarsocrural joint; 21- Proximal intertarsal (mediotarsal) joint, 21a- talocentral joint, 21b- calcaneoquartal joint; 22- Distal intertarsal (centrodistal) joint; 23- Tarsometatarsal joint.

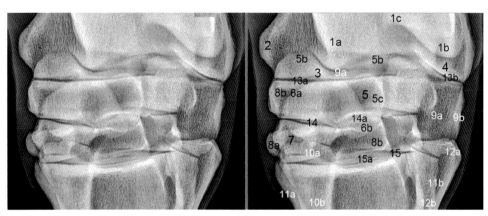

Fig. M.6 **Dorsoplantar radiographic view of the left distal tarsus.**

Talus: 1- Trochlea of the talus, 1a- medial trochlear ridge, 1b- lateral trochlear ridge, 1c- intermediate groove; 2- Distal tubercle; 3- Head of the talus;

Calcaneus: 4- distolateral part;

Distal tarsus: 5- Central tarsal bone, 5a- plantaromedial elevation, 5b- plantar margin, 5c- plantar tubercle; 6- First tarsal bone, 6a- proximomedial margin, 6b- plantar lobe; 7- Second tarsal bone; 8- Third tarsal bone, 8a- medial tubercle; 8b- plantar tubercle; 9- Fourth tarsal bone, 9a- spongy bone, 9b- compact bone;

Metatarsus: 10- Second metatarsal bone, 10a- head, 10b- body; 11- Third metatarsal bone, 11a- medial border, 11b- lateral border; 12- Fourth metatarsal bone, 12a- head, 12b- body;

Joints: 13- Proximal intertarsal (mediotarsal) joint, 13a- talocentral joint, 13b- calcaneoquartal joint; 14- Distal intertarsal (centrodistal) joint, 14a- interosseous fossa; 15- Tarsometatarsal joint, 15a- interosseous fossa.

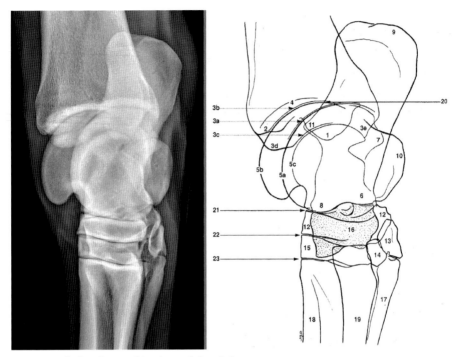

Fig. M.7 **Dorsomedial radiographic view of the right tarsus.**

Tibia: 1- Medial malleolus, 2- Lateral malleolus (distal part of the fibula); 3- Tibial cochlea, 3a- medial groove, 3b- lateral groove, 3c- intermediate ridge, 3d- dorsal extremity of the intermediate ridge, 3e- plantar extremity of the intermediate ridge; 4- subchondral bone;

Talus: 5- Trochlea of the talus, 5a- medial trochlear ridge, 5b- lateral trochlear ridge, 5c- intermediate groove; 6- Distal tubercle; 7- Proximal tubercle; 8- Head of the talus;

Calcaneus: 9- Tuber calcanei; 10- Sustentaculum tali; 11- Coracoid process;

Distal tarsus: 12- Central tarsal bone; 13- First tarsal bone; 14- Second tarsal bone; 15- Third tarsal bone; 16- Fourth tarsal bone;

Metatarsus: 17- Second metatarsal bone; 18- Third metatarsal bone; 19- Fourth metatarsal bone;

Joints: 20- Tarsocrural joint; 21- Proximal intertarsal (talocentral and calcaneoquartal) joint; 22- Distal intertarsal (centrodistal) joint; 23- Tarsometatarsal joint.

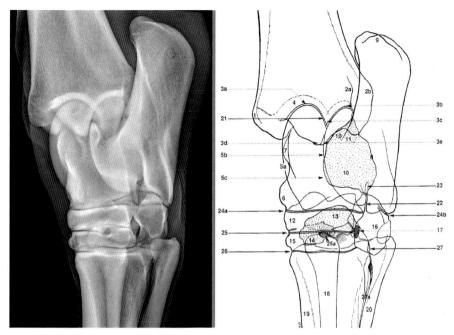

Fig. M.8 **Dorsolateral radiographic view of the left tarsus.**

Tibia: 1- Medial malleolus; 2- Lateral malleolus (distal part of the fibula), 2a- cranial lobe, 2b-caudal lobe; 3- Tibial cochlea, 3a- medial groove, 3b- lateral groove, 3c- intermediate ridge, 3d- dorsal extremity of the intermediate ridge, 3e- plantar extremity of the intermediate ridge; 4- subchondral bone;

Talus: 5- Trochlea of the talus, 5a- medial trochlear ridge, 5b- lateral trochlear ridge, 5c- intermediate groove; 6- Distal tubercle; 7- Medial articular margin of the medial trochlear ridge; 8- Lateral profile of the talus;

Calcaneus: 9- Tuber calcanei; 10- Sustentaculum tali; 11- Coracoid process;

Distal tarsus: 12- Central tarsal bone; 13- First tarsal bone; 14- Second tarsal bone; 15- Third tarsal bone; 16- Fourth tarsal bone; 17- Tarsal canal;

Metatarsus: 18- Second metatarsal bone; 19- Third metatarsal bone; 20- Fourth metatarsal bone;

Joints: 21- Tarsocrural joint; 22- Talocalcaneal joint; 23- Tarsal sinus; 24- Proximal intertarsal (mediotarsal) joint, 24a- talocentral joint, 24b- calcaneoquartal joint; 25- Distal intertarsal (centrodistal) joint, 25a- interosseous fossa; 26- Tarsometatarsal joint; 27- Intermetatarsal joint, 27a- intermetatarsal syndesmosis.

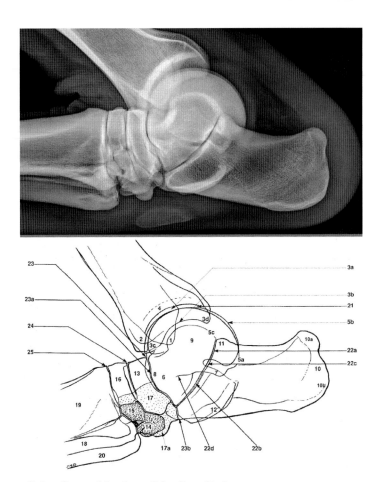

Fig. M.9 Lateromedial radiographic view of the flexed left tarsus.

Tibia: 1- Medial malleolus; 2- Lateral malleolus (distal part of the fibula); 3- Tibial cochlea, 3a- grooves, 3b- intermediate ridge, 3c- dorsal extremity of the intermediate ridge, 3d- plantar extremity of the intermediate ridge; 4- subchondral bone;

Talus: 5- Trochlea of the talus, 5a- medial trochlear ridge, 5b- lateral trochlear ridge, 5c- intermediate groove; 6- Distal tubercle; 7- Proximal tubercle; 8- Head of the talus; 9- Body of the talus;

Calcaneus: 10- Tuber calcanei, 10a- dorsal lobe, 10b- plantar lobe; 11- Coracoid process; 12- Sustentaculum tali;

Distal tarsus: 13- Central tarsal bone; 14- First tarsal bone; 15- Second tarsal bone; 16- Third tarsal bone; 17- Fourth tarsal bone, 17a- plantar tubercle;

Metatarsus: 18- Second metatarsal bone; 19- Third metatarsal bone; 20- Fourth metatarsal bone;

Joints: 21- Tarsocrural joint; 22- Talocalcaneal joint, 22a- lateral part, 22b- medial part, 22c- tarsal sinus, 22d- lateral talocalcaneal joint space; 23- Proximal intertarsal (mediotarsal) joint; 24- Distal intertarsal (centrodistal) joint; 25- Tarsometatarsal joint.

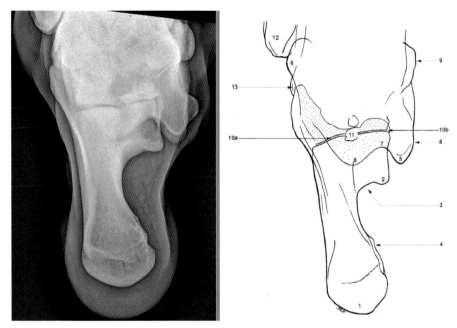

Fig. M.10 **Proximodistal radiographic view of the flexed left tarsus.**

Calcaneus: 1- Tuber calcanei; 2- Sustentaculum tali; 3- Sulcus of the lateral digital flexor tendon; 4- Insertion surface of the medial attachment of the superficial digital flexor tendon cap (medial tenocalcaneal ligament);

Talus: 5- Medial trochlear ridge; 6- Lateral trochlear ridge; 7- Intermediate groove; 8- Proximal tubercle; 9- Distal tubercle;

Talocalcaneal joint: 10- Joint space, 10a- lateral part, 10b- medial part; 11- Interosseous space communicating with the tarsal sinus;

Tibia and fibula: 12- Lateral malleolus;

Distal tarsus: 13- Fourth tarsal bone.

M.3 DISSECTED SPECIMEN

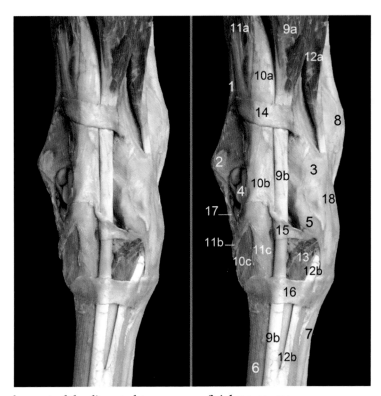

Fig. M.11 **Dorsal aspect of the dissected tarsus: superficial structures.**

1- Tibia (body); 2- Medial malleolus of the tibia; 3- Lateral malleolus (distal part of the fibula); 4- Medial trochlea ridge of the talus; 5- Lateral trochlea ridge of the talus; 6- Third metatarsal bone; 7- Fourth metatarsal bone (lateral splint bone); 8- Point of the hock (tuber calcanei covered by the cap of the superficial digital flexor tendon); 9- Long digital extensor muscle, 9a- muscle body, 9b- distal tendon; 10- Peroneus tertius muscle, 10a- fibrous muscle body, 10b- opening of distal tendon for the tibialis cranialis tendon, 10c- metatarsal branch; 11- Tibialis cranialis muscle, 11a- muscle body, 11b- tarsal (cunean) branch, 11c- metatarsal branch; 12- Lateral digital extensor muscle, 12a- muscle body, 12b- distal tendon; 13- Short digital extensor muscle; 14- Proximal (tibial) extensor retinaculum; 15- Intermediate (tarsal) extensor retinaculum; 16- distal (metatarsal) extensor retinaculum; 17- Medial collateral ligament; 18- Lateral collateral ligament.

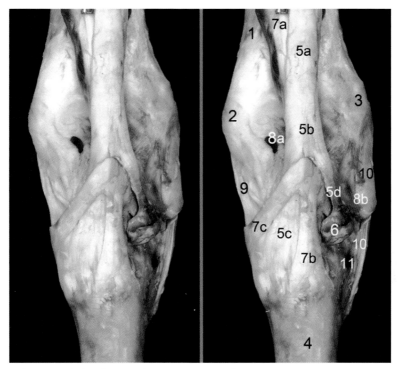

Fig. M.12 Dorsal aspect of the dissected tarsus: intermediate structures.

1- Tibia (body); 2- Medial malleolus of the tibia; 3- Lateral malleolus (distal part of the fibula); 4- Third metatarsal bone; 5- Peroneus tertius muscle, 5a- fibrous muscle body, 5b- opening of distal tendon for the tibialis cranialis tendon, 5c- metatarsal branch, 5d tarsal (quartal) branch; 6- Intermediate (tarsal) extensor retinaculum; 7- Tibialis cranialis muscle, 7a- muscle body, 7b- metatarsal branch, 7c- tarsal (cunean) branch; 8- Dorsal capsule of the tarsocrural joint, 8a- over the dorsomedial recess of the joint (opened), 8b- over the lateral trochlea ridge of the talus; 9- Medial collateral ligament; 10- Lateral collateral ligament.

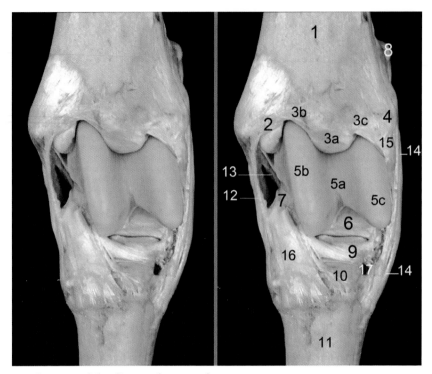

Fig. M.13 **Dorsal aspect of the dissected tarsus: deep structures.**

1- Tibia (body); 2- Medial malleolus of the tibia; 3- Tibial cochlea, 3a- medial groove, 3b- intermediate ridge, 3c- lateral groove; 4- Lateral malleolus (distal part of the fibula); 5- Trochlea of the talus, 5a- groove, 5b- medial ridge, 5c- lateral ridge; 6- Body of the talus; 7- distal tubercle of the talus; 8- Tuber calcanei; 9- Central tarsal bone; 10- Third tarsal bone; 11- Third metatarsal bone; 12- Long medial collateral ligament; 13- Short medial collateral ligament; 14- Long lateral collateral ligament; 15- Short lateral collateral ligament; 16- Talometatarsal (talocentrodistometatarsal) ligament.

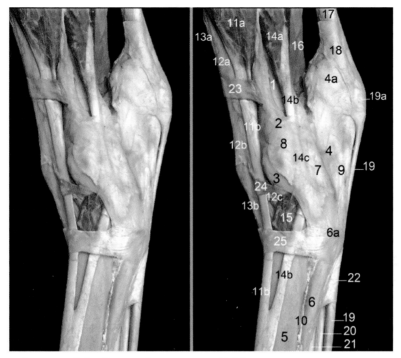

Fig. M.14 **Lateral aspect of the dissected tarsus: superficial structures.**

1- Tibia (distal metaphysis); 2- Lateral malleolus (distal part of the fibula); 3- Lateral troch-lear ridge of the talus (covered by the articular capsule of the tarsocrural joint); 4- Calcaneus, 4a- tuber calcanei; 5- Third metatarsal bone; 6- Fourth metatarsal bone (lateral splint bone), 6a-head; 7- Long lateral collateral ligament; 8- Short lateral collateral ligament; 9- Long plantar ligament; 10- Syndesmosis between the third and fourth metatarsal bones; 11- Long digital exten-sor muscle, 11a- muscle body, 11b- distal tendon; 12- Peroneus tertius muscle, 12a- fibrous muscle body, 12b- opening of the distal tendon for the tibialis cranialis tendon, 12c- tarsal (quartal) branch; 13- Tibialis cranialis muscle, 13a- muscle body, 13b- metatarsal branch; 14- Lateral digi-tal extensor muscle, 14a- muscle body, 14b- distal tendon, 14c- tendon sheath; 15- Short digital extensor muscle; 16- Lateral digital flexor muscle (main origin of the deep digital flexor tendon); 17- Common calcanean tendon; 18- Calcaneal tendon of the femoral muscles; 19- Superficial digital flexor tendon, 19a- cap of the superficial digital flexor tendon, 19b- lateral attachment (lateral tenocalcaneal ligament); 20- Deep digital flexor tendon; 21- Third interosseous mus-cle (suspensory ligament); 22- Plantar tarsal fascia; 23- Proximal (tibial) extensor retinaculum; 24- Intermediate (tarsal) extensor retinaculum; 25- distal (metatarsal) extensor retinaculum.

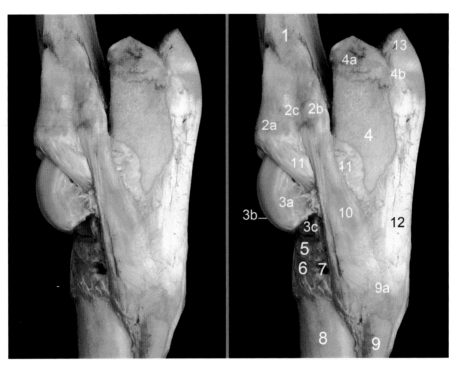

Fig. M.15 **Lateral aspect of the dissected tarsus: deep structures.**

1- Tibia (body); 2- Lateral malleolus (distal part of the fibula), 2a- cranial lobe, 2b- caudal lobe, 2c- groove of the lateral digital extensor tendon; 3- Talus, 3a- lateral trochlear ridge, 3b- medial trochlear ridge, 3c- head; 4- Calcaneus, 4a- dorsal lobe of the tuber calcanei, 4b- plantar lobe of the tuber calcanei; 5- Central tarsal bone; 6- Third tarsal bone; 7- Tarsal canal; 8- Third metatarsal bone; 9- Fourth metatarsal bone (lateral splint bone), 9a-head; 10- Long lateral collateral ligament; 11- Short lateral collateral ligament; 12- Long plantar ligament.

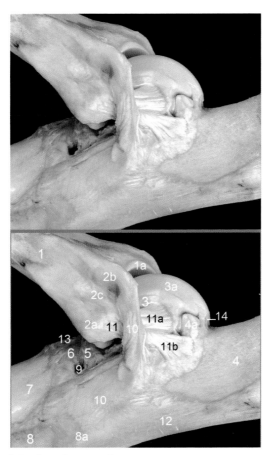

Fig. M.16 **Lateral aspect of the flexed tarsus: deep structures.**

1- Tibia (body), 1a- tibial cochlea; 2- Lateral malleolus (distal part of the fibula), 2a- cranial lobe, 2b- caudal lobe, 2c- groove of the lateral digital extensor tendon; 3- Talus, 3a- lateral trochlear ridge; 4- Calcaneus, 4a- coracoid process; 5- Central tarsal bone; 6- Third tarsal bone; 7- Third metatarsal bone; 8- Fourth metatarsal bone (lateral splint bone), 8a- head; 9- Tarsal canal; 10- Long lateral collateral ligament; 11- Short lateral collateral ligament, 11a- talean fasciculus, 11b- calcaneal fasciculus; 12- Long plantar ligament; 13- Talometatarsal (talocentrodistometatarsal) ligament; 14- Proximal talocalcaneal ligament.

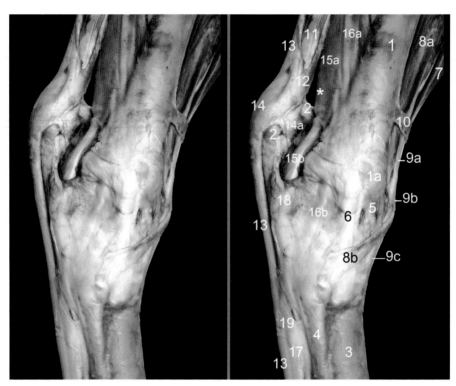

Fig. M.17 **Medial aspect of the dissected tarsus: superficial structures.**

1- Tibia (medial surface of the body), 1a- medial malleolus; 2- Tuber calcanei; 3- Third metatarsal bone; 4- Second metatarsal bone (medial splint bone); 5- Articular capsule of the tarsocrural joint; 6- Long medial collateral ligament; 7- Long digital extensor muscle; 8- Tibialis cranialis muscle, 8a- muscle body, 8b- tarsal (cunean) branch; 9- Peroneus tertius muscle, 9a- fibrous muscle body, 9b- opening of the distal tendon for the tibialis cranialis tendon, 9c- metatarsal branch; 10- Proximal (tibial) extensor retinaculum; 11- Gastrocnemius tendon; 12- Calcaneal tendon of the femoral muscles contributing to the common calcanean tendon; 13- Superficial digital flexor tendon; 14- Cap of the superficial digital flexor tendon, 14a- medial calcaneal attachment (medial tenocalcaneal ligament); 15- Lateral digital flexor muscle, 15a- muscle body, 15b- tendon (main origin of the deep digital flexor tendon); *- Tibialis caudalis muscle; 16- Medial digital flexor muscle, 16a- muscle body, 16b- tendon in its sheath; 17- Deep digital flexor tendon; 18- Flexor retinaculum; 19- Plantar metatarsal fascia.

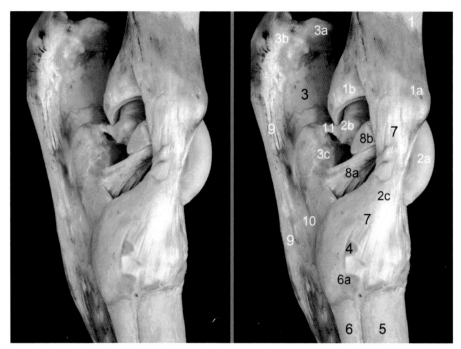

Fig. M.18 **Medial aspect of the dissected tarsus: deep structures.**

1- Tibia (medial surface of the body), 1a- medial malleolus, 1b- tibial cochlea; 2- Talus, 2a- medial trochlear ridge, 2b- proximal tubercle, 2c- distal tubercle; 3- Calcaneus, 3a- dorsal lobe of the tuber calcanei, 3b- plantar lobe of the tuber calcanei with distal insertion of the gastrocnemius tendon; 4- First tarsal bone; 5- Third metatarsal bone; 6- Second metatarsal bone (medial splint bone), 6a- head; 7- Long medial collateral ligament; 8- Short medial collateral ligament, 8a- calcaneal fasciculus, 8b- talean fasciculus; 9- Long plantar ligament; 10- Distal plantar ligament; 11- Proximomedial talocalcaneal ligament.

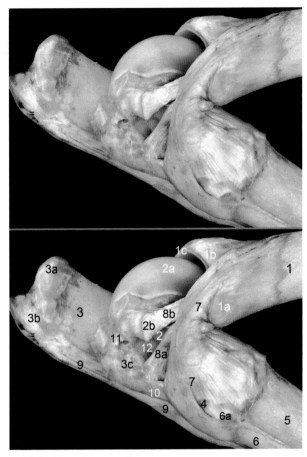

Fig. M.19 **Medial aspect of the flexed tarsus: deep structures.**

1- Tibia (medial surface of the body), 1a- medial malleolus, 1b- tibial cochlea, 1c- interme-diate ridge (caudal extremity); 2- Talus, 2a- medial trochlear ridge, 2b- proximal tubercle; 3- Calcaneus, 3a- dorsal lobe of the tuber calcanei, 3b- plantar lobe of the tuber calcanei with distal insertion of the gastrocnemius tendon; 4- First tarsal bone; 5- Third metatarsal bone; 6- Second metatarsal bone (medial splint bone), 6a- head; 7- Long medial collateral ligament; 8- Short medial collateral ligament, 8a- calcaneal fasciculus, 8b- talean fasciculus; 9- Long plantar ligament; 10- Distal plantar ligament; 11- Proximomedial talocalcaneal ligament; 12- Talocalcaneal joint space.

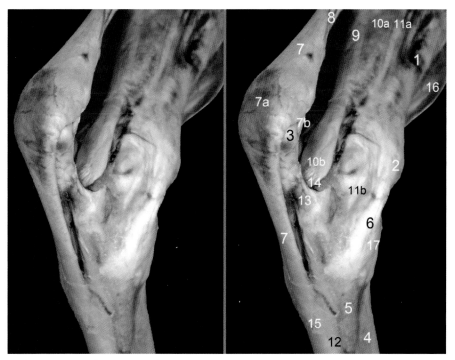

Fig. M.20 **Plantaromedial aspect of the dissected tarsus: superficial structures.**

1- Tibia (medial surface of the body); 2- Medial malleolus; 3- Tuber calcanei; 4- Third metatarsal bone; 5- Second metatarsal bone (medial splint bone); 6- Long medial collateral ligament; 7- Superficial digital flexor muscle, 7a- cap, 7b- medial attachment (tenocalcaneal ligament); 8- Common calcanean tendon; 9- Tibialis caudalis muscle and tendon; 10- Lateral digital flexor muscle, 10a- muscle body, 10b- tendon (main origin of the deep digital flexor tendon); 11- Medial digital flexor muscle, 11a- muscle body, 11b- tendon in its sheath; 12- Deep digital flexor tendon; 13- Flexor retinaculum; 14- Plantar tarsal sheath (opened); 15- Plantar metatarsal fascia; 16- Tibialis cranialis muscle; 17- Tarsal (cunean) branch of the tibialis cranialis muscle.

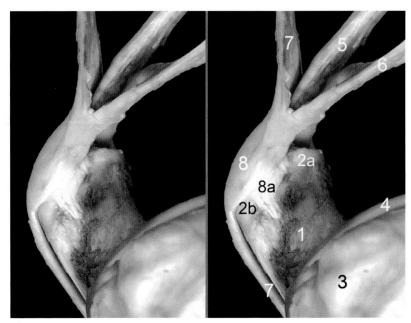

Fig. M.21 **Medial aspect of the point of the hock: common calcanean tendon.**

1- Calcaneus; 2- Tuber calcanei, 2a- dorsal lobe, 2b- plantar lobe; 3- Medial malleolus of the tibia; 4- Lateral digital flexor tendon; 5- Gastrocnemius tendon; 6- Calcaneal tendon of the femoral muscles contributing to the common calcanean tendon; 7- Superficial digital flexor tendon; 8- Cap of the superficial digital flexor tendon, 8a- medial calcaneal attachment (medial tenocalcaneal ligament).

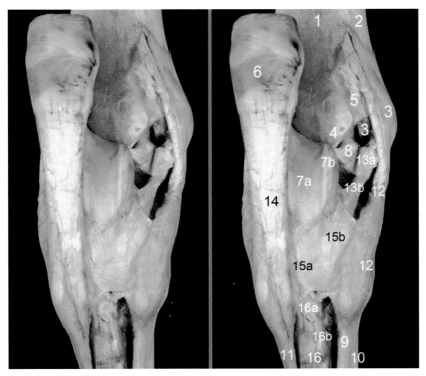

Fig. M.22 **Plantar aspect of the dissected tarsus: deep structures.**

1- Caudal surface of the tibia; 2- Medial surface of the tibia; 3- Medial malleolus, 4- Tibial cochlea; 5- Sulcus of the medial digital flexor muscle; 6- Calcaneus (plantar lobe of the tuber calcanei); 7- Sustentaculum tali, 7a- groove for the lateral digital flexor muscle, 7b- medial margin; 8- Proximal tubercle of the talus; 9- Second metatarsal bone (medial splint bone); 10- Third metatarsal bone; 11- Fourth metatarsal bone (lateral splint bone); 12- Long medial collateral ligament; 13- Short medial collateral ligament, 13a- talean fasciculus, 13b- calcaneal fasciculus; 14- Long plantar ligament; 15- Distal plantar ligament, 15a- lateral part continuing in the third interosseous muscle (suspensory ligament), 15b- medial part fusing with the long medial collateral ligament; 16- Third interosseous muscle (suspensory ligament), 16a- tarsal origin, 16b- metatarsal origin.

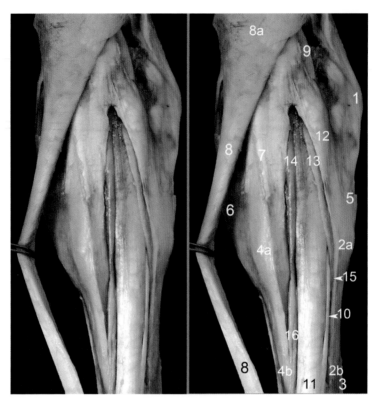

Fig. M.23 **Plantar aspect of the dissected tarsus: plantar nerves.**

1- Tibia (medial malleolus); 2- Second metatarsal bone (medial splint bone), 2a- head, 2b- body; 3- Third metatarsal bone; 4- Fourth metatarsal bone, 4a- head, 4b- body; 5- Long medial collateral ligament; 6- Long lateral collateral ligament; 7- Long plantar ligament; 8- Superficial digital flexor tendon (reclined), 8a- cap; 9- Lateral digital flexor tendon; 10- Medial digital flexor tendon; 11- Deep digital flexor tendon; 12- Flexor retinaculum; 13- Medial plantar nerve; 14- Lateral plantar nerve; 15- Medial (II) plantar common digital nerve; 16- Lateral (III) plantar common digital nerve.

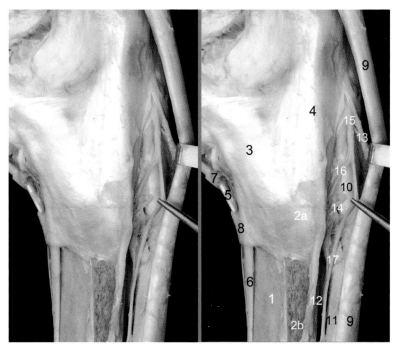

Fig. M.24 **Plantarolateral aspect of the dissected tarsus: lateral plantar nerve.**

1- Third metatarsal bone; 2- Fourth metatarsal bone, 2a- head, 2b- body; 3- Long lateral collateral ligament; 4- Long plantar ligament; 5- Long digital extensor tendon; 6- Lateral digital extensor tendon; 7- Intermediate (tarsal) retinaculum; 8- Distal (metatarsal) retinaculum; 9- Superficial digital flexor tendon (reclined); 10- Lateral digital flexor tendon; 11- Deep digital flexor tendon and accessory ligament; 12- Third interosseous muscle (suspensory ligament); 13- Flexor retinaculum (cut and open); 14- Plantar tarsal sheath (membrane and cavity); 15- Lateral plantar nerve; 16- Deep ramus; 17- Lateral (III) plantar common digital nerve.

M.4 CROSS-SECTIONS

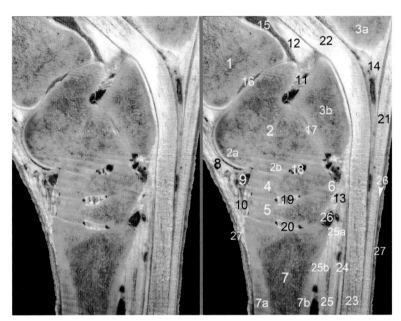

Fig. M.25 **Sagittal section of the tarsus.**

1- Tibial cochlea (distal epiphysis); 2- Talus, 2a- medial trochlea ridge, 2b- head; 3- Calcaneus, 3a- tuber calcanei, 3b- sustentaculum tali; 4- Central tarsal bone; 5- Third tarsal bone; 6- Fourth tarsal bone; 7- Third metatarsal bone, 7a- dorsal cortex, 7b- plantar cortex; 8- Dorsal capsule of the tarsocrural joint; 9- Distodorsal recess of the tarsocrural joint; 10- Talometatarsal (talo-centrodistometatarsal) ligament; 11- Proximomedial talocalcaneal ligament; 12- Proximal plantar ligament of the tarsus; 13- Distal plantar ligament of the tarsus; 14- Long plantar ligament (origin); 15- Proximoplantar recess of the tarsocrural joint; 16- Tarsocrural joint; 17- Medial talocalcaneal joint; 18- Interosseous ligament of the proximal intertarsal (talocentral) joint; 19- Interosseous ligament of the distal intertarsal (centrodistal) joint; 20- Interosseous ligament of the tarsometatarsal joint; 21- Superficial digital flexor tendon; 22- Lateral digital flexor tendon; 23- Deep digital flexor tendon; 24- Accessory ligament of the deep digital flexor tendon; 25- Third interosseous muscle (suspensory ligament), 25a- tarsal origin, 25b- metatarsal origin; 26- Plantar tarsal fascia; 27- Skin.

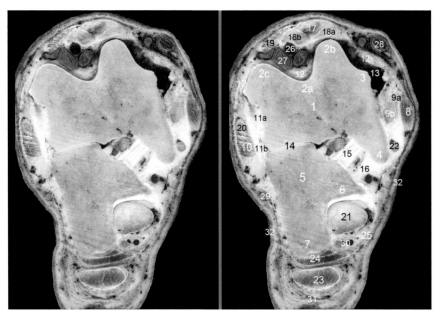

Fig. M.26 **Transverse section of the proximal tarsus. Dorsal is to the top; lateral is to the left.**

1- Talus (body); 2- Trochlea of the talus, 2a- groove, 2b- medial trochlea ridge, 2c- lateral trochlea ridge; 3- Medial articular margin of the talus articular surface; 4- Proximal tubercle of the talus; 5- Calcaneus (body); 6- Sustentaculum tali; 7- Tuber calcanei (base); 8- Long medial collateral ligament; 9- Short medial collateral ligament, 9a- talean fasciculus, 9b- calcaneal fasciculus; 10- Long lateral collateral ligament; 11- Short lateral collateral ligament, 11a- talean fasciculus, 11b- calcanean fasciculus; 12- Dorsal capsule of the tarsocrural joint; 13- Dorsomedial recess of the tarsocrural joint; 14- Lateral talocalcaneal joint; 15- Interosseous talocalcaneal ligament (proximal part); 16- Proximomedial talocalcaneal ligament; 17- Tibialis cranialis tendon; 18- Peroneus tertius tendon, 18a- metatarsal branch, 18b- tarsal (quartal) branch; 19- Long digital extensor tendon; 20- Lateral digital extensor tendon; 21- Lateral digital flexor tendon (in the tarsal sheath); 22- Medial digital flexor tendon; 23- Superficial digital flexor tendon; 24- Long plantar ligament; 25- Flexor retinaculum; 26- Dorsal pedal artery; 27- Dorsal pedal veins; 28- Medial saphenous vein (cranial root); 29- Lateral saphenous vein; 30- Plantar arteries, vein and nerves; 31- Subcutaneous tissue (swollen); 32- Skin.

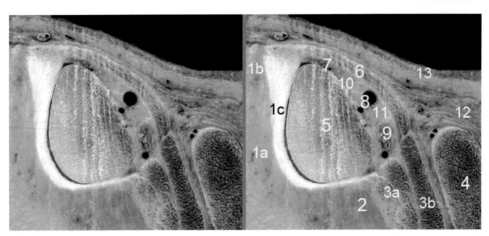

Fig. M.27 **Transverse section of the proximal tarsus; zoom on the plantar tarsal sheath. Dorsal is to the left; medial is on the top.**

1- Sustentaculum tali, 1a- groove for the lateral digital flexor tendon, 1b- medial margin, 1c- fibrocartilage; 2- calcaneus (body); 3- Long plantar ligament, 3a- dorsal layer, 3b- plantar layer; 4- Superficial digital flexor tendon; 5- Lateral digital flexor tendon (in the tarsal sheath); 6- Flexor retinaculum; 7- Tarsal sheath cavity and synovial membrane; 8- Plantar artery; 9- Plantar vein; 10- Medial plantar nerve; 11- Lateral plantar nerve; 12- Subcutaneous tissue (swollen); 13- Skin.

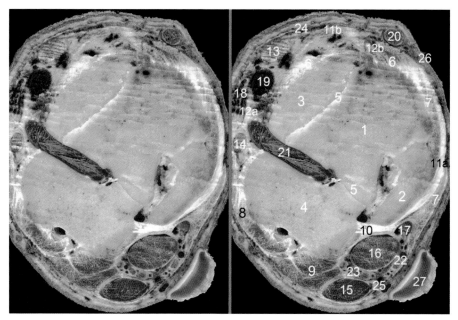

Fig. M.28 **Transverse section of the distal tarsus. Dorsal is on the top; lateral is to the left.**

1- Central tarsal bone; 2- First tarsal bone; 3- Third tarsal bone; 4- Fourth tarsal bone; 5- Proximal intertarsal (centrodistal) joint; 6- Talometatarsal (talocentrodistometatarsal) ligament; 7- Long medial collateral ligament; 8- Long lateral collateral ligament; 9- Long plantar ligament; 10- Distal plantar ligament; 11- Tibialis cranialis tendon, 11a- tarsal (cunean) branch, 11b- metatarsal branch; 12- Peroneus tertius distal tendon, 12a- tarsal (quartal) branch, 12b- metatarsal branch; 13- Long digital extensor tendon; 14- Lateral digital extensor tendon; 15- Superficial digital flexor tendon; 16- Lateral digital flexor tendon (in the tarsal sheath); 17- Medial digital flexor tendon; 18- Short digital extensor tendon; 19- Dorsal pedal artery; 20- Medial saphenous vein (cranial root); 21- Perforating tarsal vein; 22- Medial plantar artery and nerve; 23- Lateral plantar artery, vein and nerve; 24- Dorsal tarsal fascia; 25- Plantar tarsal fascia; 26- Skin; 27- Chestnut.

THE METATARSUS

N.1 PHYSICAL ASPECT

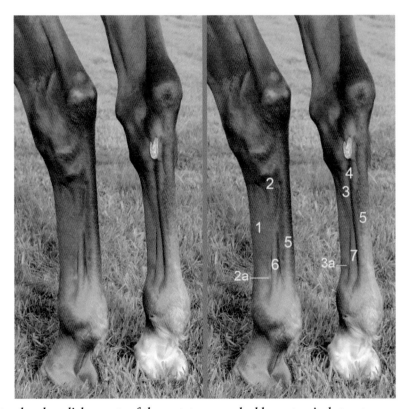

Fig. N.1 **Lateral and medial aspects of the metatarsus: palpable anatomical structures.**

1- Third metatarsal bone; 2- Lateral metatarsal (lateral splint) bone (head), 2a- distal end; 3- Medial metatarsal bone, 3a- distal end; 4- Distomedial sulcus of the hock; 5- Flexor tendons; 6- Suspensory ligament (lateral margin of the body and lateral branch); 7- Suspensory ligament (medial margin of the body and medial branch).

N.2 RADIOGRAPHIC ANATOMY

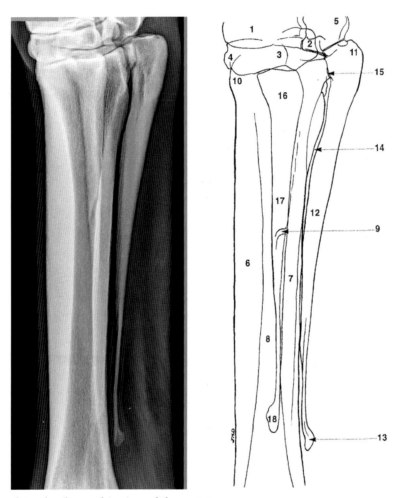

Fig. N.2 **Dorsolateral radiographic view of the metatarsus.**

Tarsus: 1- Central tarsal bone; 2- First tarsal bone; 3- Second tarsal bone; 4- Third tarsal bone; 5- Fourth tarsal bone;

Metatarsus – Third metatarsal bone: 6- Dorsomedial cortex; 7- Plantarolateral cortex; 8- Medullary cavity; 9- Vascular canal; 10- Insertion surface of the peroneus tertius tendon (metatarsal branch); **Fourth metatarsal bone:** 11- Head (insertion of the long lateral collateral ligament and long plantar ligament); 12- Body; 13- Distal extremity; 14- Third (lateral) inter-metatarsal syndesmosis; 15- Synovial lateral intermetatarsal joint; **Second metatarsal bone:** 16- Head; 17- Body; 18- Distal extremity.

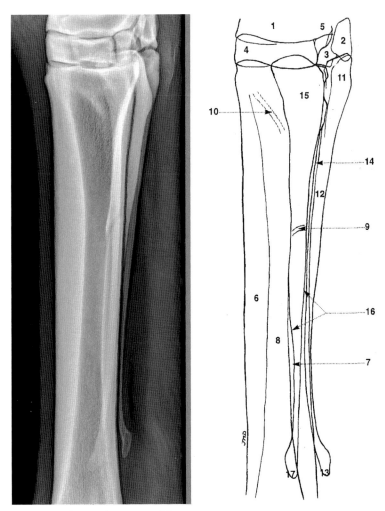

Fig. N.3 **Dorsomedial radiographic view of the metatarsus.**

Tarsus: 1- Central tarsal bone; 2- First tarsal bone; 3- Second tarsal bone; 4- Third tarsal bone; 5- Fourth tarsal bone;

Metatarsus – Third metatarsal bone: 6- Dorsolateral cortex; 7- Plantaromedial cortex; 8- Medullary cavity; 9- Vascular canal; 10- Vascular sulcus of the third dorsal metatarsal artery; **Second metatarsal bone:** 11- Head (insertion of the long medial collateral ligament); 12- Body; 13- Distal extremity; 14- Second (medial) intermetatarsal syndesmosis; **Fourth metatarsal bone:** 15- Head; 16- Body; 17- Distal extremity.

N.3 DISSECTED SPECIMEN

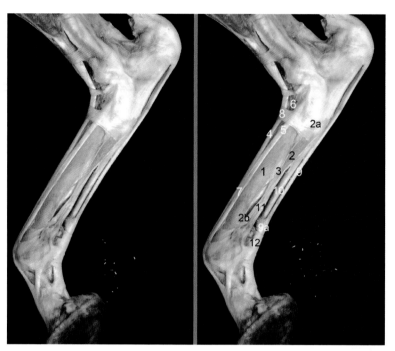

Fig. N.4 **Lateral aspect of the distal pelvic limb.**

1- Third metatarsal bone; 2- Fourth metatarsal bone (body), 2a- head, 2b- distal extremity; 3- Third (lateral) intermetatarsal syndesmosis; 4- Long digital extensor tendon; 5- Lateral digital extensor tendon; 6- Short digital extensor muscle; 7- Common tendon for the three digital extensor structures; 8- Distal (metatarsal) extensor retinaculum; 9- Superficial digital flexor tendon, 9a- manica flexoria; 10- Deep digital flexor tendon, 11- Third interosseous muscle (suspensory ligament) bifurcation; 12- Plantar annular ligament.

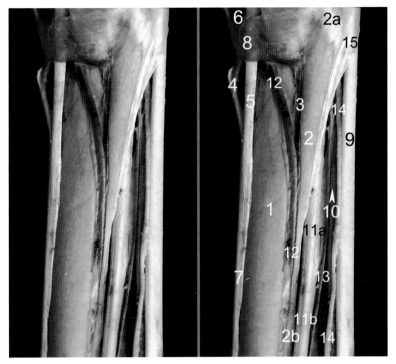

Fig. N.5 **Lateral aspect of the metatarsus.**

1- Third metatarsal bone; 2- Fourth metatarsal bone (body), 2a- head, 2b- distal extremity; 3- Third (lateral) intermetatarsal syndesmosis; 4- Long digital extensor tendon; 5- Lateral digital extensor tendon; 6- Short digital extensor muscle; 7- Common tendon for the three digital extensor structures; 8- Distal (metatarsal) extensor retinaculum; 9- Superficial digital flexor tendon; 10- Deep digital flexor tendon, 11- Third interosseous muscle (suspensory ligament), 11a- body, 11b- bifurcation; 12- Third dorsal metatarsal artery; 13- Lateral (fourth) plantar metatarsal vein (empty); 14- Lateral (fourth) plantar metatarsal nerve; 15- Plantar metatarsal fascia.

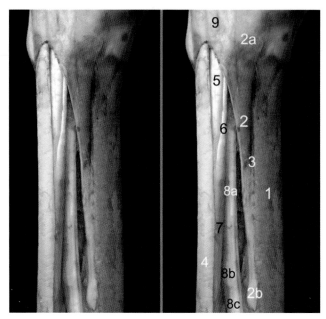

Fig. N.6 **Plantaromedial aspect of the metatarsus.**

1- Third metatarsal bone; 2- Second metatarsal bone (body), 2a- head, 2b- distal extremity; 3- Second (medial) intermetatarsal syndesmosis; 4- Superficial digital flexor tendon; 5- Lateral digital flexor tendon; 6- Medial digital flexor tendon; 7- Deep digital flexor tendon; 8- Third interosseous muscle (suspensory ligament), 8a- body, 8b- bifurcation, 8c- medial branch; 9- Plantar tarsal fascia.

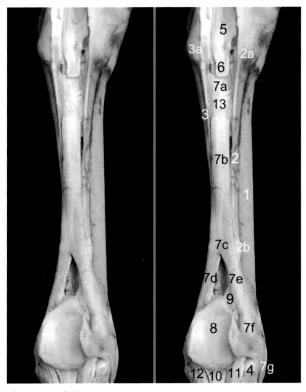

Fig. N.7 **Plantaromedial aspect of the suspensory apparatus.**

1- Third metatarsal bone; 2- Second metatarsal bone (body), 2a- head, 2b- distal extremity; 3- Lateral metatarsal bone (body), 3a- head; 4- Medial plantar eminence of the proximal phalanx; 5- Distal plantar ligament of the tarsus; 6- Accessory ligament of the deep digital flexor tendon (origin); 7- Third interosseous muscle (suspensory ligament), 7a- origin, 7b- body, 7c- bifurcation, 7d- lateral branch, 7e- medial branch, 7f- distal enthesis over the medial proximal sesamoid bone, 7g- medial extensor branch; 8- Plantar (intersesamoidean) ligament; 9- Interosseoplantar ligament; 10- Straight sesamoidean ligament; 11- Medial oblique sesamoidean ligament; 12- Lateral oblique sesamoidean ligament; 13- Deep plantar metatarsal (interosseous) fascia.

N.4 CROSS-SECTIONS

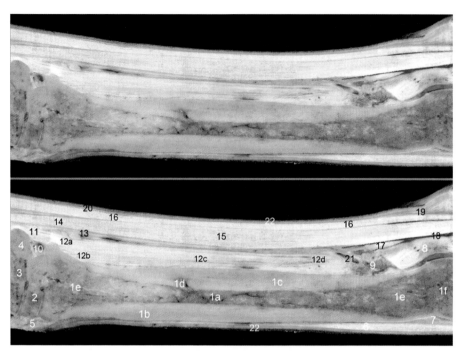

Fig. N.8 **Sagittal section of the metatarsus. Proximal is to the left.**

1- Third metatarsal bone, 1a- medullary cavity, 1b- dorsal cortex, 1c- plantar cortex, 1d- vascular foramen, 1e- spongy bone, 1f- metatarsal condyle; 2- Third tarsal bone; 3- Central tarsal bone; 4- Fourth tarsal bone; 5- Talometatarsal ligament and tibialis cranialis muscle distal insertion; 6- Long digital extensor tendon; 7- Dorsal capsule of the metatarsophalangeal joint; 8- Plantar (intersesamoidean) ligament (of the metatarsophalangeal joint); 9- Proximoplantar recess of the metatarsophalangeal joint; 10- Plantarolateral recess of the tarsometatarsal joint; 11- Distal plantar ligament of the tarsus; 12- Third interosseous muscle (suspensory ligament), 12a- tarsal component, 12b- metatarsal origin, 12c- body, 12d- bifurcation; 13- Accessory ligament of the deep digital flexor tendon; 14- Lateral digital flexor tendon; 15- Deep digital flexor tendon; 16- Superficial digital flexor tendon; 17- Manica flexoria; 18- Digital sheath cavity; 19- Plantar annular ligament; 20- Plantar metatarsal fascia; 21- Distal part of the third dorsal metatarsal artery; 22- Skin.

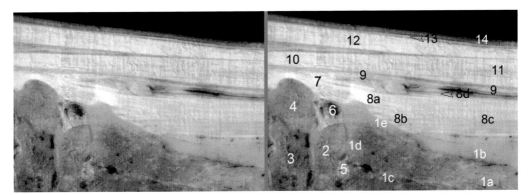

Fig. N.9 **Sagittal section of the proximal metatarsus. Proximal is to the left.**

1- Third metatarsal bone, 1a- medullary cavity, 1b- plantar cortex, 1c- spongy bone, 1d- subchondral bone; 2- Third tarsal bone; 3- Central tarsal bone; 4- Fourth tarsal bone; 5- Interosseous ligament of the tarsometatarsal joint; 6- Plantarolateral recess of the tarsometatarsal joint; 7- Distal plantar ligament of the tarsus; 8- Third interosseous muscle (suspensory ligament), 8a- tarsal component, 8b- metatarsal origin, 8c- body; 9- Accessory ligament of the deep digital flexor tendon; 10- Lateral digital flexor tendon; 11- Deep digital flexor tendon; 12- Superficial digital flexor tendon; 13- Plantar metatarsal fascia; 14- Skin.

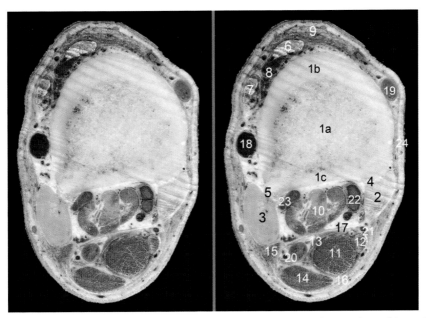

Fig. N.10 **Transverse section of the proximal metatarsus. Dorsal is to the top; lateral is to the left.**

1- Third metatarsal bone, 1a- spongy bone, 1b- dorsal cortex, 1c- plantar cortex; 2- Second metatarsal bone; 3- Fourth metatarsal bone; 4- Second metatarsal syndesmosis; 5- Third metatarsal syndesmosis; 6- Long digital extensor tendon; 7- Lateral digital extensor tendon; 8- Short digital extensor muscle; 9- Dorsal metatarsal fascia and distal (metatarsal) extensor retinaculum;

10- Third interosseous muscle (suspensory ligament, proximal part of the body); 11- Lateral digital flexor tendon; 12- Medial digital flexor tendon; 13- Distal recess of the tarsal sheath and accessory ligament of the deep digital flexor tendon; 14- Superficial digital flexor tendon; 15- Long plantar ligament (distal part); 16- Plantar (superficial) metatarsal fascia; 17- Deep plantar metatarsal (interosseous) fascia; 18- Third dorsal metatarsal artery; 19- Medial saphenous vein (cranial root); 20- Lateral common digital artery, vein and nerve; 21-Medial common digital artery and nerve; 22- Medial plantar metatarsal artery and vein; 23- Lateral plantar metatarsal vein; 24- Skin.

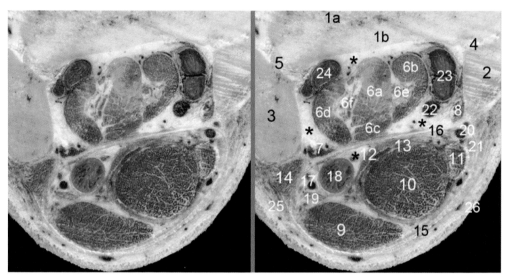

Fig. N.11 Transverse section of the proximal metatarsus focused on the plantar structures. Dorsal is to the top; lateral is to the left.

1- Third metatarsal bone, 1a- spongy bone, 1b- plantar cortex; 2- Second metatarsal bone; 3- Fourth metatarsal bone; 4- Second metatarsal syndesmosis; 5- Third metatarsal syndesmosis; 6- Third interosseous muscle (suspensory ligament, proximal part of the body), 6a- sagittal part, 6b- medial part, 6c- plantar part, 6d- lateral part, 6e- medial fat bundle (with striated muscle fibres), 6f- lateral fat bundle (with striated muscle fibres); 7- Vestigial lateral (fourth) interosseous muscle; 8- Vestigial medial (second) interosseous muscle; *- adipose connective tissue in the interosseous compartment; 9- Superficial digital flexor tendon; 10- Lateral digital flexor tendon; 11- Medial digital flexor tendon; 12- Accessory ligament of the deep digital flexor tendon; 13- Distal recess of the tarsal sheath; 14- Long plantar ligament (distal part); 15- Plantar (superficial) metatarsal fascia; 16- Deep plantar metatarsal (interosseous) fascia; 17- Lateral common digital artery; 18- Lateral common digital vein; 19- Lateral common digital nerve; 20- Medial common digital artery; 21- Medial common digital nerve; 22- Medial plantar metatarsal artery; 23- Medial plantar metatarsal vein; 24- Lateral plantar metatarsal vein; 25- Subcutaneous connective tissue; 26- Skin.

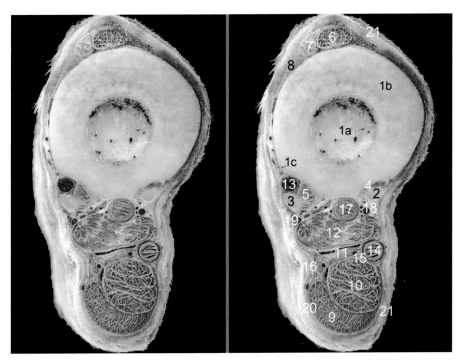

Fig. N.12 **Transverse section in the middle metatarsus. Dorsal is to the top; lateral is to the left.**

1- Third metatarsal bone, 1a- medullary cavity, 1b- dorsomedial cortex, 1c- periosteum; 2- Second metatarsal bone; 3- Fourth metatarsal bone; 4- Second metatarsal syndesmosis; 5- Third metatarsal syndesmosis; 6- Long digital extensor tendon; 7- Lateral digital extensor tendon (fused with the long); 8- Dorsal metatarsal fascia; 9- Superficial digital flexor tendon; 10- Deep digital flexor tendon (having incorporated its accessory ligament); 11- Intertendinous connective tissue; 12- Third interosseous muscle (suspensory ligament, distal part of the body); 13- Third dorsal metatarsal artery; 14- Medial common digital vein (providing the cranial root of the medial saphenous vein); 15- Medial common digital artery and nerve; 16- Lateral common digital artery (vein) and nerve; 17- Plantar metatarsal vein; 18- Medial plantar metatarsal artery; 19- Lateral plantar metatarsal artery; 20- Plantar (superficial) metatarsal fascia; 21- Skin.

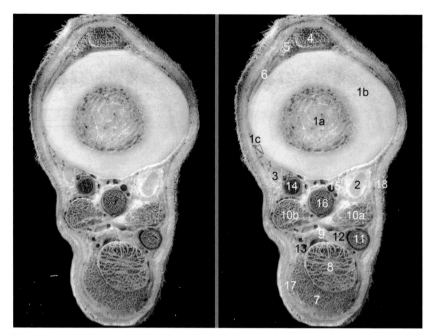

Fig. N.13 **Transverse section in the distal third of the metatarsus. Dorsal is to the top; lateral is to the left.**

1- Third metatarsal bone, 1a- medullary cavity, 1b- dorsomedial cortex, 1c- periosteum; 2- Second metatarsal bone; 3- Fourth metatarsal bone; 4- Long digital extensor tendon; 5- Lateral digital extensor tendon (fused with the long); 6- Dorsal metatarsal fascia; 7- Superficial digital flexor tendon; 8- Deep digital flexor tendon (having incorporated its accessory ligament); 9- Intertendinous connective tissue; 10- Third interosseous muscle (suspensory ligament), 10a- medial branch, 10b- lateral branch; 11- Medial common digital vein (providing the cranial root of the medial saphenous vein); 12- Medial common digital nerve; 13- Lateral common digital artery (vein) and nerve; 14- Third dorsal metatarsal artery (joining the metatarsal arteries); 15- Plantar metatarsal artery; 16- Plantar metatarsal vein; 17- Plantar (superficial) metatarsal fascia; 18- Skin.

THE DIGITAL AREA OF THE PELVIC LIMB

O.1 PHYSICAL ASPECT

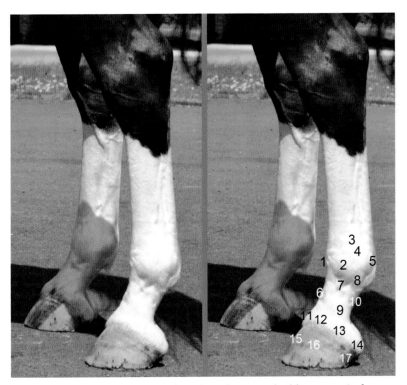

Fig. O.1 **Lateral and medial aspects of the pelvic digital area: palpable anatomical structures.**

1- Dorsal aspect of the fetlock; 2- Collateral ligament of the fetlock; 3- Plantaroproximal recess of the fetlock joint; 4- Branch of the suspensory ligament; 5- Plantar aspect of the fetlock; 6- Dorsal aspect of the pastern; 7- Extensor branch of the suspensory ligament; 8- Neurovascular fasciculus; 9- Flexor tuberosity of the middle phalanx; 10- Flexor tendons; 11- Dorsal aspect of the coronet; 12- Dorsocollateral aspect (collateral ligament of the distal interphalangeal joint); 13- Ungular cartilage; 14- Bulb of the heel; 15- Toe; 16- Quarter; 17- Heel.

O.2 RADIOGRAPHIC ANATOMY

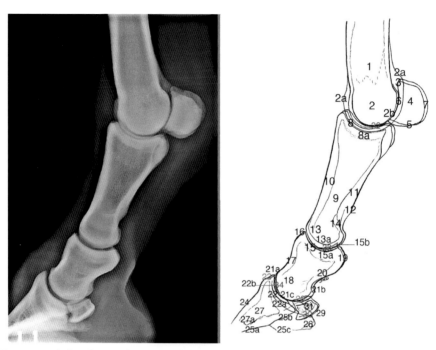

Fig. O.2 **Lateromedial radiographic view of the pelvic digital area.**

Metatarsus: 1- Distal metaphysis; 2- Metatarsal condyle; 2a- Sagittal ridge, 2b- collateral parts;

Proximal sesamoid bones: 3- Apex; 4- Body; 5- Base; 6- Articular surface; 7- Plantar margin;

Proximal phalanx: 8- Glenoid cavity, 8a- subchondral bone of the sagittal groove; 9- Medullary cavity; 10- Dorsal cortex; 11- Plantar cortex; 12- Apex of the trigonum (insertion of the oblique sesamoidean ligaments); 13- Condyle, 13a- subchondral bone of the sagittal groove; 14- Supracondylar fossa for insertion of the scutocompedal ligament (attachment of the scutum medium and through it, superficial digital flexor tendon);

Middle phalanx: 15- Glenoid cavity, 15a- subchondral bone, 15b- sagittal ridge (plantar end); 16- Extensor process; 17- Dorsal compact bone; 18- Insertion fossa of the collateral ligament of the distal interphalangeal joint; 19- Flexor tuberosity; 20- Plantar compact bone; 21- Condyle, 21a- dorsal margin of the articular surface, 21b- plantar margin of the articular surface, 21c- subchondral bone of the sagittal groove;

Distal phalanx: 22- Glenoid cavity, 22a- subchondral bone, 22b- sagittal ridge; 23- Extensor process; 24- Parietal surface; 25- Solar surface, 25a- cutaneous plane, 25b- flexor surface, 25c- semilunar line; 26- Plantar process; 27- Body of the distal phalanx, 27a- semilunar sinus;

Distal sesamoid bone: 28- Articular surface; 29- Flexor surface; 30- Plantar compact bone; 31- Spongy bone;

Joints: 32- Metatarsophalangeal joint; 33- Proximal interphalangeal joint; 34- Distal interphalangeal joint.

O.3 DISSECTED SPECIMEN

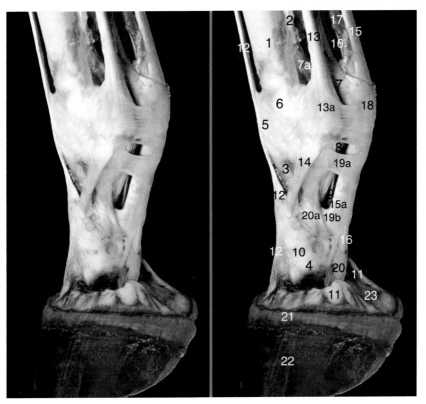

Fig. O.3 **Lateral aspect of the digital regions of the pelvic limb: superficial structures.**

1- Third metatarsal bone; 2- Fourth metatarsal bone (extremity); 3- Proximal phalanx; 4- Middle phalanx (flexor tuberosity); 5- Dorsal capsule of metatarsophalangeal joint; 6- Collateral ligament of the metatarsophalangeal joint; 7- Plantar (intersesamoidean) ligament (suprasesamoidean part), 7a- metatarsointersesamoidean ligament; 8- Oblique sesamoidean ligament; 9- Intermediate (obliquorectum) sesamoidean ligament; 10- Collateral ligament of the proximal interphalangeal (PIP) joint; 11- Ungular cartilage; 12- Long digital extensor tendon; 13- Lateral branch of the third interosseous muscle (suspensory ligament), 13a- distal enthesis; 14- Lateral extensor branch of the third interosseous muscle; 15- Superficial digital flexor tendon, 15a- (distal) branch; 16- Deep digital flexor tendon; 17- lumbrical muscle; 18- Plantar annular ligament; 19- Proximal digital annular ligament, 19a- proximal attachment, 19b- distal attachment; 20- Distal digital annular ligament, 20a- proximal attachment; 21- Periopleum; 22- Hoof wall; 23- Digital cushion.

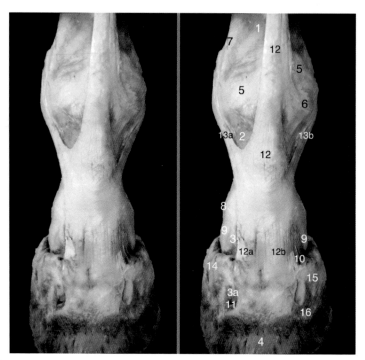

Fig. O.4 **Dorsal aspect of the digital regions of the pelvic limb: superficial structures.**

1- Third metatarsal bone; 2- Proximal phalanx; 3- Middle phalanx; 4- Distal phalanx; 5- Dorsal capsule of metatarsophalangeal joint; 6- Dorsal metatarsophalangeal fascia; 7- Collateral ligament of the metatarsophalangeal joint; 8- Collateral ligament of the proximal interphalangeal joint; 9- Collateral sesamoidean ligament; 10- Chondrocoronal ligament; 11- Distal interphalangeal joint space; 12- Long digital extensor tendon; 12a- medial lobe, 12b- lateral lobe; 13- Extensor branches of the third interosseous muscle (suspensory ligament), 13a- medial extensor branch, 13b- lateral extensor branch; 14- Medial ungular cartilage; 15- Lateral ungular cartilage; 16- Collateral fossa of the distal phalanx (insertion of the lateral collateral ligament of the distal interphalangeal joint).

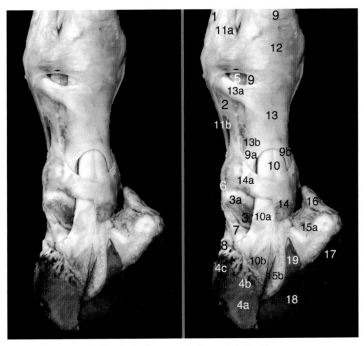

Fig. O.5 **Plantarolateral aspect of the digital area of the pelvic limb.**

1- Third metatarsal bone; 2- Proximal phalanx; 3- Middle phalanx, 3a- flexor tuberosity; 4- Distal phalanx, 4a- cutaneous plane, 4b- semilunar line, 4c- palmar process; 5- Oblique sesamoidean ligament; 6- Collateral ligament of the proximal interphalangeal joint; 7- Collateral sesamoidean ligament; 8- Ungular cartilage; 9- Superficial digital flexor tendon, 9a- lateral branch, 9b- medial branch; 10- Deep digital flexor tendon, 10a- lateral lobe, suprasesamoidean part, 10b- lateral lobe, infrasesamoidean part; 11- Third interosseous muscle (suspensory ligament), 11a- branch, 11b- extensor branch; 12- Plantar annular ligament; 13- Proximal digital annular ligament, 13a- proximal attachment, 13b- distal attachment covering the branch of the superficial digital flexor tendon; 14- Distal digital annular ligament (cut to show the lateral lobe of the deep digital flexor tendon), 14a- proximal attachment; 15- Digital cushion, 15a- collateral part, 15b- sagittal (cuneal) part; 16- Ungular cartilage; 17- Parietal corium of the inflex part of the hoof wall (bar); 18- Solar corium; 19- Corium of the frog.

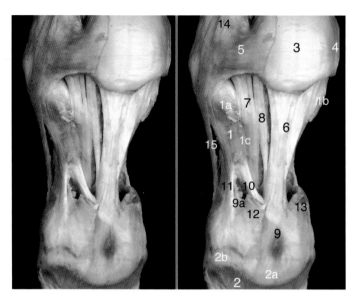

Fig. O.6 Plantarolateral aspect of the hind pastern: sesamoidean ligaments.

1- Proximal phalanx, 1a- lateral plantar eminence, 1b- medial plantar eminence, 1c- trigonum of the proximal phalanx (medial margin); 2- Middle phalanx, 2a- sagittal part of the flexor tuberosity, 2b- Collateral part of the flexor tuberosity; 3- Plantar (intersesamoidean) ligament (sesamoidean part); 4- Insertion of the plantar annular ligament (cut); 5- Collateral sesamoidean ligament; 6- Straight sesamoidean ligament; 7- Oblique sesamoidean ligament; 8- Intermediate (obliquo-rectum) sesamoidean ligament; 9- Middle scutum, 9a- scutocompedal ligament; 10- Axial palmar ligament of the proximal interphalangeal joint; 11- Abaxial palmar ligament of the proximal interphalangeal joint; 12- Lateral branch of the superficial digital flexor tendon; 13- Medial branch of the superficial digital flexor tendon; 14- Lateral branch of the third interosseous muscle (suspensory ligament); 15- Lateral extensor branch of the third interosseous muscle.

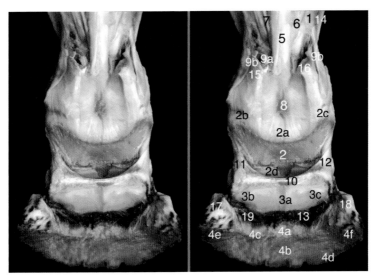

Fig. O.7 **Plantar aspect of the pelvic foot.**

1- Proximal phalanx; 2- Middle phalanx, 2a- sagittal part of the flexor tuberosity, 2b- lateral collateral part of the flexor tuberosity, 2c- medial collateral part of the flexor tuberosity; 3- Distal sesamoid bone, 3a- sagittal ridge of the flexor surface, 3b- Lateral angle, 3c- medial angle; 4- Distal phalanx, 4a- flexor surface, 4b- cutaneous plane, 4c- semilunar line, 4d- solar border, 4e- lateral palmar process, 4f- medial palmar process; 5- Straight sesamoidean ligament; 6- Oblique sesamoidean ligament; 7- Intermediate (obliquorectum) sesamoidean ligament; 8- Middle scutum; 9- Palmar ligaments of the proximal interphalangeal joint, 9a- axial, 9b- abaxial (covered by the proximal attachment of the distal digital annular ligament); 10- Proximal sesamoidean ligament; 11- Lateral collateral sesamoidean ligament; 12- Medial collateral sesamoidean ligament; 13- Distal (impar) sesamoidean ligament; 14- Extensor branch of the third interosseous muscle (suspensory ligament); 15- Lateral branch of the superficial digital flexor tendon; 16- Medial branch of the superficial digital flexor tendon; 17- Lateral ungular cartilage (cut); 18- Medial ungular cartilage (cut); 19- Proper digital artery entering the solar canal.

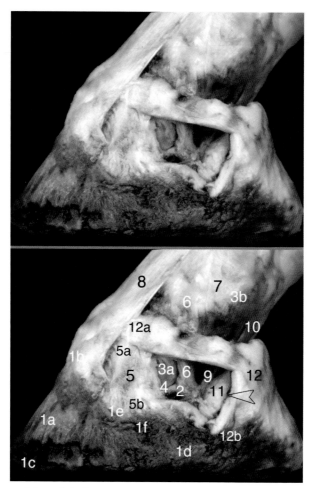

Fig. O.8 **Lateral aspect of the pelvic foot.**

1- Distal phalanx, 1a- parietal surface, 1b- extensor process, 1c- solar border, 1d- plantar process, 1e- collateral fossa for the collateral ligament, 1f- parietal sulcus; 2- Distal sesamoid bone; 3- Middle phalanx, 3a- condyle, 3b- flexor tuberosity; 4- Distal interphalangeal joint; 5- Collateral ligament of the distal interphalangeal joint, 5a- proximal insertion, 5b- distal insertion; 6- Collateral sesamoidean ligament; 7- Collateral ligament of the proximal interphalangeal joint; 8- Long digital extensor tendon; 9- Deep digital flexor tendon; 10- Distal digital annular ligament; 11- Digital cushion; 12- Ungular cartilage (with an open window in it, arrowhead), 12a- chondrocoronal ligament, 12b- chondroungular junction (ligament).

O.4 CROSS-SECTIONS

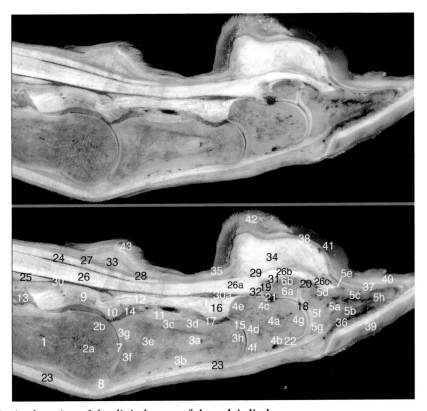

Fig. O.9 **Sagittal section of the digital areas of the pelvic limb.**

1-Metatarsal distal metaphysis; 2- Metatarsal condyle, 2a- spongy bone, 2b- subchondral bone of the sagittal ridge; 3- Proximal phalanx, 3a- medullary cavity, 3b- dorsal cortex, 3c- plantar cortex, 3d- trigonum of the proximal phalanx (distal limit), 3e- spongy bone, 3f- subchondral bone, 3g- sagittal groove of the glenoid cavity, 3h- condyle; 4- Middle phalanx, 4a- spongy bone, 4b- dorsal compact bone, 4c- plantar compact bone, 4d- subchondral bone of the glenoid cavity, 4e- flexor tuberosity, 4f- extensor process, 4g- condyle; 5- Distal phalanx, 5a- spongy bone, 5b- dorsal compact bone of the parietal surface, 5c- compact bone of the cutaneous plane, 5d- compact bone of the flexor surface, 5e- semilunar line, 5f- subchondral bone of the glenoid cavity, 5g- extensor process; 6- Distal sesamoid bone, 6a- spongy bone, 6b- compact bone of the flexor surface; 7- Metatarsophalangeal joint (MTPJ); 8- Dorsal capsule of the MTPJ; 9- Plantar (intersesamoidean) ligament; 10- Cruciate sesamoidean ligaments; 11- Oblique sesamoidean ligaments (fused in the sagittal plane); 12- Straight sesamoidean ligament; 13- Proximoplantar recess of the MTPJ; 14- Distoplantar recess of the MTPJ; 15- Proximal interphalangeal joint; 16- Middle scutum; 17- Plantar recess of the proximal interphalangeal joint; 18- Distal interphalangeal joint (DIPJ); 19- Proximal sesamoidean ligament; 20- Distal sesamoidean ligament; 21- Proximoplantar recess of the DIPJ; 22- Dorsal recess of the DIPJ; 23- Long digital extensor tendon; 24- Superficial digital flexor tendon; 25- Manica flexoria; 26- Deep digital flexor tendon, 26a- suprasesamoidean part, 26b- sesamoidean part, 26c- infrasesamoidean part; 27- Plantar annular ligament; 28- Proximal digital annular ligament; 29- Distal digital annular ligament; 30- Digital sheath synovial cavity, 30a- distodorsal recess; 31- Podotrochlear bursa; 32- Transverse ligament; 33- Ergot cushion; 34- Digital cushion; 35- Skin; 36- Parietal corium; 37- Solar corium; 38- Corium of the frog; 39- Hoof wall; 40- Sole; 41- Frog; 42- Bulb of the heels; 43- Ergot.

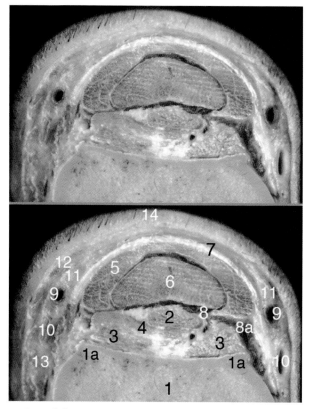

Fig. O.10 **Transverse section of the pastern of the pelvic limb at the proximal third of the proximal phalanx.**

1- Proximal phalanx, 1a- margins of the trigonum; 2- Straight sesamoidean ligament; 3- Oblique sesamoidean ligament; 4-Intermediate (obliquorectum) sesamoidean ligament; 5- Superficial digital flexor tendon; 6- Deep digital flexor tendon; 7- Proximal digital annular ligament; 8- Digital sheath cavity, 8a- collateral recess; 9- Proper digital artery; 10- Proper digital vein (collapsed); 11- Proper digital nerve; 12- Ergot ligament; 13- Connective tissue (swollen); 14- Skin.

Abdomen, 151, 162, 163
Accessoriocarpoulnar interosseous ligament, 72
Accessoriocarpoulnar joint, 52, 53, 56
Accessoriocarpoulnar ligament, 64, 85
Accessoriometacarpal ligament, 44, 63, 64, 66, 73, 76, 80, 84, 85, 87
Accessorioquartal interosseous ligament, 73
Accessorioquartal ligament, 64
Accessoriosuperficial fibers, 80, 88, 90
Accessorioulnar joint, 52, 53, 56
Accessorioulnar ligament, 64
Accessory carpal bone
    antebrachium, 35, 38, 39, 42, 44
    carpus, 49, 50, 51, 52, 53, 54, 55, 56, 57, 62, 63, 64, 68, 72
        and adjacent areas, 60, 65, 67
        anatomical structures, 74, 75, 76
        joint structures, 66
    metacarpus, 80, 84, 85
Accessory digital extensor tendon
    carpus, 59, 60, 62, 73
    metacarpus, 80, 81, 87, 88, 90, 91, 92, 93, 94, 95
    thoracic limb fetlock, 126
Accessory ligament, 193
    coxofemoral joint, 193
    deep digital flexor tendon
        antebrachium, 43
        carpus, 49, 62, 65, 66, 67, 74, 75
        distal limb, 77
        interosseous metacarpal enthesis, 89
        metacarpus, 80, 81, 82, 83, 84, 85, 87, 88, 90, 91, 95, 96, 97, 98, 264, 265, 266
        pelvic limb, 190
        suspensory apparatus, 263
        tarsus, 252
    femur, 194, 195
    lateral digital extensor tendon, 44
    superficial digital flexor tendon
        antebrachium, 43, 44, 47
        carpus, 68, 70, 71, 76
        metacarpus, 83
Accessory ligament sulcus, in pubis, 173
Acetabular area, 183, 184
Acetabular labrum, 180, 192
Acetabulum, 172, 173, 174, 191, 192
Adductor brevis muscle, 199
Adductor magnus muscle, 196, 197, 199, 220
Alar foramen, 132, 135, 136
Anconeus muscle, 39, 42

Antebrachial bones, 50, 52, 53, 54, 55, 56, 57
Antebrachial cephalic vein, 35
Antebrachial fascia
    antebrachium, 40, 45, 46, 47
    carpus, 63, 65, 67, 68, 69, 70, 71, 76
    elbow, 25, 32
        and brachium, 26, 28
    shoulder and brachium, 7, 8, 10, 11
Antebrachial interosseous space, 2, 21, 23, 29
Antebrachial muscle, 7, 10, 11, 32
Antebrachial radioulnar syndesmosis, 29
Antebrachiocarpal joint, 50, 51, 53, 54, 55, 56, 57, 61, 71, 74, 75
Antebrachioradial ligament, 71, 72, 74, 75
Antebrachium, 19, 35, 38, 39, 40, 45, 46, 47
    and carpus, 42, 43, 44
    and distal thoracic limb, 37
    on flexed limb, 36
    in flexion, 41
    lateral sulcus of, 36
Aorta, 160, 165, 167, 169, 180, 181, 182, 183, 198
Aponeurosis, 8
Arachnoid, 149
Articular process joint
    caudal cervical area, 140
    caudal thoracic area from T12 to T18, 153
    cervical area at level of C3–C4 intervertebral joint, 147, 148, 149
    cranial part of lumbar vertebral column, 158, 159
    fourth cervical vertebra, 139
    lumbar area
        between fifth and sixth lumbar vertebrae, 169, 170
        between second and third lumbar vertebrae, 167, 168
    mid-thoracic area from T6 to T12, 152
    thoracolumbar area, 165, 166
    thoracolumbar junction, 157
        and lumbar area from T17 to L4, 154, 155
Articular surface, 102, 206
Atlantooccipital joint, 137, 145
Atlas wing, 131, 135, 136
Axial margin, 103, 104, 105
Axillary ansa, 146
Axillary artery, 10, 11, 12, 16, 146
Axillary nerve, 16, 146
Axillary vein, 16

Back and pelvis, 151
Basilar sinus, 137

Biceps brachii muscle
  antebrachium, 39, 40
    and carpus, 42
  elbow, 27, 31, 32
    and brachium, 19, 20, 26, 28, 30
  proximal forelimb, 1
  scapulohumeral joint, 5
  shoulder, 9
    and brachium, 8, 11
    joints, 12, 14
Biceps femoris muscle, 190, 191, 223, 224, 227, 228
  pelvis, 171, 181, 195, 196
  femoral area (thigh), 199
  stifle, 218, 219, 220
Bicipital bursa, 8, 9, 12, 14, 16, 26
Biventer capitis muscle, 147, 148
Brachial artery, 10, 11, 12, 39, 42
  (humeral) artery, 28
Brachial fascia, 7, 8, 32
Brachialis muscle, 1, 7, 8, 11, 16, 17, 25, 26, 30, 32, 35, 40
Brachial muscle(s), 7, 10, 11, 12, 14, 19, 20, 28, 32
Brachial plexus, 144, 146
Brachial sulcus, 2, 37
Brachiocephalicus muscle, 1, 7, 14, 17, 19, 20, 131, 133, 134, 137, 141, 142, 144, 147
Brachium, 7
  and elbow, 19, 20, 26, 28, 30
Brain stem (medulla oblongata), 137

Caecum, 154, 155
Calcaneal fasciculus, 243, 245, 246, 249, 253
Calcaneal tendon, 241, 244, 248
Calcanean cap, 190, 223, 224, 225
Calcanean fasciculus, 253
Calcaneoquartal joint, 232, 233, 234, 235
Calcaneus
  dissected crus, 223
  dissected tarsus, 241, 242, 245, 249
  fibula, 222
  flexed tarsus, 243, 246
  left tarsus, 231, 232, 233, 235, 236, 237
  pelvic limb, 190
  pelvis and femoral region, 197
  point of the hock, 248
  proximal tarsus, 253, 254
  tarsus, 252
    right tarsus, 234
  tibia, 222
Capitis ligament, 195
Carina, 2
Carpal bone(s), see individual carpal bones
Carpal canal, 35, 49, 50, 70, 71, 72, 73, 88
Carpal canal sheath cavity, 74, 75, 76, 87, 88
Carpal sheath, 47, 63
Carpometacarpal joint, 50, 51, 52, 53, 54, 55, 56, 57, 61, 74, 75, 78, 79, 86, 87, 96, 97
Carpus, 47, 61, 62, 63, 64, 66, 68, 69, 71, 72, 73, 74, 75, 76, 80
  and adjacent areas, 59, 60, 65, 67
  common palmar ligament of, 83, 85, 96, 97

  dorsal capsule of, 95, 96
  joint structures, 66
  lateral collateral ligament of, 35, 39, 84, 85, 87
  medial collateral ligament of, 83, 84, 85, 87
  palpable anatomical structures, 49
Cauda equina, 184, 185, 187, 188
Caudal angle, 3, 11
Caudal antebrachial interosseous artery, 46
Caudal antebrachial interosseous vein, 46
Caudal arteries, 183
Caudal articular process, 138, 139, 152, 153, 154, 165
Caudal cervical area, 140
Caudal circumflex artery, 16
Caudal circumflex vein, 16
Caudal cortex
  femur, 203
  humerus, 4, 23
  radius, 23, 46, 52, 56, 74, 75
  tibia, 203, 227, 228
  ulna, 23
Caudal cruciate ligament, 202, 203, 206, 208, 214, 215, 216, 219, 220
Caudal crural septum, 227, 228
Caudal epigastric artery, 183
Caudal femoral artery, 219
Caudal femoral cutaneous nerve, 183, 184
Caudal femoral muscles, 189, 196
Caudal femoral vein, 219, 225, 227, 228
Caudal femorotibial membrane, 219
Caudal gluteal artery, 180, 181, 182, 188
Caudal gluteal nerve, 183, 184
Caudal gluteal vein, 180, 181, 182
Caudal horn, 211, 214, 216, 217, 218, 220
Caudal humeral circumflex vein, 14
Caudal intercondylar area, 202, 203, 204, 205, 206, 208, 209, 217, 220
Caudal margin
  of femur, 203, 206, 208
  of radius, 51
  of scapula, 3, 14, 15
  of tibia, 203, 205, 206, 208
  of ulna, 23
Caudal mesenteric artery, 182, 183
Caudal muscles, 1, 183
Caudal obliquus capitis muscle, 141
Caudal pectoral nerve, 146
Caudal ramus, of pubis, 173, 174, 180, 195
Caudal thoracic area, from T12 to T18, 153
Caudal tibial area, 221
Caudal tibial artery, 227, 228
Caudal tibial vein, 227
Caudal vena cava, 169, 182
Caudal vertebrae, 171, 183
Caudal vertebral incisura, 139, 140
Caudal vertebral notch, 152, 154, 155, 165
Caudolateral cortex
  of femur, 209
  of radius, 57
  of tibia, 203, 208, 209

Caudolateral margin, of tibia, 209
Caudolateral meniscotibial ligament, 202, 214, 216
Caudomedial cortex
    of femur, 208
    of tibia, 203, 208
Caudomedial margin, of tibia, 208
Caudomedial meniscotibial ligament, 202, 214, 216, 220
Central intercondylar area, 204, 205, 206, 208, 209
Central tarsal bone, 231, 232, 233, 234, 235, 236, 240, 242, 243, 252, 255, 258, 259, 264, 265
Centrodistal joint, 231, 232, 233, 234, 235, 236, 252, 255
Cephalic vein, 14, 20, 32, 46, 47, 49, 65, 68, 71, 72, 73, 76, 84
Cephalic vein pathway, 67
Cerebellar cavity, 132
Cerebellomedullaris cistern, 137
Cerebral cavity, 132
Cerebrum, vermis of, 137
Cervical area
    at C3–C4 intervertebral joint, 147, 148, 149
    deep structures, 144
    intermediate structures, 142, 143
    superficial structures, 141
Cervical muscles, 7, 131, 138, 139
Cervical superficial artery, 7
Cervical vertebral column, 4, 5
Cervicoauricular muscles, 137
Chestnut, 35, 49, 189, 229, 230, 255
Chondrocompedal ligament, 117, 120, 121
Chondrocoronal ligament, 120, 272, 276
Chondroungular junction, 276
Cleidobrachialis muscle, 7, 141
Cleidocephalicus muscle, 7, 141
Collateral fossa, 207, 209
Collateral sesamoidean ligament, 117, 118, 120, 123, 272, 273, 274, 276
Collateral ulnar artery, 32, 42, 46, 47, 71, 72, 73, 74, 75, 76
Collateral ulnar vein, 32, 46, 47, 71, 72, 73, 74, 75, 76, 96, 97
Common calcanean tendon, 190, 191, 195, 196, 197, 212, 221, 223, 226, 229, 230, 241, 247
Common carotid artery, 147
Common fibular nerve, 196, 199, 226
Common iliac vein, 180, 181, 182, 187, 188
Common proximal tendon, 212, 218, 223
Compact bone, 233
Complexus muscle, 133, 143, 147, 148
Condyle, 102, 103, 111, 115, 270
Connective tissue, 64, 278
    adipose, 90, 96, 97, 98, 266
    intertendinous, 267, 268
    sagittal, 90
    subcutaneous, 266
Coracobrachialis muscle, 11, 12, 16, 17, 28
Coracobrachialis proximal tendon, 16
Coracoid process, 3, 4, 5, 6, 30, 231, 234, 235, 236
Coronal artery, 124, 125
Coronal corium, 10, 114, 115, 116, 118, 124, 125, 128, 129
Coronal cushion, 115, 116, 118, 124, 125, 128, 129
Coronal vein, 124, 125

Coronet, 77, 99, 114, 115, 189, 269
Coronoid fossa, 21, 22, 23, 24, 31
Costal arch, 145, 151, 161
Costal cartilage, 2
Costal fovea, 153
Costotransverse muscle, 166
Coxal bones, 176
Coxofemoral joint, 189, 191, 192, 193, 194, 195
Cranial angle, 3
Cranial antebrachial interosseous artery, 46
Cranial antebrachial interosseous vein, 46
Cranial articular fossa, 132
Cranial articular process, 138, 139, 140, 152, 153, 154, 165
Cranial articular surface, 135, 136
Cranial border, 4, 17
Cranial cervical areas, 133, 134
Cranial cortex, 4, 203
Cranial cruciate ligament, 214, 215, 216, 219, 220
Cranial crural muscles, 201
Cranial crural septum, 227, 228
Cranial face
    patella, 203, 206, 208
    ulna, 23
Cranial femoral muscles, 189
Cranial gluteal artery, 180, 181, 182, 183, 186, 188
Cranial gluteal nerve, 183, 184
Cranial gluteal vein, 180, 181, 186
Cranial horn, 211, 213, 215, 216
Cranial humeral circumflex artery, 11, 12, 14, 28
Cranial intercondylar area, 202, 203, 204, 205, 206, 208, 209
Cranial intervertebral incisura, 175
Cranial margin
    of atlas, 135, 137
    of scapula, 3, 131
    of thigh, 151
Cranial pectoral nerves, 146
Cranial ramus, 172, 173, 174
Cranial tibial area, 221
Cranial tibial artery, 227, 228
Cranial tibial muscle, 224
Cranial tibial vein, 226, 227
Cranial vertebral incisura, 139, 140
Cranial vertebral notch, 152, 154, 155, 165
Craniolateral cortex, of femur, 208
Craniolateral meniscotibial ligament, 202, 213, 215, 216, 218
Craniomedial meniscotibial ligament, 202, 215, 216, 217
Croup, 151, 171, 189, 191
Cruciate sesamoidean ligament, 122, 123, 124, 125, 129, 277
Crural fascia, 195, 220, 223, 225, 227, 228
Crus, 189, 221, 227, 228
Cutaneous muscles, 31, 32
Cutaneous omobrachialis muscle, 1, 13, 16, 19, 32
Cutaneous trunci muscle, 13, 151
Cutaneous veins, 35
Cutaneus colli muscle, 147

Deep brachial artery, 11, 14, 28
Deep brachial veins, 14
Deep cervical fascia, 133

Deep circumflex iliac artery, 180, 181, 182, 183, 194, 198
Deep circumflex iliac vein, 182
Deep digital flexor muscle, 7, 8, 25, 26, 32, 36, 37, 38, 41, 42, 43, 44, 46, 47, 60, 63, 69, 74, 75, 76
Deep digital flexor musculotendinous junction, 71
Deep digital flexor tendon, 43, 66, 85, 100, 261, 263, 265, 266, 276
    carpus, 49, 62, 65, 67, 71, 72, 73
    dissected tarsus, 241, 244, 247, 250, 251, 252
    distal limb, 77, 99
    left distal interphalangeal joint, 111
    left distal sesamoid bone, 112
    left distal thoracic limb, 118
    left fetlock, 99
    left foot, 108, 109
    left forelimb, 80, 81
    metacarpophalangeal joint, 101, 102
    metacarpus, 87, 88, 90, 91, 92, 93, 94, 95, 96, 97, 98
    metatarsus, 260, 262, 264, 265, 267, 268
    pastern and foot, 125
    pelvic limb, 190, 260, 271, 273, 277, 278
    right digital area, 121, 123
    right forelimb, 82, 83
    right thoracic limb digital area, 117, 120
    thoracic limb, 126, 127, 128
        digital area, 124
Deep femoral artery, 183
Deep fibular (peroneal) nerve, 226, 227, 228
Deep palmar arch, 88, 89, 96, 97
Deep plantar metatarsal (interosseous) fascia, 263, 265, 266
Deep ramus
    of radial nerve, 26, 32, 39
    of tarsus, 251
    of ulnar nerve, 84
Deltoid muscle, 8
Deltoid tuberosity, 1, 2, 3, 4, 19, 26, 30
Deltoideus muscle, 1, 7, 13, 16, 19, 20, 25, 156
Dens, 132, 136
Dentis longitudinal ligament, 136
Diaphragm, 153, 154, 155, 167
Digastric muscle, 137
Digital cushion, 38, 108, 109, 113, 118, 120, 124, 125, 128, 129, 271, 273, 276, 277, 278
Digital flexor muscles, 22, 29
Digital flexor tendons, 189, 229, 230
Digital flexor tendon sheath, 93, 94, 95, 98
Digital sheath cavity, 124, 125, 126, 127, 129, 264, 278
Digital sheath synovial cavity, 277, 278
Digital torus, ramus of, 117, 125
DIPJ, see Distal interphalangeal joint (DIPJ)
Dissected back, 156, 161
Dissected crus, 223, 225, 226
Dissected stifle, 210, 211, 212, 213, 214, 216
Dissected tarsus, 238, 239, 240, 241, 242, 244, 245, 247, 249, 250, 251
Dissected withers, 156
Distal articular margin, 110, 116
Distal digital annular ligament, 41, 117, 118, 120, 121, 124, 125, 128, 129, 190, 271, 273, 275, 276, 277, 278

Distal extremity, 258, 259, 260, 261, 262, 263
Distal femur, 223
Distal (impar) sesamoidean ligament, 275
Distal interphalangeal joint (DIPJ), 108, 109, 110, 111, 112, 113, 114, 115, 116, 269, 270, 272, 276
    collateral ligament of, 118, 120, 121
    distopalmar recess of, 124, 125
    dorsal recess of, 109, 124, 125, 128, 277
    insertion fossa
        of lateral collateral ligament, 111
        of medial collateral ligament, 111
    joint space, 272
    lateral collateral fossa, 116
    lateral collateral ligament of, 122, 128
    lateral collateral recess of, 128
    medial collateral fossa, 116
    medial collateral ligament of, 128
    medial collateral recess of, 128
    proximopalmar recess of, 124, 125, 128, 277
Distal intertarsal (centrodistal) joint, 231, 232, 233, 234, 235, 236, 252
Distal limb, palpable anatomical structures, 77, 99
Distal metacarpus, 94, 95, 98
Distal metaphysis, 106, 203, 208, 270
Distal (metatarsal) extensor retinaculum, 223, 224, 238, 241, 251, 260, 261, 265
Distal palmar anastomosis, 93, 96, 98, 124, 129
Distal pastern fossa, 99
Distal pelvic limb, 260
Distal phalanx, 37, 38, 108, 109, 110, 111, 112, 113, 114, 115, 116, 118, 120, 121, 122, 124, 125, 270, 272, 273, 275, 276, 277
    collateral fossa of, 272
    lateral palmar process of, 129
    medial palmar process, 129
Distal plantar ligament, 245, 246, 249, 252, 255, 263, 264, 265
Distal radial artery, 42, 47, 65, 67, 68, 71, 72, 73, 76, 84, 87, 88
Distal ramus communicans, 84
Distal sesamoid bone, 37, 108, 109, 110, 111, 112, 113, 114, 115, 116, 118, 121, 122, 123, 124, 125, 270, 275, 276, 277
    proximal articular margin of, 128
Distal sesamoidean ligament, 121, 124, 125, 277
Distal tarsus, 229, 230, 231, 232, 233, 234, 235, 236, 237, 255
Distal thoracic limb, 37, 38, 41, 118
Distal tubercle, 231, 232, 233, 234, 235, 236, 237
Distomedial sulcus, 229, 257
Dorsal antebrachial interosseous artery, 61, 63
Dorsal arch, 132, 135, 136
Dorsal atlantoaxial ligament, 135
Dorsal atlantoaxial membrane, 135
Dorsal atlantooccipital membrane, 135
Dorsal capsule, 26, 27, 32
Dorsal cervical muscles, 138, 139
Dorsal cervical region, 131
Dorsal (common) digital extensor muscle, 7, 8, 19, 20, 25, 26, 32, 35, 36, 37, 38, 39, 40, 46, 49, 59, 60

Dorsal (common) digital extensor sheath, 71, 72, 73, 87
Dorsal (common) digital extensor tendon, 41, 47, 62, 63, 65, 70, 71, 72, 73, 80, 81, 82, 83, 87, 88, 90, 91, 92, 93, 94, 95, 96
Dorsal compact bone, 270
Dorsal cortex, 101, 102, 107, 270
Dorsal costoabdominal artery, 166
Dorsal costoabdominal nerve, 166
Dorsal costoabdominal vein, 166
Dorsal digital extensor muscle, 1, 32, 46
Dorsal digital extensor tendon, 117, 118, 119, 120, 124, 125, 126, 127, 128, 99
Dorsal hoof wall, 108, 109
Dorsal intercostal artery, 165
Dorsal intercostal vein, 165
Dorsal intermedioulnar ligament, 61
Dorsal intertransverse foramen, 176, 178
Dorsal longitudinal ligament, 136, 160, 164, 167, 168, 185
Dorsal lumbosacral intertransverse foramen, 176
Dorsal metacarpal fascia, 88, 92, 93
Dorsal metacarpophalangeal fascia, 94, 95, 126
Dorsal metatarsal fascia, 265, 267, 268
Dorsal metatarsophalangeal fascia, 272
Dorsal pedal artery, 253, 255
Dorsal pedal veins, 253
Dorsal radiointermediate ligament, 61
Dorsal sacroiliac ligament, 162, 188
Dorsal scapular artery, 10
Dorsal secondotertius ligament, 61
Dorsal supracondylar fossa, 101, 102
Dorsal tarsal fascia, 255
Dorsal tertioquartal ligament, 61
Dorsocaudal cuspid, 172, 174, 181
Dorsocollateral aspect, 269
Dorsocranial cuspid, 172, 174, 178, 181
Dorsolateral carpal fascia, 62
Dorsolateral cortex, 115, 259
Dorsolateral sacrocaudal muscle, 187, 188
Dorsomedial cortex, 258
Dorsoscapular ligament, 142, 143, 144
Dura mater, 137, 147, 148, 149, 160, 164, 167, 168, 169, 170, 185

Eighteenth rib, 154, 155, 158, 161, 166
Eighteenth thoracic vertebra (T18), 153, 157, 160, 164, 166
Elbow, 1, 31
    lateral aspect of, 27
    medial aspect of, 29
    median vein of, 32
    sulcus of, 19, 20, 35, 36
Elbow bones, 21
Elbow joint, 32, 39, 40
    dorsal capsule and recess, 41
    lateral collateral ligament of, 25, 36
    medial collateral ligament of, 28, 41
Epidural fat, 168, 170
Epidural space, 148, 149, 169, 170
Erector spinae muscle, 156, 157, 161, 166, 167, 168, 169, 170, 185, 186

Ergot, 77, 99, 100, 101, 102, 114, 115, 124, 125, 189, 277, 278
Ergot cushion, 125, 277, 278
Ergot ligament, 117, 278
Ergot ramus, 117
Extensor carpi obliquus muscle, 37, 38, 39, 40, 44, 46, 59, 60, 62
Extensor carpi obliquus tendon, 41, 42, 43, 47, 65, 66, 67, 69, 70, 71, 72, 83
Extensor carpi radialis enthesis, 87
Extensor carpi radialis muscle, 1, 7, 8, 10, 11, 19, 20, 25, 26, 28, 30, 32, 35, 36, 37, 38, 40, 41, 43, 46, 49
Extensor carpi radialis sheath, 71, 72, 73
Extensor carpi radialis tendon, 39, 47, 59, 60, 61, 62, 63, 64, 67, 69, 70, 71, 72, 73, 74, 75, 83, 96
Extensor fossa, 203, 204, 206, 207, 208, 209, 219
Extensor retinaculum, 37, 38, 39, 40, 41, 47, 59, 60, 62, 63, 67, 70, 71, 72, 73, 74, 75, 80, 87
Extensor sulcus, 202, 203, 204, 206, 208, 209, 222
External iliac artery, 180, 181, 182, 194, 198
External iliac vein, 194
External jugular vein, 147
External occipital crest, 132, 135
External occipital protuberance, 132, 135
External thoracic artery, 10
External thoracic vein, 151

Fascia latae, 181, 196
Fascicular aponeuroses, 168
Fat of mane, 141, 142, 144, 147
Fat pad, 15; see also Infrapatellar fat pad
Femoral area (thigh), 199
Femoral artery, 183, 199
Femoral condyles, 197
Femoral fascia, 181, 195, 199, 218
Femoral head, 191, 192, 193, 195
Femoral neck, 191, 192, 193, 195
Femoral nerve, 183, 184, 194
Femoral region, 189, 195, 196, 197, 198
Femoral trochlea, 197, 201, 203, 206, 208, 209, 210, 211, 213, 215, 217, 218, 219, 224
Femoral trochlear groove, 207
Femoral vein, 199
Femoropatellar joint, 207, 217, 218, 218
Femorotibial joint, 216
    lateral collateral ligament of, 226
Femorotibiopatellar joint, 189
Femur, 190, 191, 192, 193, 195, 196, 197, 199, 203, 204, 205, 206, 207, 208, 209, 211, 216, 217, 218, 220
    accessory ligament of, 194
    extensor fossa of, 212, 213, 215
    supracondylar fossa of, 213, 214
Fetlock, 114, 115, 189
    collateral ligament of, 269
    dorsal aspects of, 269
    dorsal capsule of, 99
    lateral collateral ligament of, 77, 99
    medial collateral ligament of, 99
    plantar aspect of, 269
    plantaroproximal recess of, 269

Fetlock joint
    dorsal capsule of, 80, 82, 83, 100
    and extensor tendons, 100, 101, 102
    lateral collateral ligament of, 80, 81
    medial collateral ligament of, 82, 83
Fibrocartilaginous pad, 118, 124
Fibroelastic aponeurosis, 142, 143
Fibrous non-union gap, 203, 209
Fibula, 197, 203, 204, 208, 209, 210, 211, 212, 213, 214,
    215, 216, 222, 227, 228, 237
    lateral malleolus, 238, 239, 240
Fifteenth ribs, 153
Fifteenth thoracic vertebra, 164
Fifth cervical vertebra (C5), 2, 138
Fifth lumbar intervertebral disc, 170
Fifth lumbar nerve, 170, 184, 188
    ventral ramus of, 187
Fifth lumbar vertebra (L5), 169, 170, 173, 174, 176, 177,
    180, 184, 185, 186, 198
Fifth sacral vertebra, 175
Fifth thoracic spinal process, 145
Filum terminale, 185
First caudal vertebra, 172, 174, 175
First cervical nerves
    dorsal rami of, 134
    ventral rami of, 134
First dorsal (intervertebral) sacral foramen, 175
First lumbar vertebra (L1), 155, 157, 158, 159, 160, 161,
    164, 166
    spinal process of, 154
First rib (R1), 140, 145, 147
First sacral nerve, 182, 184
First sacral vertebra (S1), 162, 163, 173, 174, 175, 176, 177,
    178, 179, 180, 182, 184, 185, 186, 187, 188
First tarsal bone, 231, 232, 233, 234, 235, 236, 245, 246,
    255, 258, 259
First thoracic vertebra, 140, 147
First ventral (intervertebral) sacral foramen, 173, 177
Flank, 151
Flavum (interarcual) ligament, 149, 159, 160, 164, 170, 185
Flexed carpus, deep structures, 61
Flexed fetlock, 105
Flexed left carpus, 57, 58
Flexed left stifle, 206
Flexed left tarsus, 236, 237
Flexed metacarpophalangeal joint, 102
Flexed right carpus, 56
Flexed right stifle, 207
Flexed stifle, 215
Flexed tarsus, deep structures, 243, 246
Flexor carpi radialis distal tendon, 42
Flexor carpi radialis muscle, 11, 20, 28, 29, 30, 35, 40, 41,
    42, 43, 46, 49, 67, 68, 69, 76
Flexor carpi radialis origin, 32
Flexor carpi radialis tendon, 44, 47, 66, 71, 72, 73, 83, 85, 87
Flexor carpi ulnaris muscle, 1, 11, 28, 29, 32, 35, 37, 38,
    41, 42, 43, 46, 47, 49, 65, 67, 68, 69, 71
Flexor carpi ulnaris tendon, 72, 83
Flexor retinaculum, 244, 247, 250, 251, 253, 254

antebrachium
    and carpus, 42, 43
    and distal thoracic limb, 37, 38, 41
    equine carpus and adjacent areas, 60, 62, 64, 65, 66,
        67, 68, 69, 70, 71, 72, 73, 74, 75, 76
    metacarpus, 80, 81, 82, 83, 84, 85, 88, 90, 91, 96, 97
Flexor tendons, 103, 257, 269
Flexor tuberosity, 103, 115, 269, 270, 273, 274, 275
Foot, 114, 115, 189
Foramen magnum, 132, 136, 137
Fourth cervical nerve, 147, 148, 149
Fourth cervical vertebra (C4), 138, 139, 145, 147,
    148, 149
    cranial articular process of, 147, 148, 149
    transverse process of, 147, 148
    vertebral head of, 147, 148, 149
Fourth lumbar intervertebral disc, 185
Fourth lumbar nerve, 184
Fourth lumbar vertebra (L4), 154, 155, 172, 176, 184,
    185, 197
Fourth metacarpal bone
    antebrachium and distal thoracic limb, 37, 38
    carpus, 49, 50, 51, 52, 53, 54, 55, 56, 57, 58, 59, 60, 61,
        62, 64, 65, 66
    distal limb, 77, 99
    flexed metacarpophalangeal joint, 102
    left distal thoracic limb, 118
    left fetlock and pastern, 100, 103, 106
    left metacarpophalangeal joint, 119
    metacarpus, 78, 79, 80, 81, 84, 85, 86, 87, 88, 90, 91,
        92, 93, 94
Fourth sacral vertebra, 173
Fourth tarsal bone, 231, 232, 233, 234, 235, 236, 237, 252,
    255, 258, 259, 264, 265
Fovea capitis, 21, 22, 191
Fovea dentis, 132, 136
Frog, 38, 108, 113, 114, 115, 116, 118, 124, 125, 277, 278
    corium of, 124, 125, 129, 273, 277, 278
    sulcus of, 109, 114, 115

Gastrocnemius muscle, 190, 197, 212, 217, 218, 219, 220,
    221, 223, 224, 225, 226
Gastrocnemius tendon, 190, 223, 224, 227, 228, 244, 245,
    246, 248
Gemelli muscle, 194
Genu lateral proximal artery, 220
Genu lateral proximal vein, 220
Genu middle artery, 220
Glenohumeral fascicules, 14, 15
Glenoid cavity, 2, 3, 4, 5, 6, 14, 15, 17, 101, 102, 103, 104,
    105, 106, 270
Glenoid incisura, 3, 5
Glenoid labrum, 15, 17
Gluteal fascia, 156, 167, 169, 181, 190, 195, 196
Gluteofemoralis muscle, 171, 181, 190, 191, 195, 196, 197,
    199, 220
Gluteofemoralis tendon, 212
Gluteofemoral muscle, 210, 218
Gluteus accessorius muscle, 188, 192, 197

Gluteus medius muscle, 156, 161, 167, 169, 171, 180, 181, 183, 184, 186, 187, 188, 190, 191, 195, 196
Gluteus muscle fibers, 179
Gluteus profundus muscle, 197
Gluteus superficialis muscle, 171, 181, 190, 191, 195, 196
Gracilis muscle, 180, 181, 183, 184, 198, 199, 219
Greater trochanter, 171, 193, 194, 195, 196, 197
Grey matter, 164, 185
Guttural pouch, 132

Haustra, 155
Heel, 108, 124, 125, 269
    bulb of, 110, 269, 277, 278
Hind pastern, sesamoidean ligaments, 274
Hip, 171, 189
Hock, 189, 221, 229, 230, 248, 257
Hoof, 114, 115, 116
Hoof wall, 37, 38, 41, 77, 99, 110, 113, 114, 115, 116, 118, 124, 125, 128, 129, 271, 277, 278
Humeral condyle, 2, 21, 22, 23, 26, 29, 31
Humeral trochlea, 24
Humeroantebrachial joint, 24
Humeroantebrachial joint space, 21, 29, 32
Humerus, 2, 3, 4, 5, 6, 12, 14, 15, 17, 21, 22, 23, 24, 32, 37, 38, 39, 41, 42, 43, 44
Hyoid, 132

Iliac face, 173, 178
Iliac fascia, 162, 163, 180, 181, 194, 198
Iliac muscle, 162, 169, 180, 181, 183, 184, 187, 188, 194, 198
Iliac wing, 178, 186, 187, 188
Iliacofemoral artery, 183, 192
Iliacofemoral vein, 192
Iliacus muscle, 192
Iliocostalis cervicis muscle, 144
Iliocostalis lumborum muscle, 166
Iliocostalis thoracis muscle, 142, 143, 144, 156, 157, 161
Iliocostal ligament, 163
Iliolumbar artery, 183, 186, 187
Iliolumbar ligament, 177
Iliolumbar vein, 186, 187
Iliopsoas muscle, ramus for, 194
Ilium, 169, 172, 173, 174, 192, 193, 198
Ilium body, 172, 173, 174, 180, 191
Ilium crest, 172, 173, 174
Ilium neck, 172, 173, 174, 177, 180, 184, 191
Ilium wing, 172, 173, 174, 177, 180
Infrapatellar fat pad, 203, 206, 212, 217, 218, 219
Infraspinatus fossa, 2, 3, 9, 13
Infraspinatus muscle, 1, 7, 8, 13, 16, 17, 141, 156
Infraspinatus tendon, 16, 26
Insertion fossa
    of collateral ligaments of distal interphalangeal joint, 108, 109, 110, 270
    of lateral collateral ligament, 21, 24, 111, 113, 114, 115
    of medial collateral ligament, 24, 111, 114, 116
    of scutocompedal ligament, 115
Insertion tuberosity, 3
Interarcual space, 170, 176

Intercondylar eminence, 202, 203, 206, 208, 209
Intercondylar fossa, 203, 204, 206, 208, 209, 215, 216, 220
Intercondylar line, 203, 206, 209, 216, 220
Intercondylar tubercle, 202
Intercostalis externus muscle, 142, 143, 144
Intercostal muscle(s), 145, 156, 157, 161, 162, 163, 166
Intercostal nerve, 145, 162, 163
Intermediate carpal bone, 50, 51, 52, 53, 54, 55, 56, 57, 58, 61, 72, 74, 75
Intermediate groove, 231, 232, 233, 234, 235, 236, 237
Intermediate (obliquorectum) sesamoidean ligament, 271, 274, 275, 278
Intermediate patellar ligament, 210, 211, 218, 219
Intermediate sesamoidean ligament, 122, 124, 125, 127
Intermediate (tarsal) extensor retinaculum, 223, 224, 238, 239, 241, 251
Intermediate tuberculum, 5, 6
Intermedioulnar interosseous ligaments, 72
Intermedioulnar joint, 58
Intermetacarpal syndesmosis
    fourth, 79
    second, 50, 51, 53, 54, 55, 67, 78, 82, 83, 86, 87, 88, 90, 91, 92, 93, 94
    third, 50, 51, 53, 54, 57, 59, 60, 62, 64, 80, 81, 86, 87, 88, 89, 90, 91, 92, 93, 94
Intermetatarsal joint, 235, 258
Intermuscular sulcus, 191
Internal iliac artery, 180, 181, 182, 187, 198
Internal inguinal ring, 183
Internal pudendal artery, 183
Internal vertebral plexus, 147, 148, 149, 166, 168, 169, 170
Interosseopalmar ligament, 98, 263
Interosseous face, 103, 104, 105, 114
Interosseous fascia, 91, 92, 233, 235
Interosseous muscle, 65, 66, 74, 75, 77, 82, 83, 84, 86, 87, 88
Interosseous muscle (suspensory ligament), 64, 67, 80, 81, 85
Interosseous muscle (vestigial), 88
Interosseous sacroiliac ligament, 175, 178, 179, 186, 187, 188
Interosseous space, 21, 237
Interosseous talocalcaneal ligament, 253
Intersesamoidean space, 105
Interspinal ligament, 145, 158, 159, 160, 161, 164, 167, 168, 169, 170, 185
Interspinal space, 153, 154, 155
Intertendinous connective tissue, 267, 268
Intertransverse foramen, 169
Intertransverse ligament, 157, 159, 167
Intertransverse lumbosacral joint, 173, 175, 178, 179
Intertransverse muscle, 157, 167
Intertransverse synostosis, 173
Intertranversarii muscles, 147, 148
Intertubercular sulcus, 14, 30
Intervertebral disc(s), 140, 147, 148, 149, 154, 155, 164, 166, 167, 168, 169, 184, 159, 160, 165
Intervertebral foramen, 138, 139, 140, 148, 149, 152, 153, 154, 155, 158, 159, 165, 166, 167, 168, 169, 170, 172

Intervertebral symphysis, 173
Intervertebral thoracic nerve, 165
Intervertebral vein, 165
Intramuscular aponeuroses, 167, 228, 168, 169
Ischiatic arch, 172, 173, 174, 183
Ischiatic spine, 172, 174
Ischium, 172, 173, 174, 191, 192, 193, 196, 197
Ischium body, 172, 173, 174, 180
Ischium table, 172, 173, 174, 180, 191
Isolated patellar apparatus, 210

Joint capsule, 14
Joint cavity, 15, 17
Jugular sulcus, 131
Jugular vein, 141, 144

Lacertus fibrosus, 11, 32, 40
Larynx, 132
Lata fascia, 190, 195, 199
Lateral (acetabular) ramus, 172, 173, 174
Lateral antebrachial cutaneous nerve, 25
Lateral chondrosesamoidean ligament, 128
Lateral collateral fossa, 103, 104, 105, 110, 114, 115, 116
Lateral collateral ligament, 22, 35, 118, 210, 212, 213, 214,
    219, 220, 238, 239
  of carpus, 39, 44, 49, 59, 60, 61, 62, 63, 64, 65, 66, 71,
    72, 73, 80, 84, 85, 87
  of elbow joint, 7, 8, 9, 25, 26, 27, 31, 32, 36, 39
  of femorotibial joint, 226
  of fetlock joint, 77, 80, 81, 99, 126
  of interphalangeal joint, 103, 114, 115, 122, 128
  of metacarpophalangeal joint, 95, 103, 104, 105, 114,
    115, 119, 122
Lateral collateral sesamoidean ligament, 121, 122, 123,
    126, 128, 275
Lateral common digital artery, 265, 266, 267, 268
Lateral common digital nerve, 265, 266, 267, 268
Lateral common digital vein, 265, 266, 267, 268
Lateral compact bone, 111
Lateral cortex, 103, 104, 105
Lateral cutaneous femoral nerve, 198
Lateral digital extensor muscle, 35, 36, 37, 38, 39, 40, 46,
    49, 59, 60, 190, 212, 223, 224, 227, 228, 238, 241
Lateral digital extensor tendon
  antebrachium, 47
  carpus, 61, 62, 63, 65, 66, 71, 72, 73
  distal limb, 99, 118
  hock, 230
  metacarpus, 80, 81, 84, 87, 88, 90, 91, 92, 93, 94, 95
  metatarsus, 261, 265, 267, 268
  pelvic limb, 260
  right digital area, 122
  tarsus, 251, 253, 255
  thoracic limb fetlock, 126
Lateral digital flexor muscle, 190, 212, 218, 220, 223, 224,
    225, 226, 227, 228, 241, 244, 247, 249
Lateral digital flexor tendon, 229, 232, 237, 248, 250, 251,
    252, 253, 254, 255, 262, 264, 265, 266
Lateral dorsal metacarpal artery, 87, 88

Lateral epicondyle, 2, 21, 23, 24, 26, 27, 37, 103, 115
Lateral femoral circumflex artery, 183
Lateral femoral condyle, 203, 204, 206, 207, 208, 209,
    212, 213, 214, 215, 216, 218, 219, 220, 222
Lateral femoral epicondyle, 204, 212, 213, 220
Lateral femoral septum, 199
Lateral femoropatellar ligament, 210, 212
Lateral femorotibial joint, 213, 218
Lateral (fourth) plantar metatarsal nerve, 261
Lateral (fourth) plantar metatarsal vein, 261
Lateral heel, 116
  bulb of, 128
  coronal corium, 116
Lateral intercondylar tubercle, 204, 205, 206, 208, 209,
    215, 216
Lateral malleolus, 222, 224, 226, 229, 230, 231, 232, 234,
    235, 236, 237, 241, 242, 243
Lateral meniscus, 210, 212, 213, 214, 215, 216, 220
Lateral meniscus ligament, 218
Lateral metacarposesamoidean ligament, 95
Lateral metatarsal bone, 257, 263
Lateral oblique sesamoidean ligament, 80, 85, 118, 119,
    121, 122, 127, 129, 263
Lateral palmar common digital artery, 76, 88, 90, 91,
    92, 93
Lateral palmar common digital nerve, 84, 88, 90, 91, 92,
    93, 94
Lateral palmar common digital vein, 76, 88, 90, 91, 92,
    93, 94
Lateral palmar eminence, 104, 105, 106, 107
Lateral palmar metacarpal artery, 88, 89, 90, 91, 92, 93
Lateral palmar metacarpal vein, 88, 89, 90
Lateral palmar process, 114, 115
Lateral parapatellar fibrocartilage, 210
Lateral patellar ligament, 201, 203, 206, 208, 210, 212,
    214, 218, 219
Lateral plantar artery, 255
Lateral plantar metatarsal artery, 267
Lateral plantar metatarsal vein, 265, 266
Lateral plantar nerve, 250, 251, 254, 255
Lateral plantar vein, 255
Lateral proper digital artery, 84, 126, 127, 128, 129
Lateral proper digital nerve, 84, 126, 127, 128, 129
Lateral proper digital vein, 126, 127, 129
Lateral proper palmar digital artery, 95, 96, 98
Lateral proper palmar digital nerve, 95
Lateral proper palmar digital vein, 95
Lateral proper palmar digital vessels, 99
Lateral proximal sesamoid bone, 85, 99, 104, 105, 106,
    107, 122, 126, 129
Lateral rectus femoris muscle area, 172
Lateral sacral crest, 174, 175, 176
Lateral saphenous vein, 226, 227, 253
Lateral short sesamoidean ligament, 129
Lateral solar canal, 116
Lateral styloid process, 60, 63, 64
Lateral talocalcaneal joint, 253
Lateral (III) plantar common digital nerve, 250, 251
Lateral thoracic nerve, 146

Lateral thoracic vein, 1
Lateral tibial condyle
    dissected crus, 223, 224
    dissected stifle, 210, 211, 212, 213, 214, 216, 218, 220
    femorotibial joint, 216
    fibula, 222
    flexed stifle, 215
    left stifle, 203, 204, 205, 206, 208, 209
    left tibial plateau, 202
    tibia, 222
Lateral trochlear ridge, 204, 207, 208, 213, 215, 218, 237
Lateral tuberosity, 21, 22, 23, 24, 27
Lateral ungular cartilage, 99, 117, 120, 121, 122, 123, 128, 129, 272, 275
Lateral (venous) ungular plexus, 128, 129
Lateral vertebral foramen, 132, 135, 136
Latissimus dorsi muscle, 1, 7, 10, 11, 12, 13, 151, 156, 161
Left acetabulum, 162, 163
Left caudal gluteal artery, 183
Left coxal bone, 180
Left distal interphalangeal joint, 111
Left distal sesamoid bone, 112, 113
Left distal tarsus, 233
Left distal thoracic limb, 118
Left ear, 133, 134, 145
Left eighteenth rib, 156, 163
Left equine carpus, 50, 51, 54, 55
Left external iliac artery, 183
Left femoral region (thigh), 198
Left femur, 172
Left fetlock, 104, 107
    and pastern, 100, 103, 106
Left fifteenth rib, 162, 163
Left foot, 108, 109, 110
Left iliac crest, 179
Left ilium, 162, 163, 176, 195
Left ilium neck, 183
Left internal iliac artery, 183
Left ischium, 162, 163, 176, 194, 195
Left lumbosacral articular process joint, 176
Left lumbosacral intertransverse joint, 176, 184
Left major psoas muscle, 162, 163
Left metacarpophalangeal joint, 101, 119
Left minor psoas muscle, 162, 163
Left obturator foramen, 162
Left obturator internus muscle, 180, 181
Left pelvis, 198
Left pubis, 162, 163, 195
    cranial ramus of, 180
Left sacral tuber, 179
Left sacroiliac joint, 162, 163, 176, 184
Left sacrosciatic ligament, 163, 180, 183, 184
Left sciatic nerve, 162, 163
Left stifle, 203, 204, 205, 208, 209
Left tarsus, 231, 232, 235
Left tibial plateau, 202
Left tuber coxae, 180
Left weight-bearing foot, 116
Lesser trochanter, 193, 195

Limbic corium, 125
Liver, 153, 154, 155
Long digital extensor muscle, 190, 212, 218, 219, 220, 223, 224 225, 226, 227, 228, 238, 241
Long digital extensor muscle body, 218
Long digital extensor tendon, 251, 253, 255, 260, 261, 264, 265, 267, 268, 271, 272, 276, 277
Longissimus atlantis muscle, 133, 134, 141, 143, 144, 147, 148
Longissimus capitis muscle, 133, 134, 137, 141, 143, 144, 147
Longissimus cervicis muscle, 142, 143, 144, 147, 148
Longissimus muscles, 156
Longissimus thoracis muscle, 142, 143, 144, 156, 161
Long lateral collateral ligament, 240, 241, 242, 243, 250, 251, 253, 255
Long medial collateral ligament, 240, 244, 245, 246, 247, 249, 250, 253, 255
Long plantar ligament, 241, 242, 243, 245, 246, 249, 250, 251, 252, 253, 254, 255, 265, 266
Longus colli muscle, 138, 139, 140, 147, 148
Lumbar area, 151, 154, 155
    between fifth and sixth lumbar vertebrae, 169, 170
    between second and third lumbar vertebrae, 167, 168
Lumbar artery, 169, 170, 183
Lumbar nerve, 167, 168, 169
Lumbar spine, 173, 174, 180, 180, 183
Lumbar vein, 167, 168, 169, 170
Lumbar ventral intervertebral foramen, 173
Lumbar vertebrae, 176; see also individual lumbar vertebra
Lumbar vertebral bodies, 162, 163
Lumbar vertebral column, 158, 159
Lumbosacral disc (L6 disc), 162, 163
Lumbosacral intertransverse joint, 177, 186, 187
Lumbosacral intertransverse ligament, 177
Lumbosacral intervertebral disc, 177, 180, 182, 183, 184, 198
Lumbosacral intervertebral foramen, 178, 179
Lumbosacral junction, 185, 186
Lumbosacral truncus, 182, 192
Lumbosacral trunk, 183, 184
Lumbosacroiliac area, 176
Lumbosacroiliac junction
    passing through first sacral vertebra (S1), 188
    passing through sixth lumbar vertebra (L6), 187
Lungs, 152, 153, 154, 155
Lymphatic vessels, 126

Major ischiatic foramen, 163
Major psoas muscle, 162
Major sciatic incisura, 172, 173, 174
Major trochanter, 191, 192
Major tuberculum, 1, 5, 6, 8, 16, 17, 26, 30
Mamillary process, 152, 153, 154, 167, 170, 176
Mandible, 131, 132, 141, 145
Mane, 131
    fat of, 141, 142, 144, 147
    skin of, 133, 134

Manica flexoria, 38, 41, 83, 95, 96, 98, 118, 124, 190, 260, 264, 277
Manubrium, 2, 20
Masseteric region, 131, 133, 134
Masseter muscle, 141
Medial angle, 207
Medial chondrosesamoidean ligament, 128
Medial collateral fossa, 103, 104, 105, 106, 114, 115, 116
Medial collateral ligament
 of carpus, 41, 42, 43, 44, 49, 59, 61, 65, 66, 67, 68, 69, 71, 72, 73, 83, 84, 85, 87
 of dissected stifle, 210, 211, 214, 219
 of distal interphalangeal joint, 128
 of elbow joint, 22, 29, 31, 32, 40, 41, 42, 43, 44
  and brachium, 28, 30
 of fetlock joint, 82, 83, 99, 126
 of hock, 230
 of metacarpophalangeal joint, 95, 103, 104, 105, 114, 115, 120
 of proximal interphalangeal joint, 114, 115
 of shoulder and brachium, 11
 of tarsus, 238, 239
Medial collateral sesamoidean ligament, 121, 122, 123, 126, 128, 275
Medial common digital artery, 265, 266, 267
Medial common digital nerve, 265, 266, 267, 268
Medial common digital vein, 267, 268
Medial compact bone, 111
Medial cortex, 103, 104, 105
Medial digital flexor muscle, 190, 225, 244, 247, 249
Medial digital flexor tendon, 227, 228, 250, 253, 255, 262, 265, 266
Medial dorsal metacarpal artery, 87, 88
Medial epicondyle, 2, 21, 23, 24, 29, 103, 115
Medial femoral circumflex artery, 183
Medial femoral condyle, 203, 204, 206, 207, 208, 209, 210, 211, 214, 215, 216, 217, 219, 220, 222
Medial femoral epicondyle, 204, 210, 211, 214
Medial femoropatellar ligament, 210, 211
Medial femorotibial joint, 211, 217, 219
Medial heel, bulb of, 118, 128
Medial iliac lymph nodes, 169, 194
Medial intercondylar tubercle, 204, 205, 206, 208, 209, 215, 216, 217, 219
Medial malleolus, 222, 224, 229, 231, 232, 234, 235, 236, 244, 245, 246, 247, 249, 250
Medial meniscus, 20, 202, 208, 210, 211, 214, 215, 216, 217, 220
Medial metacarposesamoidean ligament, 95
Medial metatarsal bone, 257
Medial oblique sesamoidean ligament, 41, 82, 83, 85, 120, 121, 122, 123, 127, 129, 263
Medial palmar common digital artery, 84, 88, 90, 91, 92, 93, 94
Medial palmar common digital nerve, 84, 88, 90, 91, 92, 93, 94
Medial palmar common digital vein, 88, 90, 91, 92, 93, 94
Medial palmar eminence, 104, 105
Medial palmar metacarpal artery, 88, 89, 90, 91, 92, 93

Medial palmar metacarpal vein, 88, 89, 90, 91, 92, 93
Medial palmar process, 114, 115, 116
Medial parapatellar fibrocartilage, 210, 211, 217
Medial patellar ligament, 201, 203, 206, 210, 211, 217, 218, 219
Medial plantar artery, 255
Medial plantar metatarsal artery, 265, 266, 267
Medial plantar metatarsal vein, 265, 266
Medial plantar nerve, 250, 254, 255
Medial proper digital artery, 84, 117, 126, 127, 128, 129
Medial proper digital nerve, 84, 117, 126, 127, 128, 129
Medial proper digital vein, 117, 126, 127, 129
Medial proper palmar digital artery, 95
Medial proper palmar digital nerve, 95
Medial proper palmar digital vein, 95
Medial proper palmar digital vessels, 99
Medial proximal sesamoid bone, 78, 79, 83, 85, 99, 104, 105, 106, 107, 121, 126, 129, 263
Medial radioulnar ligament, 29, 32
Medial ramus, 172, 173, 174
Medial rectus femoris muscle area, 173
Medial saphenous vein, 227, 228, 253, 255, 265, 266, 267, 268
Medial solar canal, 114, 116
Medial talocalcaneal joint, 252
Medial tenocalcaneal ligament, 237, 244, 248
Medial tibial condyle, 202, 203, 204, 205, 206, 208, 209, 210, 211, 214, 215, 216, 220, 222
Medial trochlear ridge, 204, 207, 208, 211, 213, 215, 216, 217, 218, 235, 237
Medial (II) plantar common digital nerve, 250
Medial ungular cartilage, 41, 99, 117, 120, 121, 122, 123, 128, 129, 272, 275
Medial (venous) ungular plexus, 128, 129
Median aponeurosis, 180, 181, 183
Median artery, 11, 28, 32, 39, 40, 42, 46, 47, 68, 71, 72, 73, 76
Median nerve, 11, 12, 16, 28, 32, 39, 42, 46, 47, 68, 71, 72, 73, 146
Median sacral crest, 174, 175, 176, 181, 195
Median vein, 32, 40, 42, 46, 47, 68, 71
Mediocarpal joint, 50, 51, 52, 53, 54, 55, 56, 57, 61, 74, 75, 78, 79
 palmarolateral recess of, 63
Mediotarsal joint, 235
Medullary cavity, 102, 103, 115, 258, 259, 270
Menisci (meniscus), 203, 204, 209
Meniscofemoral ligament, 214, 216, 219, 220
Metacarpal bones, see individual metacarpal bones
Metacarpal condyle, 101, 102, 103, 104, 105, 106, 114, 126
Metacarpointersesamoidean ligament, 119, 124
Metacarpophalangeal fascia, 117
Metacarpophalangeal joint (MPJ), 94, 95, 100, 101, 102, 103, 104, 105, 106, 107, 114, 115, 117, 119
 collateral ligament of, 117
 collateral sesamoidean ligament of, 119
 distopalmar recess of, 124, 125
 dorsal capsule of, 94, 96, 118, 120, 124, 125, 126
 dorsal network of, 95

dorsal recess of, 117, 124, 126
joint capsule of, 106
lateral collateral ligament of, 95, 103, 104, 105, 114, 115, 118, 119, 122
lateral collateropalmar recess of, 129
medial collateral ligament of, 95, 103, 104, 105, 114, 115, 120
medial collateral sesamoidean ligament, 120
palmar network of, 95
proximopalmar recess of, 94, 95, 96, 98, 117, 119, 124, 129
Metacarposesamoidean joint, 100, 101, 102
Metacarposesamoidean joint space, 126, 129
Metacarposesamoidean ligament, 94
Metacarpus, 100
    and adjacent areas, 83
    distal third, 93
    left forelimb, 78, 79, 80, 81, 84, 85
    middle third, 91, 92
    right forelimb, 82, 83
    sagittal section of, 96
Metaphysis, spongy bone of, 101, 102, 104
Metatarsal condyle, 270, 277
Metatarsal distal metaphysis, 277
Metatarsal retinaculum, 229, 230
Metatarsointersesamoidean ligament, 271
Metatarsophalangeal joint (MTPJ), 264, 270, 271, 272, 277
    collateral ligament of, 271, 272
    distoplantar recess of, 277
    dorsal capsule of, 277
    proximoplantar recess of, 277
Metatarsus, 189, 231, 232, 233, 234, 235, 236, 258, 259, 261, 262, 264, 270
    distal third of, 268
    palpable anatomical structures, 257
Middle cervical area, 138
Middle genu artery, 219, 220
Middle metatarsus, 267
Middle phalanx, 271
Middle scutum, 122, 123, 124, 125, 274, 275, 277
Minor sciatic incisura, 172
Minor tuberculum, 5, 6, 12, 17, 30
MPJ, *see* Metacarpophalangeal joint (MPJ)
MTPJ, *see* Metatarsophalangeal joint (MTPJ)
Multifidus aponeuroses, 158
Multifidus cervicis muscle, 144, 147, 148
Multifidus colli muscle, 134
Multifidus fascia, 158, 161, 166, 167, 168, 169
Multifidus muscle, 157, 159, 161, 165, 166, 167, 168, 169, 170, 185, 187, 188
Multifidus muscle fasciculi, 158
Muscle ramus, 16, 26, 184
Musculocutaneus nerve, 146

Neck
    palpable anatomical structures, 131
    and thorax, deep structures, 145
Nerve ramus, 157
Neurovascular anastomosis, 99

Neurovascular fasciculus, 269
Ninth rib, 152
Nuchal area, 132, 133, 134, 137
    deep structures, 135
    vertebral canal opened, 136
Nuchal crest, 135
Nuchal ligament, 133, 134, 137, 141, 142, 143, 144, 145, 147, 148
Nuchal region, 131

Oblique sesamoidean ligament(s), 270, 271, 273, 274, 275, 277, 278
Obliquus capitis caudalis muscle, 133, 134, 144
Obliquus capitis cranialis muscle, 133, 134, 137
Obliquus externus abdominis muscle, 161
Obliquus internus abdominis muscle, 161, 183
Obturator artery, 180, 181, 182, 183, 186
Obturator externus muscle, 162, 163
Obturator foramen, 172, 173, 174, 191, 194
Obturator internus muscle, 184, 186, 188, 192, 194, 195
Obturator muscles, 195
Obturator nerve, 182, 183, 184, 198
Obturator sulcus, 172
Obturator vein, 180, 181
Occipital bone, 132, 136, 137
    basilar part of, 136, 137
    nuchal face of, 135, 136
Occipital condyles, 132, 136
Occipital vein, 137
Oesophagus, 138, 139, 147
Olecranon, 2, 7, 8, 21, 22, 23, 24, 26, 27, 29, 31, 35, 36
Olecranon fossa, 2, 21, 23, 24, 26, 27, 29, 37
Olecranon recess, 32
Olecranon tuberosity, 25, 27, 29
Omohyoideus muscle, 141, 147
Omotransversarius muscle, 7, 13, 16, 17, 133, 134, 141, 142, 144, 147, 156

Pad, 114, 115
Palmar (intersesamoidean) ligament, 80, 81, 82, 83, 85, 95, 96, 98, 100, 101, 102, 118, 119, 122, 123, 124, 125, 126, 129
Palmar annular ligament, 80, 81, 82, 83, 84, 96, 98, 117, 118, 120, 124, 125, 126
Palmar common digital artery, 73
Palmar common digital vein, 73
Palmar compact bone, 111, 112, 113
Palmar cortex, 101, 102, 107
Palmar eminence, 101, 102
    sagittal fossa between, 101
Palmar fetlock, 113
Palmar ligament, 37, 38, 41
Palmar margin, 102, 103, 104, 105
Palmar metacarpal artery, 74, 75, 94, 95, 96, 98, 117
Palmar metacarpal fascia, 62, 65, 67, 76, 80, 81, 82, 83, 88, 90, 91, 92, 93, 94, 95, 97
Palmar metacarpal vein(s), 74, 75, 94, 95, 96, 98, 117
Palmarolateral recess, 73
Palmaromedial cortex, 78, 115

Palmarosagittal recess, 71
Palmar supracondylar fossa, 101, 102, 106
Parietal corium, 108, 109, 113, 114, 115, 115, 116, 118,
    124, 125, 128, 129, 273, 277, 278
Parotid gland, 137
Parotidoauricular muscle, 137
Parotid region, 131, 133, 134
Pastern, 114, 115, 189
    and foot, 125
    of pelvic limb, 278
    dorsal aspect of, 269
Patella, 181, 190, 191, 195, 196, 197, 198, 201, 203, 204,
    206, 207, 208, 209, 210, 212, 214, 218, 223
Patellar apparatus, 211
Patellar fascia, 217, 218, 219
Patellar ligaments, 203
Pectineus muscle, 180, 181, 184, 193, 194, 195, 198, 199
Pectoralis ascendens muscle, 1
Pectoralis descendens muscle, 1, 7, 14, 19, 20, 25
Pectoralis profundus (ascendens) muscle, 7, 10, 12, 16, 17,
    19, 151
Pectoralis transversus muscle, 7, 10, 20, 32, 46
Pectoral muscles, 31, 32
Pelvic bones, 172, 173, 174
Pelvic digital area, 270
    palpable anatomical structures, 269
Pelvic foot, 275, 276
Pelvic limb, 190, 273, 277
    palpable anatomical structures, 189
    superficial structures, 271, 272
Pelvic symphysis, 162, 163, 172, 173, 174, 183, 184, 194,
    195, 198
Pelvis, 163, 171, 173, 174, 180, 189
    and connected bones, 172
    dorsal part, 178
    and femoral region (thigh), 195, 196, 197
    muscles and nerves, 184
    superficial structures, 181
    vessels and nerves, 182, 183
Penis, 198
Perforating tarsal vein, 255
Periopleum, 271
Perioplic corium, 125
Periosteum, 268
Peroneus tertius distal tendon, 255
Peroneus tertius muscle(s), 190, 197, 212, 218, 219, 220,
    223, 224, 227, 228, 229, 230, 238, 239, 241, 244
Peroneus tertius tendon, 253, 258
Phrenic nerve, 144, 146
Pie mater, 149
PIPJ, see Proximal interphalangeal joint (PIPJ)
Plantar annular ligament, 190, 260, 264, 271, 273, 274, 277
Plantar artery, 253, 254
Plantar compact bone, 270
Plantar cortex, 270
Plantar (intersesamoidean) ligament, 263, 264, 271, 274, 277
Plantar metatarsal artery, 268
Plantar metatarsal fascia, 244, 247, 261, 264, 265, 268
Plantar metatarsal vein, 267, 268

Plantar nerve, 225, 253
Plantar (superficial) metatarsal fascia, 265, 266, 267
Plantarolateral cortex, 258
Plantaromedial cortex, 259
Plantar tarsal fascia, 241, 252, 255, 262
Plantar tarsal sheath, 247, 251
Plantar tubercle, 236
Plantar vein, 253, 254
Podotrochlear bursa, 125, 128, 277, 278
Popliteal artery, 219, 220
Popliteal face, 203, 208, 209
Popliteal fossa, 209, 215
Popliteal line, 222
Popliteal notch, 202, 203, 208, 214, 216
Popliteal vein, 219, 220
Popliteus muscle, 212, 213, 214, 216, 217, 218, 219, 220, 223
Popliteus tendon, 214, 215, 216, 218
Prepubic tendon, 162, 163, 183, 193, 194
Promontorium, 180, 182, 183, 184, 185
Promontory, 173
Proper digital artery, 278
Proper digital nerve, 278
Proper digital vein, 278
Proximal (tibial) extensor retinaculum, 223, 224, 238,
    241, 244
Proximal articular margin, 116
Proximal brachium, 15
Proximal deep palmar arch, 74, 75
Proximal digital annular ligament, 80, 82, 83, 117, 118,
    120, 124, 125, 127, 129, 190, 271, 273, 277–278
Proximal epiphysis, 22
Proximal forelimb, 1, 2
Proximal interphalangeal joint (PIPJ), 100, 103, 106, 108,
    109, 110, 114, 115, 116, 117, 270, 274, 275, 276, 277
    abaxial palmar ligament of, 118, 120, 121, 122, 123
    axial palmar ligament of, 120, 121, 122, 123
    collateral ligament of, 120, 121, 122, 271, 272, 273
    dorsal recess of, 124, 125, 127
    lateral collateral ligament of, 103, 114, 115, 118
    medial collateral ligament of, 103, 114, 115
    palmar recess of, 124, 125
Proximal intertarsal (centrodistal) joint, 255
Proximal intertarsal (mediotarsal) joint, 231, 232, 233,
    234, 235, 236
Proximal intertarsal (talocentral) joint, 252
Proximal metacarpus, 86, 87, 88, 90, 97
Proximal metaphysis, 12, 21, 23, 24, 30, 265
Proximal metatarsus, plantar structures, 266
Proximal pelvic limb, superficial anatomical structures, 191
Proximal sesamoid bone(s), 77, 78, 79, 80, 82, 100, 101,
    102, 103, 114, 189, 270
Proximal sesamoidean ligament, 109, 111, 112, 121, 122,
    123, 124, 125, 128, 275, 277
Proximal sesamoid ligament, 108
Proximal talocalcaneal ligament, 243
Proximal tarsus, 253, 254
Proximal tubercle, 231, 232, 234, 236, 237
Proximomedial talocalcaneal ligament, 245, 246, 252, 253
Proximopalmarolateral recess, 71

Psoas major muscle, 166, 167, 168, 169, 170, 180, 181, 182, 183, 184, 186, 187, 188, 194, 198
Psoas minor muscle, 165, 166, 167, 169, 170, 180, 181, 182, 183, 184, 187, 188, 194, 198
Psoas minor muscle tubercle, 172, 173, 180
Psoas minor tendon, 187, 188
Pubis, 172, 173, 174, 180, 184, 191, 193
Pubis body, 173, 180
Pubis pecten, 173, 180, 183
Pudendoepigastric trunk, 183
Pulvinus, 101, 102

Quadratus femoris muscle, 197
Quadriceps femoris muscle, 180, 181, 183, 191, 194, 197, 198, 199, 201, 217, 223
    vastus lateralis of, 195, 196
Quarter, 269

Radial (antebrachial) condyle, 50, 51
Radial carpal bone, 50, 51, 52, 53, 54, 55, 56, 57, 58, 61, 72
Radial nerve, 14, 16, 146
    deep ramus of, 26, 32, 39
Radial styloid process, 50, 51
Radial tuberosity, 21, 22, 23, 24, 27
Radiointermediate interosseous ligaments, 72, 74, 75
Radiointermediate interosseous space, 51
Radiointermediate joint, 58
Radiolucent space, 103
Radioulnar interosseous space, 43
Radioulnar joint, 21, 23
Radioulnar joint space, 22, 32
Radioulnar space, 23
Radioulnar syndesmosis, 27, 43
Radioulnar synostosis, 46, 50, 54
Radius, 2, 21, 22, 23, 24, 29, 40, 41, 42, 57, 59, 71, 74, 75
    distal metaphysis, 47, 53, 54, 55, 56, 60, 61, 62, 63, 64, 66, 67, 68, 69, 70, 83
    lateral tuberosity, 25, 37, 38, 39
    proximal epiphysis of, 29, 44
    proximal metaphysis, 43
    proximolateral tuberosity of, 19, 35, 36
    radial tuberosity, 41
    styloid process, 65, 69
Ramus communicans, 68, 71
Rectus abdominis muscle, 151, 183, 193, 194
Rectus capitis dorsalis major muscle, 134, 137
Rectus capitis dorsalis minor muscle, 134, 137
Rectus capitis lateralis muscle, 137
Rectus capitis ventralis muscle, 137
Rectus femoris muscle, 162, 183, 192, 193, 194, 195, 197, 198, 199, 217
Renal arteries, 182
Retractor costae muscle, 161
Rhomboideus cervicalis muscle, 10, 156
Rhomboideus cervicis muscle, 7, 141, 143, 144, 147
Rhomboideus muscle, 142
Rhomboideus thoracis muscle, 7, 10, 156
Rib, 142, 143, 144
Right acetabular area, 162

Right acetabulum, 180
Right articular process, 178
Right articular process joint, 174
Right caudal gluteal artery, 183
Right coxal bone, 180
Right digital area, after removal of flexor tendons, 121
    and straight sesamoidean ligament, 122
    and straight and lateral oblique sesamoidean ligaments, 123
Right dissected crus, 224
Right eighteenth rib, 162, 163
Right equine carpus, 52, 53
Right external iliac artery, 183
Right femoral nerve, 162, 163
Right femur, 162, 163, 172
Right fifteenth rib, 162, 163
Right iliac crest, 178
Right iliopsoas muscle, 162, 163
Right ilium, 162, 176
Right ilium neck, 178, 179, 185
Right internal iliac artery, 183
Right intertransverse lumbosacral joint, 180
Right ischium, 176, 194
    medial ramus of, 180
Right lumbosacral articular process joint, 174
Right lumbosacral intertransverse joint, 176
Right major ischiatic foramen, 162
Right minor psoas muscle, 162, 163
Right obturator internus muscle, 180, 181
Right pubis, 198
    caudal ramus of, 180
Right sacral tuber, 178
Right sacral wing, 180
Right sacroiliac joint, 176, 180
Right sacrosciatic ligament, 180, 182
Right scapulohumeral joint, 4
Right sciatic nerve, 162, 163
Right stifle, palpable anatomical structures, 201
Right tarsus, 234
Right thoracic limb digital area, 117, 120
Right tibia, 172
Right tuber coxae, 155, 178, 185
Right tuber ischiadicum, 176
Roof
    of abdomen and pelvis, 162
    of pelvis, bones and ligaments, 177

Sacral (vertebral) canal, 178, 179
Sacral artery, 183
Sacral canal, 174, 184, 185, 187
Sacral crest, 172
Sacral foramen, 172
Sacral tuber, 171, 172, 174, 187, 191, 197
Sacral wing, 173
Sacroiliac fat, 178, 179
Sacroiliac joint, 172, 173, 174, 176, 177, 179, 186, 187, 188
Sacroiliac ligament, 177
Sacrosciatic ligament, 192, 197
Sacrum, 163, 171, 172, 173, 174, 175, 176, 180, 183, 197

Sagittal fossa, 51
Sagittal groove, 101, 102, 103
Saphenous artery, 198, 220
Saphenous nerve, 183, 184, 198, 199
Saphenous vein, 198, 199, 219, 221, 225, 230
Sartorius muscle, 180, 181, 198, 199
Satellite arterial ramus, 25
Scalenus medius muscle, 144
Scalenus ventralis muscle, 144
Scapula, 2, 3, 4, 5, 6, 11, 13, 14, 15, 16, 17, 30, 156
    spine of, 2, 141
Scapular circumflex vein, 14
Scapulohumeral joint, 3, 4, 5
Sciatic nerve, 183, 184, 192
    muscle rami of, 196
Scutocompedal ligament, 115, 270, 274
Scutum, 102
Second (medial) intermetatarsal syndesmosis, 259, 262
Second cervical nerve, ventral rami of, 134
Second dorsal (intervertebral) sacral foramen, 175
Second intermetacarpal syndesmosis, 83, 86, 87, 88, 90,
    91, 92, 93, 94
Second lumbar intervertebral disc, 158
Second lumbar vertebra (L2), 154, 155, 158, 159, 167, 168
Second metacarpal bone, 86, 87, 88, 90, 91, 92, 93, 94, 99,
    100, 103, 106, 189, 231, 232, 233, 234, 235, 236, 244,
    245, 246, 247, 249, 250, 258, 259, 262, 263, 265, 266,
    267, 268
Second metatarsal syndesmosis, 265, 266, 267
Secondometacarpal ligament, 86
Secondotercer interosseous space, 55
Secondotertius interosseous ligaments, 73
Secondotertius interosseous spaces, 73
Secondotertius joint, 58
Second sacral nerve, 182, 184
Second sacral vertebra, 184, 198
Second tarsal bone, 231, 232, 233, 234, 235, 236, 258, 259
Second thoracic vertebra, 147
Second ventral (intervertebral) sacral foramen, 177
Semilunar plica, 155
Semilunar sinus, 116, 270
Semimembranosus muscle, 171, 180, 181, 183, 191, 195,
    196, 199, 220
Semispinalis capitis muscle, 133, 134, 137, 141, 142, 143,
    147, 148
Semitendinosus muscle, 171, 181, 190, 191, 195, 196, 197,
    199, 225, 227, 228
Semitendinosus muscle body, 224
Serratus dorsalis caudalis muscle, 161
Serratus dorsalis cranialis muscle, 142
Serratus ventralis cervicis muscle, 10, 156, 141, 142, 143
Serratus ventralis thoracis muscle, 1, 10, 142, 143, 144, 151
Sesamoidean ligaments, 100, 101, 102
Sesamoidophalangeal space, 104, 105, 106, 107
Seventeenth rib, 157
Seventeenth thoracic vertebra (T17), 154, 155, 160, 164, 165
Seventh cervical vertebra (C7), 2, 4, 5, 140, 145, 146
Shoe, 114, 115
Short digital extensor muscle, 224, 238, 241, 260, 261, 265

Short digital extensor tendon, 255
Short lateral collateral ligament, 240, 241, 242, 243, 253
Short medial collateral ligament, 240, 245, 246, 249, 253
Short sesamoidean ligament, 123
Shoulder, 7, 13
    cranial margin of, 131
Shoulder joint, 14, 17, 18
Shoulder joint area, 12
Shoulder muscles, 7, 10, 11, 12, 13
Sixteenth thoracic vertebra (T16), 164
Sixth cervical vertebra (C6), 4, 5, 140, 144, 146
    ventral ramus of, 144
Sixth intervertebral disc, 185
Sixth lumbar nerve (L6), 162, 163, 169, 170, 172, 173, 176,
    177, 180, 182, 184, 185, 186, 187
    dorsal ramus of, 187
    ventral ramus of, 188
Sixth thoracic vertebra (T6), mid-thoracic area from, 152
Skin folds, 102
Skin, mane of, 133, 134
Soft tissue(s), 100, 101, 102, 103, 104, 105, 106, 108, 109,
    110, 111, 112, 114, 115, 116, 203, 204, 208
Solar canal, 111, 275
Solar corium, 124, 129, 273, 277, 278
Solar margin, 109, 110, 115, 116
Sole, 38, 108, 109, 114, 115, 116, 118, 124, 129, 277, 278
    corium of, 118
Soleus muscle, 190, 228
Sphenoid bone, 132
Spinal cord, 147, 148, 149, 160, 164, 166, 167, 168, 169,
    170, 184, 185
Spinal process, 139, 152, 153
Spinal ramus, 165
Spinalis cervicis muscle, 147, 148
Spinalis thoracis muscle, 143, 144, 156
Splenius muscle, 133, 134, 137, 141, 142, 143, 147, 156
Spongy bone, 101, 102, 103, 104, 105, 106, 107, 111, 112,
    113, 114, 115, 204, 233, 265, 266, 270
Sternocephalicus muscle, 131, 141, 142, 144, 147
Sternohyoideus muscle, 147
Sternothyroideus muscle, 147
Sternum, 2
    manubrium of, 20
Stifle, 189, 217, 218
    passing through femoral condyles, 220
    passing through intercondylar fossa of femur, 219, 220
Stifle plica, 151
Stifle proximal to patella, 218
Straight sesamoidean ligament, 80, 82, 83, 85, 108, 118,
    120, 121, 123, 124, 125, 127, 129, 263, 274, 275, 277, 278
Striated muscle fibres, 228
Stylohyoideum, 132
Subchondral bone, 112, 113, 154, 204, 207, 209, 231, 236,
    265, 270
Subclavia artery, 146
Subclavius muscle, 1, 7, 10, 13, 14, 16, 17, 156
Subclavius nerve, 146
Subcutaneous connective tissue, 266
Subcutaneous tissue, 127, 253, 254

Subdural (subarachnoidean) space, 149, 160, 164, 167, 168, 170, 185
Subextensor recess, 218, 219
Subpopliteal recess, 218, 219
Subscapular artery, 10, 11, 12, 13, 16
Subscapular fossa, 5, 13
Subscapularis muscle, 11
Subscapular muscle, 10, 12, 13, 16, 17
Subscapular nerves, 146
Subscapular vein, 13, 16
Suclavius muscle, 141
Sulcus intertubercularis, 3, 4, 5, 5, 16
Superficial aponeurosis, 156, 157, 161, 167, 169
Superficial digital flexor muscle, 27, 32, 41, 42, 43, 44, 46, 69, 74, 75, 197, 218, 219, 223, 224, 247
Superficial digital flexor musculotendinous junction, 47, 71
Superficial digital flexor tendon cap, 237
Superficial fibular (peroneal) nerve, 226, 227, 228
Superficial ungular plexus, 117
Supracondylar crest, 2, 21, 22, 23, 24, 26, 27, 37
Supracondylar fossa, 197, 203, 208, 209, 270
Suprascapular artery, 10, 17
Suprascapular nerve, 8, 17, 146
Suprascapular rami, 16
Suprascapular vein, 17
Supraspinal ligament, 145, 153, 156, 157, 158, 160, 161, 164, 167, 168, 169
Supraspinatus fossa, 2, 3, 8, 13
Supraspinatus muscle, 1, 7, 8, 10, 11, 12, 13, 14, 16, 17, 141, 156
Suspensory apparatus, 263
Suspensory ligament, 257, 269
    extensor branch of, 269
Sustentaculum tali, 229, 231, 232, 234, 235, 236, 237, 249, 252, 253, 254
Symphysial face, 173
Synovial fossa(e), 22,109
Synovial lateral intermetatarsal joint, 258
Synovial membrane, 254
Synovial space, 3, 4, 5, 6
Synovial sulcus, 112

Tail, 171, 181, 195, 196
Talean fasciculus, 243, 245, 246, 249, 253
Talocalcaneal joint, 231, 235, 236, 237
Talocalcaneal joint space, 246
Talocentral joint, 233, 234, 235
Talocentrodistometatarsal ligament, 240, 243, 252, 255
Talometatarsal ligament, 240, 243, 252, 255, 264
Talus, 190, 197, 222, 237, 242, 243, 245, 246, 252, 253
    lateral trochlea ridge of, 238, 241
    medial articular margin of, 253
    medial trochlea ridge of, 238
    proximal tubercle of, 249, 253
    trochlea of, 229, 230, 231, 232, 233, 234, 235, 236, 240, 253
Tarsal canal, 235, 242, 243
Tarsal flexor muscles, 229, 230

Tarsal sheath cavity, 254
Tarsal sinus, 235, 237
Tarsocrural joint, 229, 230, 231, 232, 234, 235, 236, 239, 244, 252, 253
Tarsometatarsal joint, 231, 232, 233, 234, 235, 236, 252, 264, 265
Tarsometatarsal junction, 229
Tarsus, 189, 252, 258, 259
    distal plantar ligament of, 252, 263, 264, 265
    proximal plantar ligament of, 252
Temporal bone, 132
Temporal muscle, 135
Tenocalcaneal ligament, 247
Tensor fascia latae muscle, 151, 161, 171, 180, 181, 183, 187, 188, 190, 191, 195, 196, 198
Tensor fasciae antebrachii muscle, 10, 11, 16, 28, 32
Teres major muscle, 10, 11, 12, 13, 16, 26, 28
Teres minor muscle, 8, 9, 16, 17
Teres minor proximal tendon, 13
Tertioquartal interosseous ligament, 73
Tertioquartal interosseous space, 73
Tertioquartal joint, 58
Thigh, 151, 189
Third carpal bone, 96, 97
Third cervical vertebra (C3), 138, 147, 148, 149
    caudal articular process of, 147, 148, 149
    vertebral fossa of, 147, 148
Third dorsal (intervertebral) sacral foramen, 174
Third dorsal metatarsal artery, 259, 261, 264, 265, 266, 267, 268
Third intermetacarpal syndesmosis, 87, 88, 89, 90, 91, 92, 93, 94
Third intermetatarsal syndesmosis, 258, 260, 261
Third interosseous metacarpal enthesis, 89
Third interosseous muscle (TIOM), 84, 87, 88, 106, 114, 115, 129, 189, 272, 273, 274, 275
    distal limb, 99
    left fetlock, 104, 105, 126
        and pastern, 100, 103, 127
    left metacarpophalangeal joint, 101, 102, 119
    muscle body, 91, 92
    muscle branches, 101, 102
    metacarpus, 90, 91, 92, 93, 94, 95, 96, 97, 98
    metatarsus, 261, 262, 264, 265, 266, 267, 268
    pelvic limb, 190, 260, 273
    right digital area, 121, 122, 123, 129
    tarsus, 240, 249, 251, 252
    thoracic limb, 117, 118, 120
    suspensory apparatus, 263
    (suspensory ligament), 37, 38, 41, 43, 49, 64, 65, 66, 67, 75, 77, 80, 81, 82, 83, 85, 86
Third lumbar nerve, 184
Third lumbar vertebra (L3), 155, 158, 167, 168, 173, 174, 176
Third metacarpal bone, 37, 38, 40, 87, 88, 89, 90, 91, 92, 93, 94, 95, 97, 98, 99, 100, 101, 102, 103, 104, 105, 106, 107, 114, 117, 118, 119, 120, 124
    palmar recess of, 97
Third metacarpal condyle, 125, 129

Third metatarsal bone, 189, 190, 223, 224, 231, 232, 233, 234, 235, 236, 238, 239, 240, 241, 242, 243, 244, 245, 246, 247, 249, 250, 251, 252, 257, 258, 259, 260, 261, 262, 263, 264, 265, 266, 267, 268, 271, 272, 273
Third metatarsal syndesmosis, 265, 266, 267
Third rib, 147
Third sacral nerve, 182
Third sacral vertebra (S3), 177, 182, 180, 184, 185
Third tarsal bone, 231, 232, 233, 234, 235, 236, 240, 242, 243, 252, 255, 258, 259, 264, 265
Third trochanter, 171, 193
Third ventral (intervertebral) sacral foramen, 173
Thirteenth rib (R13), 145
Thoracic area, 151
Thoracic limb digital area, 124, 129
Thoracic limb fetlock, 126
Thoracic limb foot, 128
Thoracic limb pastern, 127
Thoracic muscles, 7, 10
Thoracic spinalis, 156
Thoracic structures, 4, 5
Thoracic vertebra, 2
Thoracodorsal artery, 10, 11, 12, 16
Thoracodorsal nerve, 146
Thoracodorsal vein, 16
Thoracolumbar area, 165
    between last thoracic vertebra and first lumbar vertebra, 166
Thoracolumbar articular process joint, 157
Thoracolumbar fascia, 142, 156, 157, 161, 166, 167, 181, 195, 196
Thoracolumbar interspinal ligament, 157
Thoracolumbar junction, 154, 155, 157, 158
Thoracolumbar vertebral column, 160, 164
Thorax, 2, 3, 151
Throat, 131
Tibia, 197, 201, 203, 204, 205, 206, 208, 209, 211, 213, 214, 215, 216, 220, 221, 222, 223, 225, 227, 228, 231, 232, 234, 235, 236, 237, 241, 242, 243, 244, 245, 246, 247, 250
    caudal surface of, 249
    extensor fossa of, 213
    extensor sulcus of, 212, 213, 218
    medial malleolus of, 230, 238, 239, 240, 248
    medial surface of, 249
Tibial cochlea, 222, 231, 232, 234, 235, 236, 240, 245, 246, 249, 252
Tibial crest, 203, 206, 208, 209, 211
Tibial nerve, 196, 199, 219, 225, 227, 228
Tibial (proximal) extensor retinaculum, 226
Tibial retinaculum, 229, 230
Tibial tubercle, 214
Tibial tuberosity, 195, 201, 202, 203, 204, 206, 208, 209, 210, 211, 212, 213, 215, 216, 217, 218, 222, 224, 226
Tibialis caudalis muscle, 227, 228, 244, 247
Tibialis caudalis tendon, 247
Tibialis cranialis muscle, 190, 197, 212, 218, 220, 226, 227, 228, 229, 230, 238, 239, 241, 244, 247, 264
Tibialis cranialis tendon, 238, 239, 241, 244, 253, 255

Tibiofibular joint, 204, 209, 213, 214, 222
TIOM, see Third interosseous muscle (TIOM)
Toe, 269
Trachea, 138, 139, 140, 147
Transverse cubital artery, 32, 39
Transverse cubital vein, 32
Transverse foramen, 135, 136, 139
Transverse ligament, 277, 278
Transverse process, 138, 152
Trapezius muscle, 1, 7, 141, 142, 151, 156
Triceps brachii muscle, 1, 7, 8, 10, 11, 12, 13, 14, 16, 19, 20, 25, 26, 28, 32, 35, 36, 151, 156
Tricipital line, 2, 5, 26
Trigonum, 102, 278
Trochanteric bursa, 192
Trochanteric fossa, 191, 195
Trochlea groove, 208
Trochlear incisura, 22, 23
Tuber calcanei, 231, 232, 234, 235, 236, 237, 238, 240, 244, 247, 248, 252, 253
Tubercle, 206
Tuber coxae, 151, 161, 163, 171, 172, 173, 174, 181, 190, 191, 195, 196, 197, 198
Tuberculum supraglenoidale, 2, 3, 4, 5, 6, 8, 14, 30, 140
Tuber ischiadicum (ischiatic tuberosity), 171, 172, 173, 174, 180, 191
Tuber olecrani, 2
Tuber sacrale, 151
Tunica flava abdominis, 161
Twelfth thoracic vertebra (T12), 152, 153

Ulna, 2, 11, 21, 22, 23, 24, 29, 32, 38, 37, 39, 41, 42, 43, 44, 46, 54, 55, 57, 61
    distal epiphysis of, 50, 52, 53, 56
    styloid process of, 49
Ulnar carpal bone, 50, 51, 52, 53, 54, 55, 56, 57, 58, 61, 72
Ulnar collateral artery, 11, 16, 28
Ulnar collateral vein, 16
Ulnaris lateralis distal tendon, 66
Ulnaris lateralis long tendon, 76
Ulnaris lateralis muscle, 1, 7, 8, 9, 19, 22, 25, 26, 32, 35, 36, 37, 38, 39, 43, 46, 49, 59, 60, 62, 63, 64, 65, 74, 75
Ulnaris lateralis muscle body, 29
Ulnaris lateralis musculotendinous junction, 47, 70–71
Ulnaris lateralis tendons, 72
Ulnaris lateralis, 27
Ulnar nerve, 11, 16, 28, 32, 42, 46, 47, 71, 72, 73, 74, 75, 76, 146
    deep ramus of, 84
    palmar ramus of, 76, 84, 97
Ulnar styloid process, 50, 51
Umbilical artery, 183
Ungular cartilage(s), 77, 121, 122, 123, 128, 129, 269, 271, 273, 276

Vascular canal, 258, 259
Vascular channels, 116, 209
Vascular foramen, 78
Vascular sulcus, 259

Vastus intermedius muscle, 199
Vastus lateralis muscle, 181, 197, 199, 220
Vastus medialis muscle, 183, 198, 199, 217
Ventral arch, 132, 136
Ventral cervical region, 131
Ventral condylar fossa, 132, 137
Ventral crest, 132
Ventral intertransverse foramen, 177, 178
Ventral longitudinal ligament, 159, 160, 163, 164, 167, 169, 180, 183, 184, 185
Ventral lumbosacral intertransverse ligament, 187
Ventral ramus, 133, 170, 184
    eighth cervical nerve, 146
    fifth cervical nerve, 146
    first thoracic nerve, 146
    second thoracic nerve, 146
    seventh cervical nerve, 146
    sixth cervical nerve, 146
Ventral sacroiliac ligament, 186, 187, 188
Ventral tubercle, 132
Ventrocaudal cuspid, 172, 174, 178, 180, 181, 172, 178, 180, 181
Vertebral arch, 138, 139, 140, 152, 153, 154, 155

Vertebral artery, 148
Vertebral axis, 131
Vertebral body, 136, 138, 139, 140, 152, 153, 154, 155
Vertebral canal, 132, 136, 138, 166, 167, 168, 170, 184, 185
Vertebral column, 2
Vertebral foramen, 139, 140, 147, 148, 149, 152, 153, 154, 155
Vertebral fossa, 132, 138, 139, 140, 152, 153, 154, 155
Vertebral head, 138, 139, 140, 152, 153, 154, 155
Vertebral pedicle, 136
Vertebral symphysis, 139, 140, 152, 153, 154, 155
Vertebral vein, 148
Vestigial lateral (fourth) interosseous muscle, 266
Vestigial medial (second) interosseous muscle, 266

Weight-bearing left distal limb, 114, 115
White matter, 185
Withers, 151

Xiphoid process, 2
Xyphoid area, 151

Zygomatic arch, 135